D0146594

Implementing
Shared Governance
CREATING A PROFESSIONAL ORGANIZATION

Implementing
Shared Governance
CREATING A PROFESSIONAL ORGANIZATION

TIM PORTER-O'GRADY, EdD, RN, CS, CNAA, FAAN

Principal
Tim Porter-O'Grady, Inc.
Atlanta, Georgia

Illustrated

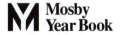

Mosby
Year Book

St. Louis Baltimore Boston Chicago London Philadelphia Sydney Toronto

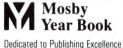
Mosby
Year Book
Dedicated to Publishing Excellence

Executive Editor: N. Darlene Como
Associate Developmental Editor: Brigitte Pocta
Project Manager: Peggy Fagen
Designer: Jeanne Wolfgeher

Printed in the United States of America.

Mosby-Year Book, Inc.
11830 Westline Industrial Drive
St. Louis, MO 63146

International Standard Book Number 0-8016-6318-0

92 93 94 95 96 CL/MY 9 8 7 6 5 4 3 2 1

Contributors

Cindy C. Campbell, RN, MSN
Chief Operating Officer
Memorial Hospital at Gulfport
Gulfport, Mississippi
Affiliated Dynamics, Inc.
Atlanta, Georgia

David G. Crocker, Esq.
Attorney at Law
Early, Lennon, Fox, Thompson, Peters,
and Crocker
Kalamazoo, Michigan

Susan H. Cummings, RN, MSN
Director for Quality, Education, and
Research
Sharp Memorial Hospital
San Diego, California

Beth E. Foster, RN, MSN, CNAA
Vice President for Patient Care Services
Borgess Medical Center
Kalamazoo, Michigan

R. Michael Kirkpatrick, Esq.
Attorney at Law
Early, Lennon, Fox, Thompson, Peters,
and Crocker
Kalamazoo, Michigan

JoEllen Goertz Koerner, RN, MS,
FAAN
Vice President, Patient Care
Sioux Valley Hospital
Sioux Falls, South Dakota

Vicki D. Lachman, RN, PhD, CS, CNAA
President
VL Associates
Philadelphia, Pennsylvania

Laura Lentenbrink, RN, MS-N, JD, CNA
Administrative Director
Borgess Medical Center
Kalamazoo, Michigan

Jim O'Malley, RN, MSN, CNAA
Vice President, Patient Services
Sharp Memorial and Sharp Cabrillo
Hospitals
San Diego, California

Tim Porter-O'Grady, EdD, RN, CS,
CNAA, FAAN
Senior Partner
Affiliated Dynamics, Inc.
Principal
Dr. Tim Porter-O'Grady, PC
Atlanta, Georgia

Sheila Smith, RN, MSN
Assistant Vice President, Nursing
Childrens Hospital Medical Center
Cincinnati, Ohio

Jaynelle F. Stichler, RN, DNS, CNAA
Executive Director, Women's Services
Sharp HealthCare
San Diego, California

To health care leaders, in all the places
where health care is delivered,
striving to prepare for an uncertain future.

Preface

The rate of change affecting the delivery of health services is almost overwhelming. Nursing leaders are struggling to keep up with the demands of a constraining and changing health care system. The direction of the future is uncertain and, in many ways, frightening.

In the past, the script was clearer and the players and their prescribed roles were more certain. With changes in the economic and social variables affecting health care, those certainties no longer exist. As the cost of health care continues to rise dramatically, providers and payers work out what and how services will be offered and how they will be paid for.

The agenda for the future is unwritten and wide open. There are no longer prescribed rules and relationships that are not subject to question or change in some way. What was once considered sacred is now history. What sense can be made of all this? What is nursing's role as we sort through the uncertainties of the future? If there is no established script, who will write a new script, and what part will nurses play in its unfolding?

All of these questions drive the nursing profession as it seeks to build a new identity and determine its place in a changing health care system. Whatever the answer to the above questions, nurses need to create a forum for discussion and establish mechanisms that will facilitate the profession's response to whatever demands emerge. Nurses will have to be able to direct their own responses, make critical decisions about their role, and assume newer responsibilities in a changing service framework. Indeed, nurses may have to play a major role in defining the framework within which nursing and health services will be offered in the future.

To be able to set the agenda and control their future, nurses of tomorrow will need to be prepared and skilled in providing leadership in a diffuse and multidisciplinary setting. They will find themselves in increasingly decentralized and noninstitutional settings. They must be able to assertively articulate their roles and expectations, manage their own practice, give direction in the application of health care, and establish a truly professional relationship with colleagues both within and outside the profession.

Preparation for the leadership role in nursing cannot simply be a unilateral process. Nurses must, in good measure, join in a common effort to advance the profession keeping in mind the best interests of those they serve. In every place where nurses practice together, a framework for interaction, policy formation, clinical standards, and nursing initiatives must be established and operated effectively. Nurses must be able to present an image of collaborative and collective commitment to health care and join with other leaders in health care to write and live out a new script that can better serve those who come to the health professions for services. Also, nurses must join with other caregivers in a collaborative coalition to deliver health care in new ways. The old hierarchies which prescribe roles and authority that are more exclusionary than inclusive will no longer work. Nurses in all arenas of practice want to play an increasing role in the decisions affecting what they do and how they do it. As the women's movement matures and influences workplace relationships, a demand for greater participation and ownership is unfolding.

Ten years ago the concept of shared governance took form in a very few institutions across the United States. Nursing service thinkers and leaders began the struggle to create a new organizational model that better fit the needs of a professional, knowledge-based worker. Also, the unique needs of nurses, most of whom are women, needed to be addressed in an organizational imperative that respected the history and unique character of nursing. Since that time, over 1000 hospitals initiated professional governance models, often called shared governance models, in an effort to create a truly professional nursing staff. The goal, at that time, was to get nurses more invested in their work and profession and to strengthen nursing in the workplace in ways that would empower it as a profession and retain the interest of its members. Shared governance activities soon became the outcome of the recommendations of the various commissions and study groups looking at nursing and assessing its needs. More data have been generated in the past few years to validate shared governance as an effective organizational model, and other disciplines in the health care field are interested in applying its concepts to their own interests and needs. Indeed, it has become a vehicle for building the collaborative interdisciplinary relationships that will be models for the future of health care delivery.

During the years that I have been associated with shared governance, people from a wide variety of settings and from different countries have asked if there are certain principles of implementation that can be applied, regardless of the specific models that may be developed. Since all who have implemented shared governance in one form or another have been creating and learning the process at each step along the way, the underlying principles for implementation have been slow in emerging and are just now being clarified.

This book is designed to articulate the principles and processes associated with the implementation of shared governance, regardless of the setting or the model chosen. It focuses not on the step-by-step processes but on the underlying characteristics of implementation that will affect all who seek to develop shared governance, regardless of their approach. In this way, the book provides a useful reference to validate the process of shared governance and to assist in the evaluation of progress. It alerts the planner and implementer to problems, concerns, and developmental issues that invariably will emerge.

While this book provides insight and advice regarding the entire process of shared governance implementation, the planner and implementer of shared governance may need additional references to successfully unfold a professional practice and governance model. The *Shared Governance Implementation Manual* (Porter-O'Grady, Mosby–Year Book Inc, 1992), which was developed as a companion to this book, provides practical, step-by-step guidance regarding the implementation of shared governance. Together the books offer a complete resource to facilitate implementation of a shared governance model.

One caveat must be mentioned at the outset and will again appear throughout this book. Shared governance is a vehicle for change, growth, and empowerment for the profession and the professional; it is not an end in itself. It serves as a vehicle for creating and managing change and preparing a desired future. It is not *the* future. When shared governance has moved the profession of nursing along the way toward a preferred future, it will have done its work. Newer and more appropriate organizational and professional configurations will undoubtedly evolve. This is as it should be. Shared governance is, however, an essential passage along the road to the future maturing of the nursing profession. All nursing organizations will, in one form or another, need to experience its impact. To the extent that this book facilitates that passage, it will have accomplished the goal of its authors.

Tim Porter-O'Grady

Contents

It ought to be remembered that there is nothing more difficult to take in hand, more perilous to conduct, or more uncertain in its success, that to take the lead in the introduction of a new order of things. Because the innovator has for opposition all those who have done well under the old conditions, and lukewarm defenders among those who may do well under the new.

Machiavelli
The Prince

1   *A Conceptual Basis for Shared Governance*

Jaynelle F. Stichler

A new age has dawned in the management of the professional worker. The superstructure of the bureaucratic organization is undergoing a tremendous metamorphosis with new norms for managerial and employee behavior. Contemporary management scholars indicate that companies demonstrating excellence are replacing traditional bureaucratic structures with governance structures that emphasize employee participation and involvement (Naisbitt, 1982; Naisbitt and Aburdene, 1985; 1990). Organizations are recognizing the positive significance of systems that grant professional employees the responsibility and accountability for governing issues directly related to their professional practice. Organizational charts are flattening with the elimination of multiple layers of bureaucratic structures. Emphasis is placed on direct interaction between the manager and the worker who delivers the service to the customer or who makes the product manufactured by the company. Successful and progressive organizations have shifted to a collaborative style of management in which management and employees work as teams or in partnership to realize the mission and values of the organization and the goals of production or service.

NEW CHALLENGES IN HEALTH CARE AFFECTING NURSING

Hospitals have exemplified the traditional bureaucratic superstructure for centuries, but current demands in health care have challenged core bureaucratic beliefs. Health care costs have continued to spiral upward despite federal mandates for their control or reduction. Hospitals that have not responded to competitive pricing in a managed care market have been closed or acquired by other, more financially successful health care systems. "Quality" health care often remains undefined, elusive, and even unaffordable.

The retention and recruitment of professional nurses and the importance of their satisfaction with their role have never been so critical. Health care employees, and specifically nurses, have become a valuable yet scarce commodity as the nursing shortage continues to escalate. American Hospital Association survey data indicate that the registered nurse vacancy rate for hospital nurses rose to 12.66% in 1989; this represented a 2% increase over the December 1988 rate of 10.6% (American

Organization of Nurse Executives, 1990). Increased acuity in hospitalized patients and increased technologic interventions require continuous and sophisticated monitoring and assessment by professional nurses. Shorter lengths of stay involving intensive plans of care and extended services after hospitalization also increase the demand for nurses. Nurses are the health care professionals best prepared to provide the coordination of patient care from home to hospital and back to home. At a time when the health care system most needs the expertise of nurses, many are leaving the profession. The shortage of nurses is evidenced by vacancies in nursing positions, job dissatisfaction in the work force, lack of organizational commitment, high turnover rates, and a diminished number of applicants to colleges of nursing. With fewer nurses to employ, some hospitals resort to using more expensive "registry nurses" when available, resulting in higher salary rates per patient visit, increased difficulty in competing for managed care contracts, and decreased profits. When replacement registry nurses are not available, hospital administrators have occasionally been forced to restrict or discontinue services, creating financial disaster for some health care organizations.

Several explanations for the nursing shortage have been offered. Career opportunities outside nursing are available to contemporary women, whereas in the past, women's career options were often limited to nursing or education. Lack of prestige and status in the nursing profession, poor remuneration for the level of education required, scope of responsibility and workload, and unsatisfactory working conditions deter young women and men from selecting a nursing career and create professional dissatisfaction and turnover among experienced nurses. Lack of autonomy and control in decisions affecting the professional practice of nursing; poor interpersonal relationships with management and other health care providers; and lack of recognition and reward for professional expertise have also been cited as reasons for disillusion with the nursing role (Bream and Schapiro, 1989; Nursing Shortage Poll Report, 1988; Office of the Inspector General, 1989).

Currently, managing personnel costs is critical to an organization's overall financial viability, but hospitals are expending major financial resources to obtain staffing through registries, to finance expensive recruitment campaigns, and to provide costly orientation programs. Nursing managers and administrators additionally are consumed by the need to retain the personnel they have and to assure their commitment to their organization.

The American Hospital Association in conjunction with other commissions, associations, and foundations has reviewed the status and image of nursing for the past three decades (National Commission on Nursing, 1981). From the myriad published public testimonials of nurses and the study findings of the commissions, several recurrent themes have been cited as critical factors leading to role dissatisfaction. These factors include (1) lack of participation in decisions affecting patient care and the practice of nursing, (2) inadequacy in the systems for delivery of care, and (3) negative interprofessional relationships, specifically with physicians and hospital administration.

Publications from numerous groups commissioned to study nursing have recommended a spirit of collaboration and collegiality among health care providers and involvement of nurses in decisions affecting nursing practice and patient care to support the vital role of nurses as members of the health care team (Department of Health and Human Services, 1988; Lysaught, 1970; National Commission on Nursing, 1982). Magnet hospitals and other organizations that have been most successful in recruitment and retention efforts have facilitated development of organizational cultures and climates that foster autonomy, accountability, and educational growth in professional practice (Department of Health and Human Services, 1988). In a professional atmosphere of mutual trust and collegiality, nurses are active on multidisciplinary committees, governance and planning councils, and career advancement programs. Many of these hospitals encourage joint practice models as recommended by the American Nurses Association and the American Medical Association as a method of enhancing nurse-physician relationships and improving the coordination of patient care (National Joint Practice Commission, 1981). Terms such as professional networks, partnerships, interdisciplinary teams and committees, and shared governance are the hallmarks of many health care organizational mission and value statements that encourage the development of a culture that recognizes the unique and necessary contribution of each of its employees and professional groups. Although nearly three decades have passed and some progress has been made in meeting these goals, realization of collaborative practice in health care organizations still is not the norm.

What is necessary to build commitment, job satisfaction, and professionalism among nurses? What changes are needed to attract bright, articulate college students to the profession? Health care organizations are struggling with such questions without realizing that the solution may require the same metamorphosis identified by other businesses and industries. Decades of empirical studies of other industries and disciplines have demonstrated the positive effect that participation in decision making has on the professional worker's job satisfaction, but this finding has yet to be implemented in many health care organizations.

Successful health care executives are beginning to realize that cost-effective, quality service is delivered by a team of professionals who have internalized the zeal for quality patient care, who are committed to the organization, and who are empowered to practice their profession without unnecessary restraint. Nurses empowered to practice their profession must participate in any decision that affects the professional practice or the delivery of care to patients. Shared governance as described and defined by Porter-O'Grady and Finnigan (1984), Pinkerton and Schroeder (1988), and others is founded on this premise.

The implementation and operationalization of shared governance requires establishment of a partnership between the nurse and the manager to work together to meet the goals of the organization. Traditional hierarchies that place position and power between the employee and the manager are replaced by a collaborative relationship in which both parties share in fulfillment of the common goal of providing cost-effective, quality patient care. By valuing and operationalizing the concept of collaborative management in health care organizations, organizational frameworks such as shared governance can be developed that encourage management and staff partnerships, enhance the professionalism of the organization, and promote role satisfaction among the professionals.

MANAGEMENT AND STAFF RELATIONS

Traditional managerial functions placed emphasis on planning, organizing, staffing, directing, and controlling (Rowland and Rowland, 1980). Contemporary authors describe the necessity for a new style of management. Naisbitt and Aburdene (1990) state that more successful organizations are replacing authoritarian organizational structures with new cultures that espouse belief in the cultivation and nurturance of employees interested in the right to participate in the organization. Hierarchical organizational charts are replaced with networking systems delineating more lateral and collaborative relationships. Naisbitt and Aburdene (1985) indicate that employees not only want to participate in the planning, decision making, entrepreneuring, and quality assurance efforts, but they also want to share in the profit of the company. Quality performance, productivity, and creativity are rewarded with new compensation systems, incentive programs, and employee stock-option plans. These authors believe that the quality of work-life is critical to today's employee, and the astute manager realizes that the more satisfied worker is more productive, needs less supervision, and provides a higher quality of service. Naisbitt and Aburdene (1990) indicate that most employees want to make a "difference" and want to be recognized as important to the overall success of the organization.

Similarly, other contemporary authors writing about the pursuit of excellence in organizations espouse the importance of building commitment to the organization and excitement about the service to the customer. An emphasis on the professionalism of the organization can be best obtained by a management and corporate culture that emphasizes human interaction and participation (Deal and Kennedy, 1982; Hickman and Silva, 1984). Peters and Waterman (1982) indicate that more successful corporations have a "loose-tight" structure—although there is control and discipline, the organization and culture support autonomy in the worker, which enhances creativity and innovativeness. Discipline is a set of shared values that provide the framework upon which autonomy can be developed.

Benveniste (1987) describes ways of "professionalizing the organization" and indicates that a management style that promotes consensus building rather than a bureaucratic structure is essential to organizational effectiveness and the motivation and satisfaction of the professional worker. He suggested several organizational models that will result in a more "professional" organization. Most of the models entail increasing the professional employee's involvement in decision making, planning, and other work of the organization. The dual governance system that Benveniste describes is similar to the shared governance system described by Porter-O'Grady and Finnigan (1984). In these models of dual or shared governance, specific decision-making responsibilities and authorities are delegated to a professional group(s) for issues relative to professional practice.

Unfortunately, some pitfalls of collaborative styles of management are often ignored by scholars. Although Benveniste indicates that collaborative management structures enhance professionalism within the organization, he warns that the scope of the delegated authority to professionals should remain narrow, well-defined, and task-oriented because some professionals do not possess strong managerial skills. He also cautions that dual governance structures may lead to disagreements between management and staff regarding the right of professionals to be involved in all decisions, including those that often are irrelevant to professional practice. Benveniste describes the disadvantages of dual/shared governance as: (1) increased bureaucracy because of elaborate committee work, (2) increased costs associated with employee time expended in participation, and (3) turf battles regarding the propriety of decisions. Benveniste warns that once dual governance systems are implemented, the formally organized groups of staff could quickly convert to unions if true collaborative efforts fail or if the system is dismantled by management without staff consent.

MANAGEMENT STYLES AND JOB SATISFACTION

Several possible frameworks for understanding and managing organizations are described by Bolman and Deal (1984), but the human resource framework seems most applicable to the discussion of employee involvement in organizational governance. The human resource approach emphasizes interpersonal relationships, individual involvement and participation, and organizational democracy. Hierarchical structures and traditional rules of communication are eliminated, thus leading to a matrix style of management dependent on networking, informal coalition building, and cooperative teamwork. Within this framework more employee involvement in planning, decision making, and governance is fostered. The authors indicate that this "people-oriented" style of management leads to increased creativity, involvement in day to day operations, and commitment to the organization.

Although not supported by empirical data, the thoughts of contemporary writers are built on the foundations of earlier works of organizational researchers and theorists. In early organizational research, employee satisfaction was linked to both individual and organizational variables (Taylor, 1911). Maslow (1954) theorized that self-actualization, the highest level of fulfillment, could not be realized until other more basic needs were satisfied in hierarchical order. This theory is important to nursing because it recognizes that the advancement of the profession is first dependent on the satisfaction of more basic needs such as the assurance of appropriate work loads (physiologic), provision of job security (safety), promotion of partnerships and team development (social), and demonstration of appreciation and recognition (esteem) for nursing's contribution to health care.

Herzberg's (1968) two-factor theory hypothesized that satisfaction was not the opposite of dissatisfaction on a single continuum but rather that satisfaction was the result of motivational factors including recognition, advancement, achievement, the work itself, increased responsibility, and other rewards. He further suggested that the absence of these factors did not cause dissatisfaction, but that dissatisfaction was caused by a different set of hygiene factors such as interpersonal relationships among organizational members, work conditions, pay, and security. Herzberg's two factors compare with the five hierarchical needs described by Maslow (1954). The motivators relate to Maslow's higher-order needs, and the hygiene factors relate to the lower-order needs. With this framework, a collaborative management style could be considered as a hygiene factor that would need to be met before job satisfaction could be realized.

Lawler and Porter (1971) described a similar theory of satisfaction suggesting that satisfaction was related to extrinsic and intrinsic rewards. Extrinsic rewards referred to those provided by the organization such as pay, promotions, job security, and status; intrinsic rewards were individual acknowledgments of worthwhile accomplishments (internal satisfaction). Building on this premise, Porter, Lawler, and Hackman (1975) suggested that a reciprocal relationship existed between the individual and the organization that affected the employee's level of satisfaction, behavior, and performance. Ultimately, the reciprocal relationship between the individual and the organization affected organizational effectiveness. Porter, Lawler, and Hackman (1975) summarized the reciprocal relationship between the organization and the individual by stating that "organizations tend to motivate the kind of behavior they reward" (p. 343).

Studies linking satisfaction and dissatisfaction to performance and productivity have been neither consistent nor conclusive. In an analysis of early research on the subject, Vroom (1964) found only a few references to worker satisfaction and productivity. In a review of current literature, Tauskey (1978) purported that a stronger relationship is observed between dissatisfaction and absenteeism or turnover, which ultimately reduces organizational effectiveness, than the relationship between satisfaction and productivity. The inverse relationship between job satisfaction and turnover has also been reported extensively in nursing literature by several researchers. Hinshaw, Smeltzer, and Atwood (1987) reported that group cohesiveness, control over practice, and autonomy were predictive of job satisfaction in nursing. Job stress as measured by factors such as lack of autonomy and conflict with administration was also negatively related to job satisfaction and predicted turnover. In a similar study, Stichler (1990) reported the results of a path analytic model in which collaboration between the nurse and the physician and between the nurse and the manager predicted job satisfaction. Although both types of collaboration predicted job satisfaction, only nurse-manager collaboration predicted anticipated turnover. It appears that the absence of nurse-physician collaboration (conflict) is episodic and affects job satisfaction situationally, but not to the same degree as the chronic nature of nurse-manager conflict, which ultimately leads to thoughts of resignation. These findings suggest the importance of a collaborative style of management to enhance job satisfaction and to reduce the possibility of employee turnover.

In a correlational study, Tiffany, Cruise, and Cruise (1988) found that the degree of autonomy or discretion is positively correlated to the degree to which professionalism is perceived by the group. "As professionals practice their skills within the context of the larger society, not only must they have the knowledge specific to their practice, but they must be afforded the discretionary room necessary for the use of that knowledge" (p. 72A).

Bechtold, Szilagyi, and Sims (1980) stated that autonomy and participation in decision making affecting the work of the employee had a great influence on worker attitude and satisfaction. Similar to these findings, Stamps and others (1978) reported that nurses from three different samples rated autonomy as the most important aspect of job satisfaction. Duxbury, Henley, and Armstrong (1982) found that an organizational climate that supported professional autonomy and participation in decision making was significantly related to job satisfaction in nurses working in a neonatal intensive care unit. Similarly, Donohue (1986) found that an organizational climate that was characteristic of open and interactive communication between the deans of schools of nursing and the faculty contributed to overall job satisfaction, high morale, and increased productivity. These studies indicate the significance of autonomy, participation in decision making, and an organizational climate that fosters interactive communication as important variables in job satisfaction among specific populations of nurses.

Argyris (1962) and Herzberg (1968) studied the effects of various leadership styles of managers on the satisfaction of workers and found that styles that promoted employee involvement in decision making contributed to increased satisfaction and productivity in employees. The findings of Vroom and Yetton (1973) and Stogdill (1974) also indicate a positive relationship between participation in decision making by subordinates and job satisfaction.

Similar findings are reported by nurse researchers (Prestholdt, Lane, and Mathews 1988; Taunton, Krampitz, and Woods, 1989). The results of these studies demonstrated that nurses who were employed in units with managers who exercised authoritative leadership styles were less satisfied and less committed to staying in their jobs. The nurses reported centralized decision making, less autonomy, less individual power, and less supervisor support than other units.

The nurse administrator can play a major role in determining the extent to which nurses participate in interdependent decision making. Several researchers have discussed the positive effect of employee participation in decision making on job satisfaction (Blegen and Mueller, 1987; Vanderslice, Rice, and Julian, 1987). Buccheri (1986) reported that nurse managers are often more satisfied than their staff because of their participation in decision making and the recognition that they receive for their involvement. This study indicated that sharing information that affects the staff, providing support for their needs for influence, recognition, and communication, and allowing participation in decision making is directly related to job satisfaction.

The works of these theorists and researchers provide the foundation for contemporary and collaborative styles of management including human resource management, participative management, organizational democracy, quality circles, self/dual/shared governance, and others promoting involvement of the workers in organizational planning, decision making, quality control, and gain sharing. Reflecting trends in the development of management science, recent nursing and health care literature also suggests, documents, and provides evidence of the positive effects of employee participation in decision making affecting professional practice.

COLLABORATIVE MANAGEMENT STYLES

Fawcett (1984) indicated that a theoretical framework can provide substantive direction to the understanding of certain concepts by identification of other related concepts and potential linkages, and implication of philosophic assumptions about the concept. Shared governance is one example of a collaborative management structure. To understand the theoretical relevance of the concept of collaboration to shared governance, it is important to first define the terms and describe the attributes, antecedents, and consequences of the concept of collaboration. Collaboration and the recognition of its importance in business, education, health care, and other behavioral sciences is not new. The term *collaboration* is often used to refer to the process of working together as a team, but such a simple definition seems to minimize the significance of the process that occurs in a collaborative effort. *Collaboration* refers to a cooperative process that synthesizes and integrates the talents, resources, information, and expertise of two or more persons to accomplish a common goal (Stichler, 1989). Although some authors (Blake and Mouton, 1964) consider collaboration a method of conflict resolution, it is also considered an essential process in situations of goal interdependence (Tjosvold, 1984). Organizations are units of individuals who work interdependently for the accomplishment of the organization's missions and goals; therefore collaborative relationships between management and staff become critical for worker satisfaction and the effectiveness of the organization.

The process of collaboration is interactive and dynamic and is characterized by a balancing of power when participants have unequal status. Elements involved in collaboration include establishing parity; defining roles, responsibilities, and accountabilities of each party; resolving conflicts by negotiation and assertive behaviors; communicating horizontally rather than vertically; and participating in decision making. In a collaborative management framework, the power between management and staff is balanced or equalized by developing a matrix of communication and authority lines rather than a hierarchical authority pattern. Roles and responsibilities are defined, negotiated, and redefined according to projects, assignments, committees, and/or functions rather than vested positions. Subordinates are delegated the authority for decision making as it relates to their specific area of interest and/or professional practice. In this sense, the power inequity between management and staff is balanced for professional practice interests.

Sharing of information, cooperating and working as a team, synthesizing talents, expertise, and input, and establishing a consensus are also characteristic of the reciprocal nature of collaborative relationships. In a collaborative management framework, the organizational structure and culture would include collective bodies in which the work of the organization would be done. The talents of individuals would be integrated and synthesized in teams, councils, or committees to create outcomes that might not be realized if only the individual efforts of managers or staff were encouraged.

The process of collaboration leads to a sense of interpersonal value and a reinforcement of interdependency to accomplish the mission or goal. In collaborative relationships, the parties develop trust and respect one another and commit to work together on specific issues. Participants are selected to work on particular issues because of their skill and expertise in a certain area rather than their position in the management structure. In a collaborative management framework, management empowers the staff by granting them the privilege of making decisions in specific areas that may include specific projects, assignments, or professional practice issues. This premise is founded on the belief that given the correct information and direction, individuals will make appropriate decisions in a defined situation.

The concept of shared governance has not been explicitly defined in the literature, but the name would imply the allocation of control, power, or authority (governance) among mutually (shared) interested and vested parties. The vested parties in nursing are those who practice nursing by providing direct patient care and those who practice nursing by managing or administrating settings (hospitals or other health care environments) where clinical nursing care is provided. Both parties share a common goal—to provide quality nursing care to patients. In this sense, those who practice nursing by providing direct patient care and those who manage or administer patient care are interdependent in their goals and in their relationships.

The concept of collaboration is one of the underlying principles of shared governance and provides a conceptual framework for management styles that promote employee participation in decision making, involvement of employees in governance issues, autonomy in professional practice, and ultimately the attainment of professionalism. Two important theories, cooperation theory and social systems theory, provide insight into the concept of collaborative management styles and their importance in organizations.

Cooperation and Goal Interdependence Theory

Deutsch (1973) stated that perceived interdependence of goals significantly affects the dynamics and outcomes of social interaction. In cooperative processes, participants perceive that their goals are positively related. Recognizing that others' progress helps their own success, persons in cooperative relationships expect to give and receive assistance from others, trust others in the relationship, disclose information, feelings, and intentions, and define role expectations of one another.

In competitive relationships, people perceive their goals as negatively related. Realizing that the success of others threatens their own success, feelings of doubt, fear, frustration, and anger often lead to offerings of misleading information, acts of hostility, and minimal productivity on joint tasks.

Deutsch (1973) also postulated that independence has its own dynamics and outcomes. Persons working in an independent state see little need to establish a trusting relationship or to communicate information, since they are essentially isolated. Because collaboration is defined as a cooperative team effort to achieve interdependent goals, Deutsch's theory is important in understanding collaboration. This theory is also significant in understanding collaborative relationships in nursing because the discipline fulfills both independent and interdependent roles in its duty to society.

Deutsch's theory of cooperation (1973) can readily be applied in understanding the collaborative relationship between nurses and management, and becomes an important theory in understanding the dynamics of shared governance.

Social Systems Theory

Homans (1950) described human social behavior as a social system characterized by interactions with and without expectation of a reciprocal response. A new internal system evolves as a result of the interactions when a reciprocal response is expected. This theory also indicates that a synergistic group effect is more powerful than the efforts of each individual combined. Social systems theory is important in understanding collaboration; it describes the benefits of mutuality, reciprocity, and the synergy of the collective whole and is important in understanding the positive effects of a shared governance system.

CONCEPTS IMPORTANT TO PROFESSIONALIZING NURSING

Collaborative management is dependent on organizational cultures that espouse the belief that both management and staff must work as partners or colaborers to contribute to the success of the overall organization. A partnership arrangement would empower staff in certain areas and enhance their sense of autonomy. According to the theorists and researchers (Porter-O'Grady, 1987; Presholdt, Lane, and Mathews, 1987) the professionalization of the organization would be enhanced with the development of partnership relationships with the staff rather than the superior/subordinate relationships seen in hierarchical organizational structures. Professionalism, autonomy, and leadership style—all these concepts have been cited in business, organizational, and nursing literature as important to the professionalization of a discipline and essential to role satisfaction. It is important to explore the meaning of these concepts and their importance to nursing to understand how to incorporate them into practice.

Professionalism of Nursing

Early sociologists (Carr-Saunders and Wilson, 1933; Greenwood, 1987) who studied professional groups created a list of characteristics typical of the professional that included (1) provision of an essential service to society, (2) theoretical foundations for a specialized body of knowledge; (3) autonomy and authority over their practice, (4) a code of ethics, and (5) membership in professional organizations that socialize the participant to a specific professional culture and define standards of performance that specify desirable and predictable patterns of behavior of the professional. This list has been expanded by to others to include (6) education at institutions of higher learning, (7) scientific inquiry to expand the knowledge base, (8) emphasis on service rather than self-gain (Sims, Price, and Ervin, 1985), and (9) formal testing on competence or control of the admission to professional standing, rights, and privileges (Hall, 1968). Hall also highlighted the characteristic of "a calling" to the profession or a commitment to the work of the profession that motivates the work of the professional and is the source of satisfaction.

Management has a responsibility to nurture and defend the work and commitment of the professional in the organizational structure, which can create conflict for the manager. The professional often believes that his or her primary commitment is to the public with a secondary commitment to the organization, whereas the manager's primary commitment and responsibility is to meeting the goals of the organization. In hospital-based nursing, the hospital's goals also are to meet the needs of the community and public that it serves. However, the other organizational goals of profitability, expansion of services and facilities, and enhancement of productivity may be perceived as conflicting by the professional and the manager (who is also a member of the professional group with the goals of the profession). Although it is critical for hospitals to remain financially strong to accomplish their goals of community service, cutbacks in staffing, tightened productivity goals, and other measures to improve the economic viability of the hospital may seem contrary to the goals of professional groups in the hospital.

Traditional bureaucratic structures emphasize order, structure, and clearly defined patterns of communication operationalized through an elaborate hierarchical system. This type of structured system is highly efficient, but it does not always allow for independent decision making or interdependent relationships that are necessary for professional practice. Excessive bureaucracy and the subsequent routinization of activities often encroach on the control of professional discretion that is needed for the work of the professional and necessary for intrinsic satisfaction. Benveniste (1987, p. 23) stated, "Professionalization . . . is the substitution of discretionary roles for routinized roles."

Managers are taught to have a global and organizational perspective of problems, whereas professionals are often more narrowly focused in areas where their specialized skills and knowledge are useful. Although discretion is necessary for professionalism, management is still required to exercise some control over the work and outcomes of the organization. Issues of professionalism, scope of responsibility, and lines of authority often become clouded and add to role confusion and conflict.

The subordinate status and dependent role of nursing has contributed to the discipline's failure to be recognized as a profession. Porter-O'Grady and Finnigan (1984) indicate that the very values of bureaucracy, with goals of order and control, may actually prevent the occurrence of professional behavior. Hospitals may espouse a belief and value of the professional role of the nurse, but the organizational design itself may prevent true professional development and create conflict and frustration. Organizations that are matrixed for multiple-level involvement in planning, networking, and communication enhance the professional development of the staff. Any organizational structure that places accountability and authority for practice issues at the level of the professional practitioner rather than with management will also promote professionalism.

Unfortunately, some nurses are unwilling to assume the responsibility for professional involvement and participation in decision making. Their commitment to the organization is limited with per diem affiliations and task orientation to their work assignment rather than a commitment to the "calling" of the profession. Porter-O'Grady (1987) purports that "true professionals exhibit an inherent ownership of the role manifested in the work of the profession" (p. 282). Professionalization of an organization requires management to relinquish some control of issues related to professional practice, but it also requires professionals to be willing to accept responsibility and accountability for their own practice.

Professionalization of the organization is the professionals' responsibility. It requires cooperation as new roles are defined and sensitive issues about authorities and accountabilities are clarified. Professionalism of the organization will lead to more collaborative relationships between staff and management, because communications are opened in the process, status differences are minimized when issues are resolved with input from both managers and highly skilled, motivated professionals, and commonalities in direction and goals become clear.

The intent of a shared governance system in a hospital is to enhance the professionalism of nursing (Peterson and Allen, 1986). Similar to the writings of Benveniste (1987), authors supporting a shared governance system for nursing suggest that a restructuring of the organization is essential for nursing to develop as a profession and that it is necessary because nursing is a profession.

Autonomy

One essential component of a professional discipline is the establishment of mechanisms for self-regulation and governance. The concept of autonomy is important in understanding the necessity for collaborative management structures in professionalizing nursing and promoting role satisfaction and retention. Simply stated, autonomy is the freedom to make choices or to choose a course of action without external controls. The word autonomy is derived from the Greek words, "autos" (self) and "nomos" (rule) and implies control over one's self and destiny (Dempster, 1990). Historically, the term has been used to denote self-functioning and self-directedness. In developmental theories, autonomy is used to describe a stage of development in which the child begins to exercise a sense of personal choice (Erickson, 1963).

Professional behavior is predominantly intellectual and based on a theoretical foundation unique to the science. The right to participate in decisions affecting one's professional practice is central to the concept of autonomy and has been a source of both interprofessional and intraprofessional conflict in nursing. Nurse-physician and nurse-management conflict has stemmed from disagreement over the right of the nurse to participate as a partner and/or colleague in decisions affecting the care of assigned patients and in decisions affecting the professional practice of nursing within the organizational context.

The history of American nursing has been steeped in bureaucratic structure. Although major strides have been accomplished in the professionalism of nursing, concern continues regarding the lack of autonomy in professional practice and true participation in decision making. Traditional bureaucratic organizational structures have limited the staff nurse's participation in decisions affecting professional practice and have delegated that authority solely to administrative nurses or to a few advanced clinicians. Policies and procedures developed by nursing for patient care are often written by administrative nurses and ratified by the medical staff structure. Care delivery systems are designed by nonpractitioners to meet the financial goals of the organization and may be unrealistic or negatively impair the quality of patient care. Orders are given by other professionals to be followed by nurses, rather than an interdisciplinary team planning care (which would consider the perspective and input from each professional group caring for the patient). Consequently, nursing as a profession is known for its lack of autonomy and is considered by some to have semiprofessional status because of this lack of control and discretion in decision making.

To function autonomously within organizations, nurses must be granted the authority to define the scope of practice, the goals and subsequent responsibilities, and the specific role functions and domains of practice. The professional group must also have the power to influence the organization in matters related to its professional practice. According to Aydelotte (1983) ". . . the degree of professional autonomy . . . depends on the effectiveness of the group's efforts at governance. Without governance, there is no autonomy. Without autonomy, full professional status is unattainable" (p. 632).

Other scholars suggest the concept of autonomy incorporates the sense of competence (Flathman, 1987; Haworth, 1986), self-mastery (Lindley, 1986), and individualism and independence (Christman, 1989). Autonomy in professional practice cannot be realized without competence, nor the ability to exercise discretion without the proficiency to anticipate the consequence of one's decisions. Other dimensions of autonomy have been described as cooperation, interdependence, self-determination, sanctioning or vesting, and mature participation (Curtin, 1982; 1987). The roles that nurses fulfill are independent, dependent, and interdependent. Autonomy is an important concept to be realized for professionalism to develop, although complete autonomy may not be completely achieved (McKay, 1983; Stichler, 1989).

The professionals' desire for autonomy, self-organization, and increased discretion in their work has been studied and discussed critically in the last decade. The quality of life movement (Meltzer and Nord, 1981; Toch and Grant, 1984), participative management (Scanlon, 1948; Toch and Grant, 1984), and shared governance proponents all discuss the enhancement of autonomy of the professional practitioner as benefits to management. The positive effects of participation in decision making by the professional in practice issues have also been studied and reported extensively (Kanter, 1977; Loveridge, 1988; Mann and Jefferson, 1988; Metzger, 1989; Prescott, Dennis, and Jacox, 1987). Although the literature has abundant references to the importance of autonomy in professional practice, operationalization of this concept in the hospital and other organizations has been difficult.

The concepts of power, autonomy, and discretion are closely related. Power has been correlated with independent actions, involvement in decision making, and assumption of accountability for actions (Kalisch and Kalisch, 1982). Although there are many definitions of power, it is often defined as the ability to accomplish one's intended goals. Power is viewed as a characteristic of individuals (Beck, 1982). One is perceived as powerful when able to control important organizational resources, have possession of certain information, or is influential because of relationships with other powerful people. Power is the ability to choose and make those choices happen (French and Raven, 1959; Raz, 1986), which results in a perception of freedom and autonomy.

Issues of autonomy and authority are also interrelated. The professional desire for autonomy inevitably alters traditional managerial roles, challenges vested lines of authority, and creates potential conflicts between management and staff. Authority relates to the legitimate use of power. Benveniste (1987) suggested that organizational authority differs from professional authority and that moving more authority to the professional does not necessarily minimize the authority, responsibility, or accountability of the manager. In fact, he suggests, authority and power are increased as a result of shared tasks and responsibilities. In this sense, the benefits of shared power and authority are similar to the social systems theory discussed earlier that espouses that the synergistic group effect is more powerful than the combined efforts of individuals. The fear of losing one's power in a shared effort is a common fear and often prevents collaborative management styles from developing and evolving to full maturity.

A premise of shared governance and other collaborative management styles is that the professional makes decisions about professional matters and the work of the profession. Professional discretion is necessary to actualize this principle. Professional and managerial authorities overlap whenever managerial decisions must consider professional knowledge or when professionals must use managerial principles and authorities to perform the professional work. Benveniste (1987) suggests that managing professionals requires not only giving professionals sufficient discretion to accomplish professional tasks, but also sharing managerial tasks where professional values, knowledge, and skills are relevant. In essence, managing the professional worker requires the development of an organizational structure that not only supports and sanctions professional discretion and autonomy, but also shares decision making with management on issues affecting the practice.

Accountability is also a concept related to autonomy. The self-determination, discretion, and independent decision making inherent in autonomy also entail the accountability for one's decisions and actions. Some suggest that the degree of autonomy attained by nurses is measured in the degree of accountability of practitioners held in the public court system (Marks, 1987; Murphy, 1987).

Although these concepts have been defined, analyzed, and demonstrated as important to the job satisfaction of professional nurses, professionalization of nursing has not been actualized in many hospital settings. It appears that a new style of manager is necessary to change the cultures of organizations to embrace collaborative styles of management.

LEADERSHIP STYLES AND MANAGING PROFESSIONALS

Bureaucratic organizational structures have been the frame of reference for hospitals for centuries, and the traditional roles of management from the industrial model have been well established. Participative management, shared governance, or other models that enhance professional practice demand a new style of manager different from those characterized in more bureaucratic structures. Contemporary management scholars indicate that this new style of management is necessary to motivate professional employees who are paid for their knowledge, skill, and expertise, and not "just to get the job done."

Kotter (1990) suggests that managers in organizations may be "overeducated in management and undereducated in leadership" (p. 105), which results in their inability to move people with diverse opinions, skills, and interpersonal relationships in a similar direction to accomplish the goals of the organization. Kotter contends that interdependence is the central feature of contemporary organizations in which no one has complete autonomy, but rather employees interface because of technology, management systems, the work itself, and matrix-style management structures. These linkages and interdependencies require a leadership style that assists others to change and cope with change in an environment that is highly volatile, competitive, and fast-paced. With less emphasis on management and more on leadership skills, Kotter contends that managers must spend time aligning individuals and developing networks within the organization to help implement the vision and strategies of the organization. This process includes helping individuals to focus more globally on a new approach to an issue rather than attempting to solve a series of short-term problems. Such an approach empowers employees to think in new ways and allows discretion in solving both the short- and long-term problem.

Naisbitt and Aburdene (1990) suggest that the dominant principle of organizations has shifted from operations control to leadership that motivates people to respond quickly to change and enhances individual potential. They suggest that leaders will "inspire commitment and empower people by sharing authority" (p. 219). Successful organizations will treat employees as partners and team members in which the personal goals of the professional worker are met while accomplishing the mission of the organization.

New descriptors have been developed to represent the contemporary manager of professional organizations. Teacher, coach, facilitator, coordinator, and integrator are terms often used in current literature (Naisbitt and Aburdene, 1990; Porter-O'Grady and Finnigan, 1984). The new leadership style develops a "winning" commitment and attitude from the professional employee, and the leader is both coach and cheerleader assisting the professional to be self-managed, empowered, and better educated. Because of diminishing labor forces, the leader will need to hire employees who are highly educated and motivated to completing the job in times of uncertainty and fluctuation. Today's management emphasis is less focused on control, because uncertainty is uncontrollable, and is directed more to managing the constant and rapid change characteristic of modern organizations. Leadership requires vision and the interpersonal skills to articulate the vision. It is essential that leaders be capable of inspiring the professional rather than moving the group toward the accomplishment of the organization's goals.

Bennis and Nanus (1985) advise that organizations that manage professionals or work that is scientific and highly technical should emphasize decision making that is participative and should encourage communication of ideas from "the bottom up." All those who affect or are affected by the decision should have a voice in making the decision. Power, influence, and status should be based on participant involvement, face-to-face communication, and information sharing rather than on hierarchical position. Peer recognition should be determined by competence levels, interpersonal skills, and involvement. These themes, which Bennis and Nanus refer to as "collegial architecture," are founded on the following belief that people will do a good job if: (1) they are provided with the correct information, equipment and facilities, and procedures; (2) the vision and need have been well articulated to them; (3) the blame is not attached to failure; (4) there is shared responsibility and accountability for outcomes; and (5) managers will "lead" rather than manage and allow the employee flexibility to use individual discretion.

Kotter (1988; 1990) suggests that the new leadership does not push or pull people in the "right" direction, but rather motivates and inspires employees to achieve the vision of the organization by satisfying the basic human needs for achievement, belonging, recognition, autonomy, and self-esteem. True leaders involve people in achieving the organization's vision and work, which gives the employee a sense of control. Creating an environment in which leadership skills can be role modeled and developed in younger employees who also demonstrate leadership potential is the ultimate act of leadership and will provide the most powerful source of competitive advantage today.

Leadership for Collaborative Management Styles

The manager in a collaborative management structure such as shared governance must focus on new roles that Porter-O'Grady and Finnigan (1984) summarize as facilitating, coordinating, and integrating. Although the manager/administrator may lose some centralized decision making authority, accountability for the outcomes of the professional staff's decision making is still maintained. Because the collaborative process is the underlying framework for shared governance, the administrative team must develop collaborative group process skills to develop and consult with the nursing staff. Unequal status and power must be balanced, professional knowledge integrated, and participants valued for their contribution in order for collaborative relationships to develop and flourish. Obviously inherent in such a culture is the belief and trust that the staff will be able to complete the work necessary to accomplish the mission and goals of the organization. Consultation for critical decisions is accomplished with the chairpersons of strategic councils as well as the management team, which equalizes the power base of both groups.

Shared governance systems also affect the traditional managerial roles in hiring, promoting, disciplining, and controlling. Many organizations espousing shared governance use peer review and credentialing committees to perform the work of evaluating and controlling professional performance and privileging professional practice. Such actions provide the professional body with the authority and accountability to examine members of their profession and certify their competence, which is a hallmark of professional practice.

Interdisciplinary collaboration is essential in shared governance models as the administrative staff and council chairpersons work closely with other professionals to articulate and negotiate the needs of nursing. An essential management role is to promote interdisciplinary collaboration by planning and implementing forums for assessing and assuring quality, discussing bioethical issues, and promoting interdisciplinary communication in practice and education.

Most importantly, administrative nurses in a shared governance system should understand the domain of nursing and how the governance or management of nursing can complement and support the professional practice of nursing. By developing collaborative partnerships between the administrative and clinical nursing staff, the professionalism of nursing can be enhanced.

NEW ORGANIZATIONAL STRUCTURES IN NURSING

Bureaucracies are considered the antithesis of values related to professional functioning. Emphasis on control, order, standardization, and routinization may help measure outcomes and promote a false sense of organizational effectiveness, but it does nothing to promote the innovative thinking essential to the creation of successful organizations. To achieve full professional status, the members of the discipline must function autonomously in the governance of their own practice.

Shared Governance Models

According to Porter-O'Grady and Finnigan (1984), the professional worker needs an organizational structure that emphasizes lateral rather than hierarchical communication and relationship patterns. Such models would be more collaborative, using the expert knowledge of the professional in all issues related to professional practice. The professional's work and goals are interdependent with the management and mission of the organization. Without provision for interdependence and autonomy, the professional's practice is reduced to that of a technician who is subordinate to others and to the system. These authors relate the need for a system that delegates decision-making authority related to professional practice to the professionals within the organization. This delegated responsibility is actualized in collective forums and in independent discretionary judgments. Such action places the accountability for professional activities with the professional employees and promotes collegiality and equality in peer relationships between interdependent parties (clinical nurses and the management staff).

Recognizing that the hospital organization is an interdependent system of units whose success is dependent on the success of the whole, Porter-O'Grady and Finnigan's model of shared governance focuses on an organizational design that acknowledges this interdependence and facilitates the interaction among professionals at all levels within the organization. Shared governance reduces the emphasis on hierarchical relationships and highlights the professional's right to be involved in governance of the profession.

Shared governance is one example of a collaborative management structure and is characterized by the same dimensions seen in collaborative processes: balancing of power, reciprocating, and interpersonal valuing. Power is balanced equally between management and staff on issues related to the professional practice of nursing. Communication is facilitated by a matrix of councils or representative bodies empowered with the authority and accountability of decision making for the profession. Roles and responsibilities are clearly delineated in bylaws for the nursing divisions.

The essential structure of a shared governance system supports the work or practice of nursing and includes a network of five fundamental elements including governance or management, peer relations, professional development, practice, and quality assurance. Management assumes accountability for issues within its control, whereas the profession is accountable for the definition, delivery, and evaluation of its practice. In this sense, the dimension of reciprocating is operationalized as council, team, or committee members share information, expertise, and talents to do the work of nursing. Consensus on these issues represents the beliefs of the nursing professional group for each specific organization. Most specifically, the talents of the professional practitioners are integrated and synthesized with those of the administrative professionals to create a stronger dimension of nursing than was realized by the simple representation of the profession by administrative nurses.

Shared governance also initiates the third dimension of a collaborative management framework by granting the authority necessary for true decision making to the practitioners of the profession. There is a valuing of the nursing staff, with the realization that the work of the organization cannot be accomplished without the practitioners of nursing. As in all collaboration, a commitment to the process must occur. A commitment to shared governance must also occur at all levels in the organization for the organizational process to be successful.

In shared governance there are distinct areas in which the employee and manager have rights of final authority in decision making. The clinical nurses have authority over practice issues, and nurse managers have authority over management issues. Inherent in operationalizing shared governance is the belief and trust that employees, when given pertinent information and parameters, will make sound decisions. Because hierarchical organizational structures vest authority and control with the managerial staff, new roles emerge for the manager in a shared governance or collaborative management model.

Unionization

Bureaucratization of professional work often results in the unionization of the professional workers, since it minimizes their professional discretion and autonomy. Mercadante (1983) identified that unionization of nurses is often the result of lack of control and participation in decision making in professional practice issues, performance appraisal and promotion, and policies and procedures. Although the professional desires more control and autonomy when initially seeking assistance from an organized union, unionization of an organization often results in less individual control over professional issues. Individuals also experience less personal power because power is shared among management, union, and the individual professional practitioner. Collaborative management is minimized in a unionized organization, since the relationship between the union and the profession with the organization is often viewed as conflictual rather than cooperative or collaborative.

Participative Management

Participative management is based on the premise that involving the professional in decision making is important for role satisfaction, but the term "participation" provides for many levels of involvement. Forms of participation can include seeking advice, obtaining support, voting on decisions, or simply notifying interested parties of actions previous to implementation. The amount of participation should be determined by how essential the professional knowledge is to management or organizational effectiveness, and how important professional participation is to motivate and potentiate the professional's effectiveness. In hospitals, it is apparent that the organization's effectiveness is dependent on the professional's knowledge and expertise. It would seem apparent that a high level of participation by professional nurses would be essential.

Mercadante (1983) viewed participative management as a form of shared governance and indicated that a shared-authority model is a staff motivator and satisfier since it promotes communication between management and staff. The results of the study indicate, however, that the subjects perceived themselves as involved in decision making but that the final decisions were made by administration. In this sense, their involvement was more consultative than participatory. Mercadante offers a four-point plan to improve the perception of true participation that includes (1) goal planning with committee members, (2) recruiting committee members who wish to be actively involved, (3) eliciting suggestions and input from members and providing responsive feedback, and (4) developing joint problem-solving sessions with administration and staff nurses.

In contrast to Mercadante's belief that participatory management is a form of shared governance, Porter-O'Grady (1988) believes that the two types of management are distinctly different. Porter-O'Grady (1982) indicates that strategies to increase communication and interaction between staff and management are important but cannot replace the importance of true involvement and control over issues that govern the work activity of the employee. "Participative management by its very definition means allowing others to participate in decisions over which someone else has control" (Porter-O'Grady, 1987, p. 282).

MAKING COLLABORATIVE MANAGEMENT A REALITY IN THE WORKPLACE

Several studies (Blegen and Mueller, 1987; Hinshaw et al., 1987; McKay, 1983; Vanderslice, Rice, and Julian, 1987) have demonstrated a number of variables that affect job satisfaction, and the variables cited as predictors of job satisfaction are also essential variables for the professionalization of organizations. Because recruitment and retention resources are scarce, interventions having the greatest impact must be carefully identified and initiated. Enhancement of collaborative management styles and the development of organizational cultures that nurture professional autonomy and legitimate participation in decision making affecting professional practice are critical. Promoting collaborative management systems in a hospital is complex, and multiple strategies can be implemented.

The process of collaboration is characterized by interpersonal valuing, integration of ideas, opinions, and expertise, and a balancing of unequal power (Stichler, 1989). The collaborative manager should promote an environment or culture that demonstrates a valuing of the professional nurse and recognizes that the goals of the hospital/unit could not be realized without the professional nurse. It is recommended that the manager involve the clinical nurse in decisions that affect the professional practice of clinical nursing and in decisions that affect the delivery of patient care to enhance the development of collaborative behaviors. Implementing systems such as shared governance, participative management, joint practice models, or other similar programs enhances staff involvement and participation in decision making. These systems also provide for increased nurse-manager interaction, planning, and coordination of patient care that integrates the expert opinions of administrative and clinical nurses. A balancing of power occurs in the council model of shared governance, which fosters nurse-manager collaborative behaviors. Nurse managers generally serve on the clinical councils as consultants without voting privileges, which helps to balance the power in patient care decision making between clinical and administrative nurses. In addition, the chairpersons of each council in the shared governance system meet with an administrative director to coordinate the activities of patient care and the professional practice of nursing.

It is also recommended that career advancement programs be developed that allow those who choose to practice clinical nursing at advanced levels to be rewarded financially and with recognition of their power by expertise. Open communication between management and nurses that allows freedom of expression of concerns, criticisms, creativity, and opinions is recommended to enhance nurse-manager collaboration. Encouraging clinical nurses to be active participants in strategic planning and program implementation, quality assurance activities, scheduling on-duty time, along with providing educational offerings will promote nurse-manager collaboration in domains traditionally recognized as management. It is recommended that nurse managers move from the more traditional leadership styles and roles of management to contemporary and collaborative roles that include facilitation of patient care, integration of ideas, opinions, and expertise, and the coordination of resources including manpower and finances.

Organizational Climate and Collaborative Management

The climate of the organization characterizes the generalized "feeling" of the organization and reflects the structure and processes of the organization. Although organizational climate is relatively stable over time, the manager can influence the climate by her or his style of management. To enhance a positive organizational climate, the manager should recognize the nurse's expertise as a clinician and empower her or him to participate in decisions, actions, and planning that affect patient care or the professional practice of nursing. Minimizing bureaucracy and traditional lines of communication facilitates the development of autonomy in the professional nurse and will minimize the formal structure of the organization. Position structure can inhibit the natural creativity of a nurse who wishes to risk individual participation in changes to unit functioning or patient care. Reward and recognition by the manager of the clinical nurse's contributions to quality patient care facilitates the perception of a positive organizational climate. Leaders who demonstrate warmth, concern, and consideration will effect increased job satisfaction among the work force. It is recommended that managers maximize positive changes in the organizational climate by facilitating nurses' participation in all aspects of operations and by empowering nurses to seek creative solutions to day-to-day problems. In developing a true partnership relationship with the nursing staff rather than the traditional bureaucratic relationship, the manager can positively affect the climate of the organization and ultimately the job satisfaction of the individual nurse.

Numerous studies (Godfrey, 1978; Jacobson, 1988; Nursing Shortage Poll Report, 1988; Stember et al., 1978) have validated that an unrealistic work load has a tremendous influence on the stress level of nurses and is directly related to burnout, job dissatisfaction, and anticipated or actual turnover. Because of the importance of this variable in job satisfaction and retention, it is strongly recommended that the nurse manager be particularly attentive to ensuring realistic work loads and preserving the same when hospitals face severe economic challenges and nursing shortages. Clinical nurses and administrative nurses must work together to redefine patient care delivery systems that realistically have professional nurses performing responsibilities that must be performed by the professional and delegating palliative, comfort, or general hygiene functions to other support personnel.

"Administrative or managerial support" is a little-understood construct and can be defined differently depending on each individual's perspective. It is recommended that the manager talk with staff to better understand their perspective of support. By so doing, the manager can be better equipped to meet the employees' expectation of supervisor support and minimize the stress incurred when expectations are not met.

SUMMARY

Professional partnerships between management and the professional staff can result in organizations that value collaborative management principles and structures rather than the superior-subordinate relationship in bureaucratic structures. An integrative network promotes both interprofessional and intraprofessional consultation and collaboration that not only fulfills the employees' need for participation and ownership in organizational processes and outcomes, but also fosters collective creativity and innovativeness. The theoretical framework and the operationalization of collaborative management styles support the work of earlier organizational researchers and theorists and most specifically support contemporary writers, who suggest that organizations rich in collaborative networking rather than bureaucratic hierarchies will be the most successful.

REFERENCES

American Organization of Nurse Executives. (1990). *Nurse Executive* 2(9), 1.

Argryis, C. (1962). *Interpersonal Competence and Organizational Effectiveness,* Homewood, Ill.: Irwin Dorsey Press.

Aydelotte, M.K. (1983). Professional Nursing: The Drive for Governance. In Chaska NL, editor: *The Nursing Profession: A Time to Speak,* New York: McGraw-Hill Book Co, pp 830-843.

Bechtold, S.E., Szilagyi, A.D. and Sims, H.P. (1980). Antecedents of Employee Satisfaction in a Hospital Environment, *Health Care Management Review,* 5(1), 77-78.

Beck, C. (1982). The Conceptualization of Power, *Advances in Nursing Science,* 4(2), 1-17.

Bennis, W. and Nanus, B. (1985). *Leaders.* New York: Harper & Row.

Benveniste, G. (1987). *Professionalizing the Organization,* San Francisco: Jossey-Bass.

Blake, R.R. and Mouton, J.S. (1964). *The Managerial Grid,* Houston: Gulf Publishing.

Blegen, M.A. and Mueller, C.W. (1987). Nurses' Job Satisfaction: A Longitudinal Analysis. *Research in Nursing Health,* 10, 227-237.

Bolman, L.G. and Deal, T.E. (1984). Modern Approaches to Understanding and Managing Organizations, San Francisco: Jossey-Bass.

Bream, T. and Schapiro, A. (1989). Nurse-Physician Networks: A Focus for Retention. *Nursing Management,* 20(5), 74-77.

Buccheri, R.C. Nursing Supervision: A New Look at an Old Role. *Nursing Administration Quarterly,* 11, 11-25.

Carr-Saunders, A.M. and Wilson, P.A. (1933). *The Professions,* Oxford: Oxford University Press.

Christman, J. editor: (1989). *The Inner Citadel: Essays on Individual Autonomy.* New York: Oxford University Press.

Curtin, L.L. (1982). Autonomy, Accountability, and Nursing Practice, *Advances in Nursing Science,* 4, 7-14.

Curtin, L.L. (1987). The "Employment" of Autonomy, *Nursing Management,* 18, 9-12.

Deal, T.E. and Kennedy, A.A. (1982). *Corporate Culture: The Rights and Rituals of Corporate Life,* Reading, Mass,: Addison-Wesley.

Dempster, J.S. (1990). Autonomy in Practice: Conceptualization, Construction, and Psychometric Evaluation of an Empirical Instrument, Unpublished manuscript, San Diego.

Department of Health and Human Services. (1988). *Secretary's Commission on Nursing,* vol 1, Washington, D.C.: US Government Printing Office.

Deutsch, M. (1973). *The Resolution of Conflict,* New Haven, Conn.: Yale University Press.

Donohue, J.D. (1986). Faculty Perceptions of Organizational Climate and Expressed Job Satisfaction in Selected Baccalaureate Schools of Nursing, *Journal of the Professional Nurse,* 2, 373-379.

Duxbury, M.L., Henley, G.A. and Armstrong, G.D. (1982). Measurement of the Nurse Organizational Climate of Neonatal Intensive Care Units, *Nursing Research,* 31, 83-88.

Erickson, E. (1963). *Childhood and Society,* ed 2, New York: WW Norton.

Fawcett, J. (1984). *Analysis and Evaluation of Conceptual Models of Nursing,* Philadelphia: F.A. Davis Co.

Flathman, R.E. (1987). *The Philosophy and Politics of Freedom,* Chicago: University of Chicago Press.

French, J. and Raven, B. (1959). The Bases of Social Power. In Cartwright D, editor: *Studies in Social Power,* Ann Arbor, Mich.: Institute for Social Research, pp 259-269.

Godfrey, M.A. (1978). Job Satisfaction: or Should That Be Dissatisfaction? How Nurses Feel about Nursing. Part two, *Nursing 78,* 8(5), 105-120.

Greenwood, E. (1987). Attributes of a Profession, *Social Work* 2, 45-55.

Hall, R.H. (1968). Professionalization and Bureaucratization, *American Sociological Review,* 33, 92-104.

Haworth, L. (1986). *Autonomy: An Essay in Philosophical Psychology and Ethics,* New Haven, Conn.: Yale University Press.

Herzberg, F. (1968). One More Time: How Do You Motivate Employees? *Harvard Business Review,* 46 (Jan-Feb), 53-62.

Hickman, C.R. and Silva, M.A. (1984). *Creating Excellence,* New York: New American Library.

Hinshaw, A.S. Smeltzer, C.H. and Atwood, J.R. (1987). Innovative Retention Strategies for Nursing Staff, *Journal of Nursing Administration,* 17(6), 8-16.

Homans, G.C. (1950). *The Human Group,* New York: Harcourt, Brace & Co.

Jacobson, S.F. (1988). *Nurse Retention on High Stress Clinical Specialty Units. Nursing Resources and the Delivery of Patient Care.* Washington D.C.: U.S. Department of Health and Human Services.

Kalisch, B.J. and Kalisch, P.A. (1982). An Analysis of the Sources of Physician-Nurse Conflict. In Muff J, editor: *Socialization, Sexism, and Stereotyping,* St. Louis, Mo.: CV Mosby, pp. 221-233.

Kanter, R.M. (1977). *Men and Women of the Corporation,* New York: Basic Books.

Kotter, J.P. (1988). *The Leadership Factor,* New York: The Free Press.

Kotter, J.P. (1990). What leaders really do, *Harvard Business Review,* 90(3), 103-111.

Lawler, E.E. and Porter, L.W. (1971). The Effect of Performance in Job Satisfaction. In Connelly, J.H. Jr, Gibson, J.L. and Ivanevick, J.M. editors: *Fundamentals of Management: Selected Readings,* Austin, Texas: Business Publications, pp 110-150.

Lindley, R. (1986). *Autonomy,* Atlantic Highlands, NJ: Humanities Press International, Inc.

Loveridge, C. (1988). Contingency Theory: Explaining Staff Nurse Retention. *Journal of Nursing Administration,* 18(6), 22-25.

Lysaught, J.P. (1970). *An Abstract for Action,* New York: McGraw-Hill Book Co.

Mann, E.E. and Jefferson, K.J. (1988). Retaining Staff: Using Turnover Indices and Surveys, *Journal of Nursing Admininstration,* 18(7,8), 17-23.

Marks, D.T. (1987). Legal Implications of Increased Autonomy, *Journal of Gerontological Nursing,* 13, 26-31.

Maslow, A. (1954). *Motivation and Personality,* New York: Harper & Row.

McKay, P.S. (1983). Interdependent Decision Making: Professional Autonomy, *Nursing Administration Quarterly,* Summer, 21-30.

Meltzer, H. and Nord, W. editors: (1981), *Making Organizations Humane and Productive: A Handbook for Practitioners,* New York: Wiley.

Mercadante, L.T. (1983). A Study of Nurses' Perceptions of Participative Management. In Chaska N.L., editor: *The Nursing Profession: A Time to Speak,* New York: McGraw-Hill Book Co, pp 696-707.

Metzger, N. (1989). Making Employees Feel that They Make a Difference, *Health Care Supervision,* 7(3), 1-7.

Murphy, E.K. (1987). The Professional Status of Nursing: A View from the Courts, *Nursing Outlook,* 35, 12-15.

Naisbitt, J. (1982). *Megatrends,* New York: Warner Books, Inc.

Naisbitt, J. and Aburdene, P. (1985). *Re-inventing the Corporation,* New York: Warner Books, Inc.

Naisbitt, J. and Aburdene, P. (1990). *Megatrends 2000,* New York: William Morrow & Co.

National Commission on Nursing. (1981). *Summary of Public Hearings,* Chicago: American Hospital Association.

National Commission on Nursing. (1982). *Nursing in Transition: Models for Successful Organizational Change,* Chicago: The Hospital Research and Education Trust.

National Joint Practice Commission. (1981). *Guidelines for Establishing Joint or Collaborative Practice in Hospitals,* Chicago: National Joint Practice Commission.

Nursing Shortage Poll Report. (1988). *Nursing 88,* 18(2), 33-41.

Office of the Inspector General. (1989). Hospital Best Practices in Nurse Recruitment and Retention, *Nursing Economics,* 7(2), 98-106.

Peters, T.J. and Waterman, R.H. (1982). *In Search of Excellence,* New York: Harper & Row.

Peterson, M.E. and Allen, D.G. (1986). Shared Governance: A Strategy for Transforming Organizations, *Journal of Nursing Administration,* 16(1), 9-12.

Pinkerton, S.E. and Schroeder, P. (1988). *Commitment to Excellence,* Rockville, Md.: Aspen Publications.

Porter, L.W., Lawler, E.E., and Hackman, J.R. (1975). *Behavior in Organizations,* New York: McGraw-Hill.

Porter-O'Grady, T. (1982). What Motivation Isn't, *Nursing Management,* 13(2), 27-29.

Porter-O'Grady, T. (1987). Shared Governance and New Organization Models, *Nursing Economics,* 5(6), 281-286.

Porter-O'Grady, T. (1988). Personal communication, Aug 1, 1988.

Porter-O'Grady, T. and Finnigan, S. (1984). *Shared Governance for Nursing,* Rockville, Md.: Aspen Publications.

Prescott, P., Dennis, K., and Jacox, A. (1985). Power and Powerlessness in Hospital Nursing Departments, *Journal of Professional Nursing,* 1(6), 348-355.

Prestholdt, P.H., Lane, I.M., and Mathews, R.C. (1987). Nurse Turnover Reasoned Action: Development of a Process Model, *Journal of Applied Psychology,* 72(2), 221-227.

Prestholdt, P.H., Lane, I.M., and Mathews, R.C. (1988). Predicting Nurse Turnover, *Nursing Outlook,* 36(3), 145-147.

Raz, J. (1986). *The Morality of Freedom,* Oxford: Clarendon Press.

Rowland, H.S. and Rowland, B.L. (1980). *Nursing Administration Handbook,* Rockville, Md.: Aspen Publications.

Scanlon, J.N. (1948). Profit Sharing Under Collective Bargaining: Three Case Studies, *Industrial and Labor Relations Review,* 2, 58-75.

Sims, L.M., Price, S.A., and Ervin, N.E. (1985). *Professional Nursing Practice, The Professional Practice of Nursing Administration,* New York: Wiley.

Stamps, P.L., and others. (1978). Measurement of Work Satisfaction Among Health Professionals, *Medical Care,* 16(4), 337-352.

Stember, M.L., Ferguson, J., Conway, K., and Yingling, M. (1978). Job Satisfaction Research—An Aid in Decision Making, *Nursing Administration Quarterly,* 2, 95-105.

Stogdill, R.M. (1974). *Handbook of Leadership,* New York: The Free Press.

Stichler, J.F. (1989). Development and Psychometric Testing of a Collaborative Behavior Scale, Unpublished dissertation.

Stichler, J.F. (1990). The Effects of Collaboration, Organizational Climate, and Job Stress on Job Satisfaction and Anticipated Turnover in Nursing, Unpublished manuscript.

Stogdill, R.M. (1974). *Handbook of Leadership,* New York: The Free Press.

Taunton, R.L., Krampitz, S.D., and Woods, C.Q. (1989). Manager's Impact on Retention of Hospital Staff, Part 2, *Journal of Nursing Administration,* 19(4), 15-19.

Tauskey, C. (1978). *Work Organization: Major Theoretical Perspectus,* ed 2, Itasca, Ill.: Peacock Press.

Taylor, F.W. (1911). *Principles of Management,* New York: Harper & Brothers.

Tiffany, C., Cruise, P., and Cruise, R.J. (1988). Discretion and Professionalization: A Correlational Study, *Nursing Management,* 19(2), 71D-72P.

Tjosvold, D. (1984). Cooperation Theory and Organizations, *Human Relations,* 37, 743-767.

Toch, H. and Grant, D.J. (1984). *Reforming Human Services: Change Through Participation,* Beverly Hills, Calif.: Sage.

Vanderslice, V.J., Rice, R.W., and Julian, J.W. (1987). The Effects of Participation in Decision-Making on Worker Satisfaction and Productivity, *Journal of Applied Psychology,* 17(2), 158-170.

Vroom, V.H. (1964). *Work and Motivation,* New York: John Wiley & Sons.

Vroom, B.H. and Yetton, P.W. (1973). *Leadership and Decision-Making,* Pittsburgh: University of Pittsburgh Press.

2 A Decade of Organizational Change

Tim Porter-O'Grady

SHARED GOVERNANCE: THE CALL FOR CHANGE

It has been more than a decade since the concept of shared governance began to be implemented in nursing organizations throughout the United States. The three originating hospitals, St. Joseph's in Atlanta, St. Michael in Milwaukee, and Rose Medical Center in Denver, have not only pioneered the shared governance model but have matured in it and remain as committed to it today as when they first implemented it 11 years ago (McDonagh, 1990).

The shared governance approach to organizing and empowering the nursing profession in the workplace continues to grow in the United States at a rapid rate. More than 1,000 hospitals and health care agencies are in some phase of shared governance implementation, and more than 300 hospitals have had it in place for 5 years or longer. Data are being generated from research studies that support the efficiency, efficacy, and satisfaction of the nursing staff and leadership with the approach (Ludemann and Brown, 1989). As more data become available, generalizations can be made about the effectiveness of nurse empowerment and the satisfaction with this approach by a broad host of beneficiaries (Jones and Ortiz, 1989).

As with any "new" approach to organizing professionals and their work, much activity and energy have propelled shared governance into an identifiable, meaningful form. Although the concept has been based on solid organizational principle and theory as well as emerging notions about the professional workplace, there were no models in place for implementers to use for guidance. Rather, the "script" was written as shared governance models were unfolding.

Shared governance represents the democratic and representative principles congruent with a democratic society, but there has been little support of such approaches to empowering and organizing the professional worker in the American workplace. Other than the typical third-party collective bargaining processes, which sometimes polarize worker and workplace, there were few other models of integration and empowerment that were mutually beneficial and agreeable.

The historical role of the nurse also influenced the kind of organizational approaches that have been used in the past to manage nurses and control their work

(Henry, 1990). There was little to suggest that the individual nurse had much control over her own work, and there is much to support the fact that the nurse's role was always subjugated to the role of the physician and administrator in the hospital environment (Ashley, 1976).

There have been many changes to this scenario. The relationship between the nurse and the workplace has recently undergone assessment for dramatic and even radical change as both the health care system and its broader community undergo adjustment.

Even the research data on which much of the management process has been based have been subject to much question and reinterpretation in the past 10 to 15 years (Mintzberg, 1990). Much of the application of management and human resource theories has been based on studies conducted in manufacturing plants and industrial settings. There has been little research that reflects the unique characteristics of professional employees and the working conditions that are unique to them (Porter-O'Grady, 1986).

Only within the last three decades has there been an emerging consciousness of gender equity in the American workplace. Because of legal changes and the burgeoning number of women in the work force, much has changed with regard to the legitimate role and relationship of women and men. Some discussion regarding and attempts to create a truly equitable workplace in which gender considerations do not affect role selection or performance considerations have been initiated (Gibbs and others, 1990).

Shared governance models anticipate this reality and have served to give form to the effort to create equity in the nursing workplace and to build a model that not only represents the beliefs of equity but also provides a form and forum for the expression of the related beliefs. Much of the original impetus for organizational structuring of shared governance has subsequently been determined to be unsubstantiated. However, it should come as no shock to the reader that much of what we come to accept as gospel in health care organizations is based on a great deal of myth. The nursing leader must sort through a wide variety of behaviors, cultural values, rules, relationships and other organizational variables in order to find the truth that undergirds the behaviors of those who work in health care (Helgesen, 1990).

Because nursing organizations have seldom been successful in attaining attendant organizational support, it has been challenging to achieve generalized commitment in making workplace changes. Nurses are not accustomed to "rocking the boat" and taking control of their sector of the health care system. It can even be said that nurses historically did little to change their work status. It is surprising how prevalent this sentiment still remains among practicing nurses (del Bueno, 1990).

It can easily be said that the very nurses that organizations have prepared to be this way are practicing today. They have been socialized to behave in the most acceptable way along a path of least resistance. The truly unique and creative nurses either burn out early, slip away, or are driven away. Some of them may even become nurse managers. Childish behavior and general anger frequently emerge in the staff as such nurses act out their impotence and frustration and the organization soon can become petulant. At best, the staff become dependent, malleable, and passive, unable to act for themselves and unwilling to expend the requisite energy to change their condition. At worst, the staff become passive-aggressive, acting out their anger by sabotaging, undermining, complaining, and refusing to change their condition or circumstances.

Although these characterizations may appear extreme and unflattering, they are nonetheless true. When there is no legitimate outlet for the nursing staff to express anger and frustration, they must find alternate ways to deal with sentiments. When the organization finds the staff's feelings upsetting and challenging and cannot accept their expression and disapproves of the associated behaviors, the energy must be vented elsewhere. Thus it is directed in the only tolerated manner, which is on the self and immediate others. The ways are often violent, demeaning, and self-deprecating. This scenario creates a neurotic and codependent organization (Kets de Vries and Miller, 1984).

If classic family systems were used to assess this scenario, the dysfunctional elements would be evident. Issues of control, mental anguish, hostage holding, parent-child role behaviors, and family violence, all would be present and extreme therapeutic measures would be recommended. The nursing "family" in the nursing organization would require much dialogue and communication and a solid reformatting of relationships to determine a healthier way for the parties to interrelate and interact.

This backdrop provides the impetus to study organizational models that would change the relationship between staff and management. The dependency characteristics benefit none in the profession and therefore have no real or legitimate social value. Both the organization and the profession must mature with regard to their relationship and neither can remain unchanged. Both parties need each other, but not in ways that represent an unhealthy continuation of their past dependencies and dysfunctional behaviors. A newer model of interaction representative of an adult relationship is necessary to create a positive framework for interaction. It is in this context that shared governance takes its form and provides its meaning.

Leaders involved with shared governance have reflected on this historic conditioning and sought appropriate strategies to define a newer, healthier, and stronger relationship between the profession and the workplace (Pinkerton and Schroeder, 1988). When the concept of shared governance was being considered, it was thought that it did not have the seeds of any substantive changes in the health care system or the social system. In addition, the staff was not prepared for such a radical role and structural change and could never accomplish significant decisional process without substantial support from the appropriate manager(s).

The issue in operation relates to readiness for change. Change never can be fully anticipated or planned for; it evolves. The key to handling change is to be open to it and to find ways to work in concert with it. Participants should let its energy pull them into newer and more desirable realities. This is not always easy.

Shared governance as a concept applied to nursing developed from the above realities and circumstances. It seemed to address directly those operant behaviors in most hospitals that exemplified the nurses' greatest frustrations with the system. The concept appeared to confront the organizational beliefs that nurses often found themselves confronting. The concept of shared governance forced almost everyone to look at what they were doing, how they were doing it, and at what cost (Porter-O'Grady and Finnigan, 1984).

To ensure that the shared governance approach addressed the problem appropriately, or at least was not a retread of past models, its form was squarely centered in professional accountabilities and nonadministrative-driven values. Most management principles in the United States were the fruits of research done in industry and manufacturing plants (Witte, 1980) and are not particularly relevant to the values inherent in nursing. Nursing, on the other hand, is a knowledge profession with an emphasis on professional value formation that often puts it at odds with a workplace, the hospital, determined to shape its workers in values of its own making. When nursing education was centered in hospitals, the task was relatively easy. As nursing education moved into independent schools, the task became harder and nurses were less predisposed to manipulation of their values. Dissatisfaction and other negative responses about the relationship between nurses and their practice settings have accelerated over the past three decades.

More recent research in work settings similar to nursing's has shown that an entirely different approach is necessary for successful relationships between the work setting and the worker (Peters, 1987). Control, influence, partnership, and recognition are all terms emerging in studies of the last two great commissions studying nurses and their needs. The orientation of the hospital and other clinical centers toward the nurse has been in great need of retooling. High turnover rates and increasing demand for nursing services have created pressure for different approaches to organizing and managing the workplace that are more compatible with the character of the nursing profession and the needs of its members.

Of equal impact on the practice of nursing is change in the health care system. It is widely known that the United States is in the midst of tough economic times (Beatty, 1990). When the magnitude of the economic shortfalls is considered, they may be overwhelming. It is obvious that the health care system cannot remain exempt from the realities of constraining economics without undergoing some adjustment in its service provision (Brown and McCool, 1990). Demand for health care service has not changed; indeed it is increasing. Cost of service has not declined, even though the hospital-based portion of care has declined as a percent of the whole, and thus the needs of the consumer have not justified reductions in dollars available for health care services. Yet, reductions in hospital-directed dollars have totaled more than $10 billion in the past 4 years. Clearly, whether desired or not, reduced funding forces service changes, and nursing cannot help but be directly affected. A need to be cognizant of the economic realities affecting nursing practice has driven nursing leaders to consider how the health care dollar is apportioned, the impact on nursing, and how best to respond to any resultant changes. The important point is that nurses want to respond to their own issues and make space for themselves at the policy-making tables and no longer let others decide their economic and service fates (Haddon, 1989).

The need for partnership relationships has also emerged in the nursing value system. Understandably, nurses want to play a major role in making the decisions that affect what they do, how they do it, and the impact of their work on patients and on the health care arena. Nurses have realized that they are stakeholders in the health care enterprise and therefore should play both a policy and an implementation role in service selection and how it is provided. If the health care organization does not manage its services well and thereby suffers losses, nurses and patients suffer, too. The institution's gains and losses do not occur independently of those who provide them. Nurse providers are aware of the impact of mission, direction, and position statements that set a course for the institution for better or for worse. At best, nurses will have to work to achieve, and at worst, accept and live with the impact of these policies. As stakeholders, nurses have found that a passive stance did not ensure that service provision considerations were an integral part of decisions made that influenced patient care. As the ostensible advocate for the needs of the consumer, nurses believe it is imperative that they play a more direct and integral role in decisions that impact patient care (Burda, 1990).

It is clear that the above may be true and desirable, but nurses and nursing practice are not positioned or skilled in the processes essential to accomplish the desired roles associated with power and policy decisions. This reality is irrelevant to whether nurses can effectively make such decisions. It has more to do with the internal structures and dispositions of nursing. Can nurses legitimately be expected to both play out decisive roles and then actually do the work?

The internal dynamics of most nursing organizations do not permit a sufficiently broad base of professional involvement and investment from the professional staff to either permit staff to assume these roles, or even modify the structures and skills that would make it possible for staff to have some locus of control in these arenas. As indicated in previous texts on shared governance, history and gender have had a restrictive influence on nursing staff roles that involve influence and control. Managers, even nurse managers, have maintained this status quo. What has resulted is a passive-aggressive, dependent, clinical staff with neither interest or insight into the issues that most affect what they do (Porter-O'Grady, 1986).

This situation creates a direct conflict, and it is difficult for the nursing staff to emerge a winner. When nurse managers attempt to persuade their staffs to expand interest in their own accountability, the rewards of passive dependency moderate against nurses affirming both the energy necessary to make changes and the very value of the change itself. This, combined with the lack of insight and skill, assures that there will be limited, almost isolated, response to critical political, policy, and economic issues that directly affect what nurses do and the resources available to them.

SHARED GOVERNANCE: THE PRINCIPLES OF RESPONSE

From this context the concept of shared governance takes form. Connecting the words *shared* and *governance* is both purposeful and meaningful. Shared, because no one will get to tomorrow alone. People are inherently interdependent. Hardly anyone can do anything without impacting someone else. Shared governance recognizes this reality and, as a result, integrates unilateral action with collateral values or purposes and, through negotiation and consensus, seeks an agreeable outcome. These operational realities impact decision making and roles. There are no unilateral decisions in health care (Bocchino, 1990).

The second word, *governance,* ties the activities of the nursing profession in a given setting into the governing, ruling, decision-making processes of the entity of which nursing is a part. It indicates that as a professional discipline, nursing has a governance character with regard to its own affairs and a governance connection to the policy and directional decisions of the governing body of the entity. Such characterization is synonymous with corporate partnerships wherein each of the partners has a negotiated but defined role in both policy and the work of the enterprise. Each partner knows the extent and nature of their individual contribution and is required to exercise it because each is committed to it. Rather than being mutually exclusive processes, governance and function are correlates of each other. The essential variable in this connection, however, is that each party knows what the other party has to offer, offers it, and is thereafter accountable for what is achieved or accomplished as a result of the action. In a professional model of shared governance, the accountable professional stakeholders define their mutual and distinct relationships and contributions and collectively agree to unfold them for a purpose that is mutually beneficial and consistent with both the mission of the enterprise and the charge of the profession.

ACCOUNTABILITY

The key to the work of the parties in the work relationship is a clear understanding of the accountabilities of each of the partners. The concept of accountability is essential to the definitiveness of any productive relationship in the work context. A fuller understanding of accountability and its meaning lies at the heart of the effectiveness of any equity-based collateral work relationship. When nursing is trying to evolve into an equity-based relationship from a subordinated relationship, with all that movement implies, understanding the character of accountability becomes central to shared role definition and shared decision making.

Accountability differs from the responsibility-based processes we normally associate it with. Indeed, it has a definition that really operates in reverse of the nominal action of responsibility. Accountability within a professional context can be simply defined as the exercise of activities inherent to a role that cannot and are not legitimately controlled outside the role and for which the locus of control emanates from within the role. Conversely, responsibility is generated or delegated to the role, always has an external locus of control, is generally assigned by someone with the authority to do so, and depends on negotiation and acceptance of the delegation for fulfillment. In other words, accountability is fundamental to the role and can never be assigned away, whereas responsibility is delegated from outside the role and is, therefore, always assigned. Accountability reflects an attributed role, and responsibility reflects an assigned role. Responsibility falls within the context of the structure of the work; accountability falls within the context of the character of the work. This contrast will be rearticulated later in this chapter.

There are conditions to accountability that give form to its meaning. It is both a concept and a term that is not always characterized or used consistently. For professional accountability to operate it must meet three conditions: autonomy, authority, and control (Porter-O'Grady, 1989). The professional must have the right (autonomy) to undertake specified action, the power (authority) to implement action, and the ability to enforce (control) the action in an ongoing and consistent manner. These conditions of accountability are essential characteristics of the professional role of the nurse. Without them, much of the definition of nursing's professional role and the underpinnings of shared governance are missing. It is often difficult to shift understanding of legitimate roles and accountability in an organizational system that is structured on the premise that there is only one locus of control in the organization that it is tied exclusively to the management role. When the conditions and circumstances of professional accountability are more clearly delineated and its differences and legitimacy recognized, it becomes easier to comprehend models that, by design, purposely structure other control points in the organization and build structure on the legitimate loci of accountability.

These issues have emerged over the past few years as important foundations for professional governance models (Porter-O'Grady, 1989). In the initial years, issues of organization and operation were secondary to reactionary strategies to change an undesirable structure that produced professional impotence in the practice arena. However, there is more to organizing work than simply objecting to the status quo. Whatever is to be substituted in place of the "old" must work better, fulfill what it purports to do, and effectively alter the conditions that drove nursing leaders to consider it in the first place. The change also must reflect a set of values that drive the move to shared governance, which give the change some meaning, and connect that meaning to some useful format. This change must empower the affected group (nursing) to make the requisite change in their best interests, but not at the expense of any others, and to the net overall benefit to those who receive nursing services.

In the formative stages of the first shared governance systems, much attention was given to empowerment structures. Although structure is important, it is not as important as a solid understanding of the principles that drive shared governance. Leaders in shared governance now understand that a variety of structures can be used to house the process of self-governing activities. Attention to structure provides a format for the concept, but no structure is adequate if it does not support the principles upon which the concept is based.

Clarifying the accountabilities attendant to the professional role of the nurse is a formative activity. Professions can generally express their accountability in the following areas.

Practice

The role of any profession is related to the work it does. Its "birthright" should be found from within its work activities. As such, those activities should result from the fundamental values and beliefs that drive the work. It is presumed that the nurse knows these and can actively apply them within the context of her role. However, often the nurse does *not* know what these premises and values are and cannot identify whether her practice is consonant with them or operates in opposition to them. If she does know them, the nurse may not always be confident that she is free to act on them and that, if conflict were to emerge from her actions, that her actions would be adequately supported by the delivery system. All of these elements must operate in consonance before they can be effectively applied.

Practice is that process whereby the professional does the primary work of the profession. It is toward that work that all the activities of the organization and the profession are directed. It can be stated that both the purposes of the profession and its fundamental activity take their form in the work or practice of the individual practitioner. This accountability is fundamental and cannot be assigned or given away. It is directly attributed to the practitioner and cannot be legitimately located anywhere else in the organization. Included in this premise is all the attendant authority the practitioner needs to accomplish the requisites of the professional role and the expectations of those served by that role. In a governance model, this authority does not legitimately rest anywhere else in the organization. Included in this accountability is the right to control the following: position (job) descriptions, standards of care, performance expectations, career advancement, and interdisciplinary relationships.

Accountability for the above standards rests solely with the practicing nurse and cannot be legitimately exercised beyond that role in a shared governance system. The belief that the practitioner is ultimately accountable for defining practice is fundamental to the concept of shared governance. The challenge lies in the establishment of structures that support the practicing nurse's locus of control within this accountability.

Quality Assurance

Quality assurance is the second major element for which the nurse is ultimately accountable. The adequacy of practice cannot be assured without a clear delineation of whether that practice has actually achieved the outcomes to which it was directed. Because quality assurance is dependent on both the definition of practice and its exercise, it is a subset of the clinical role that takes its precedence in nursing practice. Again, the legitimate locus of control rests with the practitioner because it is a measure of the nursing role and is necessarily invested in the action of nursing practice for which only the practitioner can be accountable. For quality assurance to be appropriately carried out, it must be located with and in the practice context. Therefore, in shared governance, quality assurance is viewed as a clinical accountability and becomes a function of clinical work. The locus of control both for undertaking quality assurance and for assuring compliance with its requirements is a clinical function for which some structure must be attached.

It is necessary when thinking about the quality assurance function to recall that assurance of the quality of care cannot exist as a function outside the process that assures the quality of the caregiver. Both processes are quality assurance functions. Historically, however, the performance evaluation function that focuses on the practitioner has always been considered a management function. It has been assumed that the manager is the appropriate locus of control for this function. Because quality of care and quality of the caregiver are necessarily connected and essential if quality of care is to be provided, it can be asked, "How could one aspect be so distinctly clinical in focus and not the other?" Simply, it cannot. If the locus of control is in the practitioner for the quality of care delivered (and must necessarily be there if quality is to be obtained), then it is reasonable that determining the processes associated with measuring the quality of the caregiver must also be controlled by the practitioner. One is synonymous with the other; indeed, they are inseparable. Historically, they have been arbitrarily separated as a matter of institutional control, not as a legitimate expression of staff accountability. They must be rejoined if they are to be fully realized and valued in the discipline. Shared governance accomplishes this. The accountabilities that normally fall within the context of the quality assurance function are: quality of care, performance evaluation, career advancement measurement, measurement criteria development, credentialing process, and privileging mechanism. The identified accountabilities form the basis of the work of quality assurance. Mechanisms for the undertaking of quality assurance without removing it from the practice setting and the practicing nurse are essential in the shared governance accountability format.

Competence

Competence is one of the vital concerns of a profession and its members. Issues related to the ability of the members of a profession and their ability to perform the activities of the profession within the standards of the profession for those activities are often identified by those outside the profession. The definition of competence and the standards that measure it are fundamental characteristics of the nursing profession and also exist as an accountability of every member of the professional group. The ability to assure the public that those who provide nursing services are and remain competent is a central activity of the professional group. However, traditionally in nursing, responsibility for competence has often been viewed as the role of the institution's management. Again, this comprises an illegitimate exercise of accountability because if the organization really wants to obtain it, it has to be placed in the hands of those who can give it, and historically, it has been placed in the wrong hands. Because accountability can only emerge from within the practitioner's role who performs the work of the profession, accountability for that work must rest with the service provider and the authority for that must emerge from the same place.

Unfortunately, both the beliefs and behaviors necessary to support staff accountability, how they perform their role, and what they need to do it often did not include the involvement of the staff affected by the rule making. As a result staff members saw those accountabilities as though they rested outside their role, in essence belonging to someone else, and their own individual ownership for them was moderated and muted. Conversely, in shared governance it is recognized that the accountability for competence rests within the role and cannot be legitimately transferred from the nurse's role. Ownership of competency accountability, therefore, must emerge in the appropriate ways in the professional organization and structures that support it in the staff role must be created and affirmed.

There is a dual obligation in the shared governance organization in relation to competence. In a profession the obligation for competence does not solely rest with the individual practitioner. There is also a corporate obligation for the competence of the whole profession, that is manifested in the individual nurse's obligation to others in the profession to ensure that each is competent to practice the profession. There is a corporate obligation of each for the other. This accountability is manifested in the obligation to both teaching and learning processes directed to obtaining and ensuring competence. Professionals are clearly liable to maintain learning sufficient to the performance requirements of their work and necessary to the advancement of the work of the profession. At the same time they have the obligation to teach each other and to extend their colleagueship to the role of mutuality in learning by agreeing to share knowledge as well as obtain it.

Learning in the service setting has always been an expectation of every practitioner, but attention to the role of teacher for every practitioner has been less emphasized. The role of teacher has been considered more a function of skill and choice than a generalized expectation of each nurse. Indeed, functional roles have been created in nursing services for just such purposes, further deemphasizing the individual obligation to teach and creating a functional service framework (inservice educator) for the role of teacher. Rather than creating structures that accommodate the education accountability in every staff member, service leaders have created a functional framework for education that actually removes individual obligation for teaching and places it in a departmentalized function. Recent movement to competency-based unit education models is a current redirection of this process back to the clinical environment and thus into the hands of nursing staff.

The three accountability areas are fundamental to any service-based delivery of nursing care. Because they represent accountabilities common to the practice of any profession, they are often considered generic to professional work. They should, therefore, be incorporated into any clinical authority structure in the organized nursing service.

Often activities that relate to the validation of current knowledge and the production of new knowledge (as identified in the research function) are not considered part of the operations of a professional service. Previous work on shared governance (Porter-O'Grady, 1984) has not devoted much space to the issue of professional research even though it is a fundamental accountability of a service profession.

Research

Research is essential to the activities of any profession. If a service profession is to remain current and to advance the work of the profession and the service it provides to society, time must be spent in research activities. The reality, however, is somewhat removed from the principle. Research activity requires time and money. In nursing, both these resources are at a premium. Although this is true, it is also important to raise the issues of competence, growth, new knowledge, and professional equity as they relate to the public and to other disciplines. It becomes an issue of distribution of resources from a number of sources for the purpose of making clinical improvements that may change the way health care is provided and the cost associated with nursing services.

Initially, in the process of providing resources for the research function, the use of operational dollars may not be advisable or even available. However, strategies used to obtain grant funding, and foundation, corporate, or private donation programs are all appropriate to initiate a nursing research function. Because the function has not frequently been incorporated into a practice framework in most community hospital settings in the United States, it is a challenging experience to initiate. Leaders can expect that both staff and management may find it difficult to either understand or support the introduction of research activities without a period of transitional stress. Although it is likely that there may be a variety of funding opportunities in the community to subsidize nursing research, activities that support it and energize the staff with regard to its benefit should accompany any initiation effort. As more nursing organizations expand on the accountability of research in their settings, additional information regarding how to be successful in these efforts will become available. The principle of research accountability for the profession, however, is fundamental and needs to expand in the service setting if the professionalization of nursing practice is to be complete.

Management of Resources

The final arena of accountability is the management process in the governance organization and relates specifically to the management of resources. The work of nursing cannot be accomplished without the requisite resources. The organization must be equipped to deliver what it commits to—without the appropriate resources and the ongoing management of them, it is difficult to assume that anything will be accomplished. Because the above accountabilities are essential to the practice of nursing, resources directed to their fulfillment serve essentially as the context within which nursing practice takes form. Recent research has indicated that attention to the issue of resources is equal to the exercise of the work of the entity (Mintzberg, 1990). In fact, resource management is so important to the enterprise that shared governance continues to recognize it as a defined role and supports the belief that someone must fulfill the obligation of this role.

This approach differs from some recent efforts to eliminate the specific role of manager in some self-governing enterprises and to allow the staff essentially to be self-directed. In these situations, however, the role has still somehow emerged in these systems because the accountability for resources must still be attended to. Often one of the staff members assumes certain aspects of the role, becomes proficient, and is assigned that role as a functional component of his or her job. Others may take on the other resource activities, thus dividing the role among workers. What has been noted in the recent research is that it is often ineffective and poorly attended to in such arrangements and staff is often unhappy with the obligation (Dumaine, 1990).

The legitimate role of the manager then becomes highlighted. Instead of eliminating this much needed role, it would be more appropriate for the organization to clearly isolate the functional accountabilities of the role and then ensure that it fulfills the defined expectations clearly within the parameters provided for it. It should operate in relation to its accountabilities in the same way that any of the other accountabilities function in the nursing organization. Historically, the manager's role in nursing has been expanded in a way that parallels industrial structures and behaviors. The professional character of nursing "got lost" in the experience and a whole era of employee- and job-based systems and expectations arose. In effect, nursing became a vocation with all the attendant behaviors that a job orientation naturally creates. Driving this system was the ever-expanding role of the manager. The role of the staff was diminished to the same degree as the manager's role increased. The resultant problem was a highly professionalized nursing management staff and an equally highly vocationalized clinical nursing staff.

Shared governance models reconsider this equation and attempt to address it by "reprofessionalizing" the clinical staff and more clearly isolating areas for which the staff is fully accountable and areas for which the management staff is accountable. Separating these functions and distinguishing them from each other serves to clarify and assert the appropriate roles and to ensure that each party (practitioners and management) is fully invested with both the right and the opportunity to exercise its legitimate roles.

PRINCIPLES COMMON TO SHARED GOVERNANCE STRUCTURES

As shared governance has expanded across the country in recent years, principles that guide both the concept and the development of the structure have emerged. First attempts at initiating shared governance were uncertain and risky, but later activities have been clearer in both concept and design. Previous experience and good structures as well as an emerging body of knowledge have been helpful in unfolding newer approaches. The rigid adherence to existing knowledge about organizations and implementation has yielded to more flexible approaches that consider resources and culture in their design. It is becoming clearer that many of the principles that have driven industrial model organizations do not transfer adequately to an emerging parallel and collateral work system. Indeed, many of the traditional rules for organizations no longer apply (Farnham, 1989).

In such a scenario, the implementor writes the script for implementation as the structure unfolds. Satisfaction is derived from the validation of the structure, which comes from its success, and the new demands that evolve from a new structure and its impact on creating new relationships. That is not to say that there are not principles of shared governance that apply and guide the implementor in forming a model. Some basic rules of shared governance that have emerged over the years that guide both thinking and development of an effective approach to governance are listed below.

It Is Not a Form of Participatory Management

First and most important to the concept of shared governance is the recognition that shared governance is *not* a new brand of participatory management. In fact, the concept and workings of shared governance do not reflect the characteristics of participatory management at all. The shared governance process is an accountability-based approach that may change the locus of control and spread it across the roles in the discipline depending on the accountability and the legitimate location of authority for it. It assumes that there are a number of people who have fundamental accountability for defined functions in arenas of both practice and management. As explained previously, shared governance specifically recognizes five professional accountability areas: practice, quality assurance, competence, research, and management of resources, and defines the appropriate functions that attend to these accountabilities and then structures the organization to support their exercise.

It Is Not Management Driven

A second principle of shared governance is that it is not management driven. Because nursing is primarily and purposefully a practice profession, it is reasonable that the work of nursing must be at the heart of the nursing delivery system. It is also reasonable to assume that all activities that are neither direct caregiving nor related to that process are in support of it. To both logically and systematically tie the organization together, it is essential that the priorities be properly ordered. In a professional governance model, priority for authority designation must be addressed to the practitioner for those issues that directly affect what she does. This reality empowers her and provides the basis for some definitive allocation of staff-based authority and control. The staff members, therefore, are empowered to do whatever is directly necessary to them, affecting both what they do and how they do it. For the staff nurse, it is the first and final locus of control for those issues that most directly relate to her and what she does: practice, ensure quality, remain competent, and participate in the creation of new knowledge.

There Is No Single Locus of Control

A third principle relates to the shift in the locus of control. Traditional organizational principles indicated that there must be a focused locus of control for the work of the organization that takes form in the role of the manager. The manager, in both business and industry, became the central point on which the organization organized its work and obtained accountability. This role ensured that the work of the organization was accomplished and the goals of the service or section were met. The manager integrated not only outcome but also function and ensured that all was done within the context appropriate to the work.

In shared governance it is recognized that the work of a knowledge-based practice profession has no single locus of control. Indeed, in this model, a single locus of control both is alien to the processes associated with the accountability of the nurse and is not a condition conducive to the work obligations of the profession. A single locus of control can legislate against the principle of accountability identified above. If the nurse manager is identified as the sole locus of control, then it can be assured that the accountabilities identified in the practitioner's role are never addressed and thus are not appropriately fulfilled.

Differentiation of accountabilities and the appropriate designation of those accountabilities throughout the organization is necessary to the successful exercise of accountability. To clarify this, some basic distinctions must be made between responsibility and accountability. The nurse often finds that these two concepts are used interchangeably and that they are essentially assumed to basically mean the same thing. In fact, as pointed out at the beginning of this chapter, they are very different concepts.

By definition responsibility is fluid and must always be identified by someone in a preeminent role, assigned to someone in a subordinated role, accepted by the person in that role as a condition of functioning in that role, and then completed as agreed to. The person in the role must fulfill that obligation for as long as she agrees to serve the functions the role demands. It is accepted that as the person changes roles, so will the responsibilities associated with the new role change and that responsibility does not automatically transfer. Responsibility, therefore, is always externally generated, must always be assigned, and does not customarily transfer to other roles or situations.

Conversely, accountability operates in a different manner. In a professional context, there are expectations associated with the role of the professional. There are educational and social preconditions that are necessary for the profession's work. It is assumed that when a worker completes the obligations of the profession and has been incorporated into the professional body, there are essential characteristics that will attend to the exercise of that role. Those characteristics are so vital to the role that they are considered a part of the essence of that role; the role cannot unfold without them nor can it be defined without conceiving it in the context of those characteristics. They are inherent to the role and emanate from it— not to have them is not to live the role. They can be defined as the accountabilities of the role. These characteristics are attributed to it from within the role, can never be assigned, nor can they be given away. They arrive and leave with the person, even when the person leaves the function of that role for another setting or role.

The reason accountability is discussed with such intensity relates to the fact that most long-term shared governance models are based on accountability delineations. As work accelerates to create a newer model for organizing and delivering nursing care services, a solid premise for these newer models must be provided. This is especially true for governance models, which presuppose a different belief about both the worker and the work. The traditional industrial model structures represent a way of believing and working that is an outgrowth of concepts and research ensuing from manufacturing organizations and productivity models in the industrial sector, as discussed earlier in this chapter. Most of the research on which hospital organizational and management systems are based reflects similar thinking as that directed toward assembly line and production-oriented settings. Only in the last decade have concepts and research that represent professional nursing values and work begun to unfold (Hersey and Blanchard, 1989). It must be emphasized that whatever professional approaches emerge, they must not only be empowering but also be solidly based on a set of professional values that can bear the weight of organizational integrity, and incorporate the checks and balances necessary to ensure that work is both appropriately identified and performed at the level of satisfaction identified by both the worker (nurse) and the consumer (patient).

Models Should Be Based on a Clinical, Rather than Administrative, Organization

Another principle of shared governance must be considered—all designs and models should reflect a clinical base of organization rather than an administrative structure. Historically, the nursing organization has reflected administrative lines and mechanisms of authority and function in the prevailing hospital structure. This setting allowed good integration and control of nursing within both the dominant medical system and the hospital's own complementary medical service system. Because the hospital's originating purposes were strongly medically driven, most of the service structures developed in the system reflect the predominant service requirements of the medical staff. All service providers in this model were developed to accommodate this relationship, and the organizational characteristics of the hospital reflect this relationship for the most part. This structure does not assume equity of roles and reflects both the ascendant role of the doctor and the hierarchical structure of the hospital that supports it. The nurse has heretofore been a subset of both.

If nurses are to create equity in the hospital or health system, they must temper the current structure, refuting the fundamental underpinnings of the current modus operandi and much of its operating characteristics. It is not wise, however, to legislate against an inadequate structure unless it is known both why it is inadequate and what will replace it. A previous work provided a thorough discussion of why the structure is inadequate and how shared governance is an appropriate structural alternative (Porter-O'Grady, 1984). It is essential, however, that the nurse remember that the structure cannot simply be changed by noting its inadequacy and not moving toward substantive change. One of the major problems in current nursing self-governance efforts is the fact that nurse leaders, in many cases, have created the operating structure without the essential behavioral and organizational shifts, which delivers a different message to the various members of the system about the position and role of nursing in corporate as well as practice decision making.

The base of this shift and the basic principle promulgated is that nursing is primarily and wholly a clinical system. If it is to reach full tenure in the organizational system and reflect the desired equity, it must be centered squarely on what the profession is and what it does. All roles not directly involved in its work then become supportive to the work; in essence, servants to the practitioner to whom the nursing organization and its support must be directed. Anyone who does not do the direct work of the profession is therefore a servant to those who do.

This has not been the prevailing consciousness of the profession in the current health care system with its traditional management structures. Management has evolved into the caretaker and agency role, ensuring that the staff members do what they are supposed to, in the right numbers and kind, at the right time, and to the right degree of proficiency and productivity. In most current structures the manager, regardless of position within the system, acts more as the agent of the institution than as the profession's link to the necessary support and resources of the organization directed to the provision of nursing care.

This relationship is significantly altered in shared governance. The accountability of the manager is closely assessed and narrowly defined to focus on those roles and functions that directly relate to both resource provision and staff support. The manager's role, however, is not weakened in the delivery system. If anything, it is enhanced because for the first time, a clear, definitive expectation for the manager can be articulated and applied without confusion regarding roles and functions that are not properly or legitimately attendant to it.

Conversely, the staff role also becomes clearer and accountable in a much broader context. Ownership of the clinical processes becomes much more definitive as the definition of what that ownership means also becomes more distinct. Accountability becomes a solid basis on which to build the role of the nurse because all the organizational structures must reflect it. When the staff members know what their power base is and the arenas over which they have control, they develop highly effective checks and balances to ensure that the clinical values are adequately addressed.

Sorting the roles of management and staff and distinguishing the accountabilities distinct to each function is also beneficial to the manager. In the past, with industrial model beliefs and structures, the role of the manager was not so clearly distinguished from the role of the staff. Often the manager was expected to make certain that the staff fulfilled both work rules and practice requirements. Indeed, the manager has historically been the locus of control for most every function in the delivery of nursing services. In the shared governance approach, the nurse manager's role operates within a narrower frame of reference with a much clearer framework for management accountability.

Instead of an amorphous and expansive boundary to the role, a more clearly defined structure of accountability becomes essential and better defined. Focus on the fundamental role of the manager and the resource base of management emerges, freeing the manager to be more capable of investing in those activities that more directly relate to expectations for the role. The manager can then actually produce outcomes for which the role is directly accountable without the pressure of fulfilling accountabilities that can never be legitimately those of the manager. This also frees the nursing organization to better define and obtain those outcomes from the role of practitioner it could only partially obtain in the past. The staff members' accountability for their roles is directly related to the proximity of the accountability to the legitimate locus of control for its exercise. This principle also applies to the manager.

The principle of management accountability for the exercise of the role within the context of the work of the role is fundamental to shared governance success. The manager is accountable for the human, material, fiscal, support, and organizational resources of the service. In the past managers have been insulated from this expectation because it was highly ambiguous. When accountability for the role of management becomes clearer to all in the organization, the parameters that both define it and measure performance related to it become much clearer and straightforward. It remains less ambiguous to all parties that relate to it and depend on it. From this framework much clearer performance expectations can be defined and nurses can more clearly articulate their management role with other key managers, who can then act as moderators and evaluators. In a shared governance structure, it is important that each role be clearly described and understood by the individual and the staff. The management role is no exception.

SHARED GOVERNANCE STRUCTURES

There are a number of structural approaches to shared governance in the United States. In the early 1980s when the concept was first applied to hospitals, there were few principles to guide the introduction to the process. Although it was intended to empower the staff, it was not clear what that was and how the staff should be empowered. As the concept of accountability was clarified, it became the base for validating the approaches to shared governance as a part of ensuring that true empowerment was the outcome of the process. Many times, attempts to include staff in some form of participation never seemed to move them to the degree of participation anticipated. The staff's "do I gotta wanna" response often surprised and disheartened nursing leaders to the point of asking whether efforts to motivate the staff were worthwhile.

The real transfer of accountability and the attendant power changes in the staff are noted in shared governance models. When there is no real net transfer of powers there is little commitment to the process. The shell of shared governance is in place but the core action of shared governance is missing.

Some organizations have implemented the format for shared governance but little of the substance. Participatory efforts are not characteristic of real shared governance. Participation always indicates that control and authority rest elsewhere. One shared governance principle when applied to professional practice indicates that accountability only truly exists where the authority for it does; if there is no authority, there is no accountability. If authority can be second-guessed or approval for it rests elsewhere, then true authority is located in the place of final approval. This is the principle most often missing or compromised in shared governance organizations that are not complete or do not yet work as intended or hoped.

Shared governance is a trust-based system. It purports that *all* members of the nursing staff are full participants in the profession's work. The prevailing belief is that all nurses are stakeholders in the work of health care and want to do all that is possible for them to render good health services. Although the system recognizes that there are a few in the profession who do not share these values, the entire professional system should not be built to protect the receivers of health care from the indiscriminate actions of a small minority, but instead, to validate the commitment and contribution of the majority of nurses who do the lion's share of the positive work of providing health care services.

Nurses are capable and effective caregivers worthy of trust and ownership of their practice and their work. This is the belief on which the whole process of shared governance is built. The structure and its characteristics should reflect this reality. Different from the more traditional participative management approaches, shared governance is based on trust and constructs a trust-based organizational model. There must be a sense in all the leaders in the nursing service, both administrative and clinical, that all are committed to the same purposes and seek the same outcomes.

Because shared governance reflects professional values, it moves the location or positioning of the practicing staff nurse from the bottom of the hierarchy to the middle of the organization. The hard lines of the organizational pyramid are softened and rounded and a more egalitarian approach is created. In the center of the circle is the professional nurse, who by both role and location connects the organization to the service it provides. As Deming concludes, this approach builds the organization around its service provider and creates a relationship between the service provider and the client (the nurse and the patient) (Deming, 1990). All other roles related to that one must support it. In other words, all roles not directly providing service to the consumer of the service are subservient to the service provider. This approach clearly changes the character of the organizational relationships and seriously redefines all the roles in the service setting.

Shared governance models that do not reflect this key value may fail to achieve the outcomes intended by the approach. Unless there is a sincere and true shift of accountability and authority to the staff for those things that are essential to their role, there will be serious problems in obtaining the staff commitment and care outcomes expected from this approach.

There are three prevailing model approaches to shared governance that reflect these characteristics to date: congressional, unit-based (sometimes called administrative), and councilor. These approaches comprise the majority of organizational avenues undertaken by health care settings around the country. Each has a unique organizational form yet supports the common underpinnings and principles of shared governance. These models are introduced here, but they will be explored in more detail in Chapter 5.

Congressional Approach

This approach to shared governance is perhaps the model with the strongest nursing-based structure currently in operation. Its internal integrity and highly rational democratic foundation make a vigorous framework for institutional use of shared governance. The congress, made up of the entire professional body (and designated others as institutionally determined), sets the infrastructure for the profession. The congress elects or appoints from among its membership representatives who will undertake the various accountabilities and functions of the nursing profession on behalf of the congress. Accountability for the work is invested in the committees of the congress that are responsible to the congress for what is done on its behalf. Committees such as practice, quality assurance, education, management, staffing, professional issues, research, etc. are assigned control of the various accountabilities determined by the congress as essential to the work of nursing. The chairs of these committees make up the cabinet of the congress or the nursing staff. The cabinet is the locus of authority for those things that relate to the profession as a whole and all of the professional interests of the nursing staff in the institution. It is the highest executive body in the nursing service and integrates the nursing activities, and functions and deals with major issues related to mission, purposes, finances, and objectives of the nursing service. It also serves as the forum for the chief nursing officer and acts as the liaison between the corporate system and the nursing professional system. It is efficient, tightly structured, and representative and it gives strong evidence of the partnership between the profession of nursing and the organizational system. This is its strength. Its greatest weakness is that it serves nursing well but does nothing to really integrate the health care organization as a whole. It creates a strong power base for nursing but can alienate the other services and create an elitism that can be threatening to others, sometimes undermining the organization. It is also a high-risk model to other professional leadership, notably physicians, within the organization. This approach sometimes make it difficult to start but serves as an excellent transitional model when inroads have been successfully created through an alternative approach. The other two models in the nursing organization can also provide transition toward this model because of its strong internal structure and its viable political statement in the organization.

Unit-Based Approaches to Shared Governance

This approach is perhaps one of the most popular processes. It has the most immediate impact on the staff, with rewards and payoffs coming early in its implementation. It is also the least risky approach because it does not invest the entire nursing service in its implementation. It is usually begun by staff at the unit of service level and often responds to a long-determined need for more staff involvement and ownership. It is a high-ownership model because all the unit staff members are involved to some degree in its implementation or operation.

No two approaches are exactly alike. One of this approach's strengths is the cultural specificity of its application. It most uniquely represents the values of the staff and can be manifested in a range of vehicles. From self-scheduling to standards setting, and from staffing systems to salary programs, many opportunities arise for the staff in the unit-based approach, limited only by the insight, desires, and creativity of the staff. Even clinical delivery approaches and budget design can be addressed in such approaches, which can lead to an abundance of exceptional processes for how nursing work is done and its costs along with the return on the investment of the nurse.

The unit-based model's strength, however, is also its weakness. Although the unit may flourish in this context, the profession as a whole may languish. The diversity of approaches and values emanating from the unit structures may be so diverse and so culturally and unit-specific that a central theme or quality to define and characterize the nursing profession as a whole may never emerge. With this approach, often when the nursing organization attempts to gain a consensus from the various unit models, set a common agenda, or establish a common identity, their differences are so great that the various unit representatives cannot communicate effectively because their understanding of the issues and the shared governance approach may be fundamentally different. The nursing organization fails to become fully functional and ultimately serves merely as the sum of its parts rather than the parts reflecting the values of the whole.

This can best be avoided by developing a unit-based approach in conjunction with the professional model as a whole in the service setting. The service setting should determine the prevailing beliefs and values on which all shared governance activities unfold within the organization. Some attempt to control and moderate unit design should be located in an integrating authority in the service. Effort should be made not to cap the creativity and uniqueness of the unit approach. Rather, the professional authority should simply seek consistency of direction and integration of fundamental values in the process of implementation. Those issues that affect the profession as a whole in the setting should be reserved for the powers of the integrating authority so that units do not dictate practice and rules for the rest of the service or in contradiction to the intents and beliefs of the nursing organization. This approach maintains a healthy tension between the unit development and the organizational integration in a shared governance system.

Councilor Model

This model is perhaps the most frequently implemented method for shared governance. It is solidly based on the delineation of accountability and the principle of appropriate locus of control. It is an institutional model and provides for both service structuring and unit-based differentiation. It is based on an organizational script that calls for centralization of professional control and decentralization of professional accountability. It is the model with the strongest potential for expansion beyond the nursing organization to include other health professionals and workers in the health care family. It is perhaps more challenging to implement because of its solid accountability base, but it clearly creates a strong basis for both the professionalization of nursing and the behavioral change necessary to a new script for health care.

Like the other models, it requires broad-based support from the executive to the staff centers in the organization. It depends greatly on the cooperative effort of both management and staff for its success. It does not devalue any of the roles in the organization; indeed, it builds on all of the roles that have an accountability base in the nursing service. It does, however, shift the locus of control for specified accountabilities, recognizing that many legitimate accountabilities may lie outside of the scope of the management role, contrary to the traditional delineators in organizations.

The councilor model divides the nursing organization into its five key arenas of accountability: practice, quality assurance, education (competence), research, and the management of resources. It builds an organizational system and the requisite structures on the established accountabilities and spreads authority for them throughout the staff and management. It attempts to sort the activities associated with the delineated accountabilities and build the authority for them within specified councils reflecting the accountabilities, themselves. Typically, therefore, there are four to five councils that have authority over the defined accountabilities. The necessary control mechanisms are invested within the councils to assure that the activities determined as appropriate for the council are performed and that all activities related to such functions are unfolded as expected.

In most cases there are three to four clinical councils and one management council. The clinical councils reflect a character of accountability designated as specifically clinical in scope and provide only for input from the management team. Usually this is provided for minority membership on the clinical council by a management representative from the management council. The prevailing membership of these clinical councils is composed of practicing staff members, and the leadership for the councils is also selected from the practicing staff.

The role of management on these clinical groups is to provide access to information and resources necessary to support decision making within the council. Each council needs to have essential data and supporting information to make decisions; access to some data may not be available. Much key information is provided to the manager to assist in the management and control of the service's resources. That information source and network should be made available to the councils to facilitate decision formation, and entry to it can only be provided by the management leadership. The locus of control for those accountabilities determined to be clinical shifts to the staff, and management support becomes central to the exercise of the clinical authority inherent in the council's activity. Until newer models of information generation and sharing emerge in professional organizations, the manager as moderator will continue to be vitally important.

In the councilor model the manager focuses more specifically on her role in the organization. As staff members become increasingly competent in their accountabilities, the role of the manager in a broader but more specific definition of her role becomes vital to the success of the process. Newer delineators of coordination, integration, and facilitation of the work of the organization become central to the view of the work of the manager. From a narrow departmental focus with a strong operational component to a more systems-related orientation to the role of manager, newer ways of expressing and experiencing the role emerge. The concept of linkage in the organization increases in value and meaning as its application expands from the first-line manager to the executive in the nursing service. The nature of the linkage depends on the role's location in the system and demands a different set of skills and application of the role. The expectation, however, is that wherever the linkage is demanded, the manager must be clear about the role expectation and be skilled in fulfilling the role as effectively as possible. No longer are role understanding and exercise amorphous and ambiguous. Both the requisites and skills necessary to the role must be clear, readily apparent to all, and exercised with the greatest of skill. In all shared governance models, clarity of design, structure, function, and role are essential to the success of the model.

This model does not clearly define unit level activity or structure. It does not intend to prescribe those activities that should unfold at the unit level. Instead, this model seeks to provide a framework within which unit approaches can be designed to reflect both the service and culture of the unit. The only caveat that operates in this model is a constraint on those activities or approaches that may not be in concert with both the design and structure of the prevailing shared governance model. This model, therefore, provides an approach that attracts both unit level approaches with the need to integrate at the divisional or departmental level.

FORMALIZING THE STRUCTURE

There is limited reason to move toward a staff accountability-based shared governance prototype if it does not empower the staff and alter the way in which they are involved in decision making. Shared governance should change the very character of the organization and the relationships essential to its work.

Formalizing the shared governance structure and creating firm parameters for its successful operation are necessary for the system to function effectively. Both the culture and the operating system must reflect the character of the model in the way in which the organization does its work. Included must be the roles and relationships that emerge in a shared governance structure. There would be little value in implementing a shared governance approach and simply having it parallel or report to the existing reporting structure, with no substantive changes in the organization's operations. Empowerment would become merely an empty idea.

Giving empowerment substance requires a supporting structure that indicates respect for and involvement of those who have been empowered in the real decisional process. Value for this approach must be reflected in all the arenas where shared governance can have a legitimate impact. From administration and board to the other service providers, the shared governance approach should change the nature and content of the relationships entered into between nursing and the rest of the organization.

In the first instance, the nurse executive is key to this transition. She must first believe that the shared governance model has legitimacy and can function effectively to empower the profession to do what it needs to do in delivering health care services. She must be committed to the nursing role in the organization and the right of nurses to play key roles in decisions that affect patient care. This is a vital consideration in implementing shared governance.

There are some (mostly those in clinical practice) who believe that the nurse executive soon forgets her fundamental foundation in nursing when she becomes an administrator and thereby becomes an opponent. Implied in that accusation is that she is no longer sensitive to the issues that emerge from the practitioner's perspective and work experience. Generally this is not true; indeed, most nurse administrators are as sensitive to the needs of patients and nurses as anyone else. Sometimes, however, the nurse administrator's perspective related to the practitioner shifts because of differences in role and the traditional power obligations and relationships in the job.

As an administrator, the nurse executive has an obligation for the appropriate use of institutional resources and the production of sufficient revenues to maintain the viability of the health care facility. The problem, however, is that in that role, the nurse administrator owes the predominant obligation for her position and its continuance not to the nurse's exclusive support but to her colleagues in administration and members of the board of trustees. Of course, the nurse executive could not survive without the long-term support of her peers in practice, but this is really a secondary consideration. This difference in perception and expectation may create tension in her role, but it can be easily managed through the control of information and through use of traditional participatory strategies.

In the "darker" character of her role, the nurse executive has the ability to manage and control both participation and resources, including the decision-making process. If she desires, she can manage and manipulate relationships and resources for her personal viability and advantage. She can, if she wants, manage the political framework and power equation for some time without truly empowering her colleagues and peers. In some cases, she can even create a powerful dependency (or codependency) relationship within the nursing organization to both maintain her power and to accelerate her personal value. For a few more controlling personalities, in this scenario, to share power is to lose it. For others, usually more insecure administrators, getting power and keeping it is difficult enough; to share it risks too much in both personal investment and organizational change.

Although there are certainly other factors in this scenario, it is interesting that many times the largest single provider of health care services is afraid to make substantive changes in the work structures and relationships that can both benefit the profession and, therefore, patient care. Unilateral and paralyzing fear of what others would think, or how they would respond, how the medical staff feels, what other departments think, whether it would be permitted, etc., in some cases indicates the relative dependent relationship of nursing and nurses to the prevailing structures. This is true in many organizations even at a time when it is claimed nursing has the strongest and best-educated leadership available in the health care system.

Moving to shared governance is a risky enterprise. It is an effort to create a new organizational model that better serves the needs of nurses and their patients. To empower means to shift the power arrangements and to create new sources of power. The belief is that there is a net enhancement to both the nurse and the organization. Such a critical shift represents a transformation of everyone's roles and relationships, including those of the traditional manager and administrator as previously indicated in this chapter.

CREATION OF STAFF LEADERSHIP

One of the most dramatic and difficult undertakings in the development of shared governance is the culturing of leadership skills in the staff. Because shared governance is a staff-driven model, exercise of leadership skills in the various forums of decision making is not optional for the staff leadership.

Although the need for leadership is unquestionable, the availability of it in a staff that never expected to assume it in a formal way is uncertain. At times, there are those, who by predisposition or previous exposure, are strong leaders. Usually these people do not readily or freely emerge in the nursing organization. Not only do they not emerge, but staff members are often reticent to undertake the leadership role. The degree of risk and the uncertainty of the role sometimes predicate against assuming these roles.

Operating to moderate the emergence of staff leadership is the uncertainty of the shared governance process itself. Often staff members are unable to conceive an organization that would be willing to allow the staff to govern themselves. They may feel that there is a "catch" somewhere, or that some manager is waiting, ready to second-guess the exercise of staff authority and decisions. Genuine feelings of inadequacy are often present during the initial stages of shared governance implementation. It is not surprising, therefore, that many staff members are both unprepared and uncertain about assuming leadership or becoming active on shared governance forums.

A slow transition to the role of leadership with the staff combined with liberal support are essential at the outset. The staff members must trust that they are, first, respected in the role and then have a base of support available to them when needed. An orientation to the expectation of the role as either a member of a key governance group or the group's leader is often needed. Depending on the degree of authority and commitment, a training program that provides the essentials of the leadership role covering such topics as group process, group dynamics, problem solving, priority setting, consensus seeking, and agenda writing is an appropriate way to indicate solid support for the effectiveness of the leader. Time invested in the staff leader early in the developmental process will be beneficial in effective work in the governance bodies later in the process.

Lack of preparation for the role and the requisite supports are often the greatest barrier to the success of the staff leadership role in shared governance. Although some of those expenditures may appear like major commitments at the outset, they are returned to the organization in positive group output and the value of the leader to the organization.

The successful application of the leadership role in the staff is central to effective expression of power in the governance bodies. Because most decisions will be made there and the successful operation of the nursing organization depends on the work of the governance groups, both the quality of the process and outcomes of the group are critical to their viability. To facilitate this requires some sophisticated insights with regard to the culture and character of the group, its definitive work, and those processes that enable the group in its work rather than inhibit it.

Staff participation is also critical to the success of any staff model. At the outset, however, staff members will not participate in overwhelming numbers. Some have even indicated that the staff purposely stays away. This is acceptable behavior, which reflects the staff's current values and limited job-based investment in their profession and work. Most see what they do as job-directed and are dedicated exclusively to doing the work that is required, when it is required, and then returning home to the nonwork aspects of their lives, often forgetting they were ever involved in it.

Many nurses would object to this characterization of them, indicating that there are many who feel strongly about their role and are very committed to the work of the profession. This is undoubtedly true and the sentiments are valid. The focus of the above statements is related less to the dedication of the nurse and more to the structure that fails to give that dedication direction and form. If the practicing nurse sincerely wants to express professional values in a legitimate forum, she often has to leave her patient care work and move into other more significant decisional and power roles in the organization to do so. Even this scenario creates frustration and confusion, simply because as she moves further away from the work of nursing, she is both perceived to be and is actually less in touch with the practice setting.

To change this paradigm requires much work and time. Of course, the whole foundation for shared governance reflects the attempt to address this problem within the context of the organization without creating either threat or revolution. As some of nursing's more devout feminists would advocate, revolution may be exactly what is needed in the health care system (Maraldo, 1990). It is important to reflect that all parties to the venture must arrive at the future together and the continuing attempt to create ascendant responses will, over the long run, be futile.

Shared governance must use all of the available resources to create an effective delivery and governance response to the changing role and demand for the nurse. This is characteristic in the attempt to empower all the nursing roles affecting patient care. Each member of the nursing team has a primary right and obligation to participate in all the activities that focus on the delivery of nursing care services. Connecting this person in the current clinical setting to important decision making is the central theme of an effective shared governance system. It is in this effort that true staff leadership will emerge.

CLUSTERING AND UNIT TO DIVISION RELATIONSHIPS

Connecting the nurse to effective decision making is only half of the connection necessary to ensure that shared governance succeeds. Organizational and systematic connections are necessary if it is to operate effectively throughout the system. As indicated earlier in this chapter, formatting shared governance for only part of the nursing system and not integrating it with the whole can create disconnections and inadequacies in the organization. One of the main purposes of shared governance is to link members of the profession in a way in which they can have a collective role in affecting nursing decisions and activities. On the other hand, it would be inappropriate and ineffective to have large numbers of nurses in groups trying to make quick and effective decisions for the professional body as a whole. It is for this reason that group size is a major consideration in shared governance models. Because the key decisional groups must be kept small, their linkage to the organization and its components becomes increasingly important. Clustering services or units of like size and service often assists in reducing the tension of too broadly based representation on the one hand, and focuses decisions within the appropriate groups on the other. Selecting the decisional leaders from these cluster groups helps link the service clusters and entities, allowing them to feel properly represented to the key decisional forums in the organization without overwhelming them with members. Often the representative to the nursing service governance group can link that group to the cluster more directly by being selected as the chair of the cluster group and as that cluster's representative to the governance group. This approach is especially beneficial in larger hospital models (more than 300 beds) since it maintains effectiveness in the model without overwhelming its membership and drawing nursing resources away from the workplace in great numbers. In these constraining times, it is wise to select approaches that support the judicious use of nurses' time and keep them as close to their service as possible. Clustering works well to link the unit/service setting and the departments/division for effective decision making in both arenas.

SUMMARY

Much activity has unfolded over the past 10 years that has given nursing opportunity to grow in ways not previously possible. Shared governance has enabled nursing professionals to exercise great control over their practice and decisions that affect them. It has expanded the individual and corporate sense of self and contribution to the delivery of health care systems. It has done much to create in organizations the equity and parity in role, relationship, and responsibility between nurses (notably women) and hospital and health care leadership. Through it much freedom to risk, undertake creative change, alter service structures and patterns, and take control of the delivery of nursing has emerged with the resultant improvements in productivity and outcomes.

Shared governance is only the first step in a series of moves that will be necessary if the profession of nursing is to provide the leadership and set the direction necessary to retool the health care delivery system. It is simply the vehicle for starting the journey that will move nurses in that direction by establishing an organizational format that invests all its members, creates a mechanism for equity and power sharing, establishes a structure for retooling the work of nursing, and positions the nursing profession to restructure the way in which health care is delivered.

Although shared governance represents a significant step toward creating the future, it is just a first step. Newer models and arrangements must emerge that join the nursing professional with other services and professions to address broadranging service issues in a transformed health care system. Ownership of nursing and nursing practice must continue to move into nursing hands and then be repartnered with other services and service providers in equitable and meaningful ways. Empowering nursing to simply have unilateral or ascendant power becomes parochial and self-serving, and provides nothing to positively affect either those nursing serves or the profession itself.

These are exciting times for nursing. The old rules and ways are quickly passing. The future is radically different from the past. Innovative and creative efforts are necessary to change the health care system in ways that are more health giving and responsive to the health rather than the illness needs of the American society. All nurses must be involved in the effort to respond to this change. Shared governance provides the opportunity to those who seek it to fully participate as partners in creating a better, more meaningful health care system. Shared governance provides a forum to look beyond what is currently in place and to secure nursing's place in the future of health care delivery.

REFERENCES

Ashley, J.A. (1976). *Hospitals, Paternalism, and the Role of the Nurse*, New York: Teachers College Press.

Beatty, J. (1990). A Post Cold War Budget, *Atlantic Monthly*, February, 74-82.

Bocchino, C. (1990). An Interview with Stuart Altman and Uwe Reinhardt, *Nurs Econ* 8(3), 142-151.

Brown, M. and McCool, B. (1990). Health Care Systems: Predictions for the Future, *Health Care Manage Rev* 15(3), 87-94.

Burda, D. (1990). A Simmering Perception of Inequality, *Mod Healthcare*, April 23, 30-31.

del Bueno, D. (1990). Warning: Retention May Be Dangerous to Your Health, *Nurs Econ* 8(3), 239-243.

Deming, W.E. (1990). *Total Quality Management*, New York: Warner Books.

Dumaine, B. (1990). Who Needs a Boss? *Fortune*, May 7, 52-60.

Farnham, A. (1989). The Trust Gap. *Fortune*, Dec 4, 56-78.

Gibbs, N., and others. (1990). Women: The Road Ahead, *Time*, Fall, 10-82.

Haddon, R. (1989). The Final Frontier: Nursing in the Emerging Healthcare Environment, *Nurs Econ* 7(3), 155-161.

Helgesen, S. (1990). *The Female Advantage: Women's Ways of Leadership*, New York: Doubleday/Currency.

Henry, B. (1990). Nightingale's Perspective of Nursing Administration, *Nurs Health Care* 11(4), 201-209.

Hersey, P. and Blanchard, K. (1989). *Management of Organizational Behavior*, ed 6, Englewood Cliffs, NJ: Prentice-Hall.

Jones, L. and Ortiz, M. (1989). Increasing Nursing Autonomy and Recognition Through Shared Governance, *Nurs Admin Q* 13(4), 11-16.

Kets de Vries, M. and Miller, D. (1984). *The Neurotic Organization*, San Francisco, Calif.: Jossey-Bass.

Ludemann, R. and Brown, C. (1989). Staff Perceptions of Shared Governance, *Nurs Admin Q* 13(4), 47-56.

Maraldo, P. (1990). The Nineties: A Decade in Search of Meaning, *Nurs Health Care* 11(1), 11-14.

McDonagh, K. (1990). *Nursing Shared Governance,* Atlanta: KJ McDonagh Associates, Inc.

Mintzberg, H. (1990). *Mintzburg on Management,* New York: The Free Press.

Peters, T. (1987). *Thriving on Chaos,* New York: Harper & Row Publishers.

Pinkerton, S.E. and Schroeder, P. (1988). *Commitment to Excellence: Developing a Professional Nursing Staff,* Rockville, Md.: Aspen Publishers.

Porter-O'Grady, T. (1986). *Creative Nursing Administration: Participatory Management into the 21st Century,* Rockville, Md.: Aspen Publishers.

Porter-O'Grady, T. (1990). *The Reorganization of Nursing Practice: Creating the Corporate Venture,* Rockville, Md.: Aspen Publishers.

Porter-O'Grady, T. (1989). Shared Governance: Reality or Sham, *Am J Nurs,* March, 350-351.

Porter-O'Grady, T. and Finnigan, S. (1984). *Shared Governance for Nursing,* Rockville, Md.: Aspen Publishers.

Witte, J. (1980). *Democracy, Authority and Alienation in Work,* Chicago: University of Chicago Press.

3 *Redesigning the Nursing Organization*

Cindy C. Campbell

Words such as *disruptive, chaotic,* and *whirlwind* are used to describe current health care systems. In Cybernetics II theory, fluctuations are viewed as positive, expected, and the main vehicle for creating order in systems (Smith, 1984, p. 273).

CYBERNETICS II THEORY

Cybernetics II sounds like some space-age theory with no relevance to nursing; however, it is an applicable theory that affects the entire health care industry. It is a new system of thinking that expands on the traditional parameters of open systems theory (also known as Cybernetics I). One of the two principles central to this new theory is the concept of dissipative structures. Dissipative structures reflect the principle of "order through fluctuation" (Smith, 1984, p. 273). Generally, fluctuation has been viewed as a disturbance in the system. Disturbance was to always be avoided; disturbance caused problems. It was believed that fluctuations should be minimized at all cost to the system. Even the language used in systems today to describe change seems to validate that disturbances are regarded negatively. In organizations, extreme fluctuations and chaos are almost always perceived as conditions that should be slowed and "controlled." Chaos is not considered to have any positive impact on a system.

There is a cyclical nature to most things in this world. Within organizations, cycles are also present. Viewing change and fluctuations in a manner that represents them as a natural part of the cycle and a necessary part of organizational life is a necessary step before major restructure or reorganization. The energy and planning toward restructure need to flow with the cycle of change, not attempt to control the cycle. The new perspective should be that chaos produces change through a natural cycle, thus allowing opportunities to cleanse the system and move forward toward more productive means of meeting organizational goals (Smith, 1984, p. 275). Without the cycle, the system would stagnate. In addition, controlling the cycle and fighting its natural movement would disrupt and stagnate the system.

CURRENT FLUCTUATIONS IN HEALTH CARE
Staffing Fluctuations

The health care system suffers from a variety of fluctuations, none of which are part of the world's attempts to "control" health care costs. The health care system also suffers from a shortage of professionals in all fields of health care workers, especially nursing. Several studies have examined this phenomenon, and numerous suggestions have been made to organizations on how to correct the situation— how to control the losses (Aiken, 1990). Nurses and other health care professionals are leaving hospital systems. They desire numerous changes within the system to afford them the autonomy and professional opportunity they feel they need and deserve. These losses cause more disruption, which in turn causes more attempts to control the crisis situation that exists. The attempts to retain and attract nursing personnel made by some short-sighted systems include bonuses, differentials, creative weekend plans, increased use of agency personnel, etc. These "quick fix" ideas have limited value; however, independent of the acceptance and challenge of some basic system changes, they will ultimately have only short-term effectiveness. Some professional health care groups are so frustrated with the traditional systems' responses to these "fluctuations" and "disturbances" in the system that they feel the need to organize and unionize. Traditional responses from hospital administration to these attempts in the past have been to attempt to further "control" the situation—even not recognize the groups officially—a response that ultimately will not be accepted by most groups of health care practitioners.

A New Perspective on Fluctuation

In troubled organizations the average worker's frustration and emotion is doubled on the part of the average hospital chief executive officer or chief nursing executive. Such individuals are at a loss as to how to control these variables that confront them from all sides. They find themselves in the middle of what Peters so aptly calls "chaos" and recognize clearly that they must learn how to cope. It was no mistake that Peters titled his book "Thriving On Chaos"—that is the challenge (Peters, 1987). If Cybernetics II thinking were to be applied to the current health care system, the situation might be perceived differently. The new perspective might unfold in the following manner. The extreme frustration with the system proves that the system is still alive—that people are capable of caring deeply about things that affect them—that people are being afforded an opportunity to find a way to improve quality—that the chaos that many believe exists serves to convince everyone that it is time for change, time to restructure and rebuild. Would health care have ever changed its pattern of everyday existence in ineffective systems to seek radical new ways of organization if the chaos in the system had not forced it to do so? Cybernetic thinking encourages the practice of viewing turbulence and fluctuations as essential to the system's ability to ultimately survive. Survival is the finite and ultimate goal.

Resilience Versus Stability

How much change and fluctuation can the health care system withstand? At what point is it correct to plateau and stabilize? Historically, stabilization has been viewed as a positive goal for an organization. Resilience, however, may be a more appropriate goal for today's health care organization. A clarification of the difference between the terms *stability* and *resilience* as made by Holling (1976) helps understanding of this goal. Holling defines stability as the capacity of the system "to return to an equilibrium state after a temporary disturbance; the more rapidly it returns and the less it fluctuates, the more stable it is." Conversely, resilience may be viewed as a "measure of the persistence of a system and of its ability to absorb change and disturbance and still maintain the same relationship" with other entities (Holling, 1976). As Smith (1984, pp. 275-276) postulates, "with these two concepts in place it is possible to think of an entity becoming more unstable as a result of large fluctuations, but that knowing how to survive with these fluctuations makes for greater resilience in that a lot of changes can be absorbed." Resilience clearly should be the goal.

PROFESSIONAL ORGANIZATIONS
Commitment to Change

Can anyone within the health care industry clearly and objectively observe its shortcomings and offer concrete, creative solutions? Is it possible to change perspective and perceive things differently? Several experts question this possibility without significant effort. Smith (1984, p. 290) says, "Consider the task of trying to determine how the rules of grammar shape the way we think. To do this we have to use a language that is governed by those rules of grammar to explore the impact those grammatical rules have on our thinking. To really understand we would have to use a metagrammar. But that metagrammar in turn will be shaped by a meta-metagrammar and so forth." In other words, could nurse executives and others be so familiar and comfortable with the current system that it impairs their ability to think about and explore new alternatives and ideas fully and completely? It is clear that most executives have been "raised" in the current health care system and thus are hindered to some degree by that past. It is also true that it is difficult to find the time and energy to creatively explore new alternatives and structures while expending most of each workday combating the current health care environment and its constraints. However, the cycle must change. Nurse executives must find the time and energy to find a more creative and long-term answer to the system's needs. Faced with the challenge of possible bias in their current perspectives and stressed by time availability, executives must analyze the options carefully.

Today's New Organization

The demands on hospital systems are becoming increasingly complex. That complexity places unique challenges on the need to find and develop new organizational structures to address the need. How workers are integrated into the operations of any system varies, depending on the structure of the organization. The main goal of health care systems is basically the same—to meet the health care needs of the client in the most effective, efficient manner possible. Different systems organize to meet that goal differently. Today's health care systems are complex entities and as such need to coordinate their essential activities in a variety of ways. The structure of any organization basically defines the ways in which its tasks are divided and then coordinated to accomplish the work of the organization. There are several ways of coordinating an organization's work. Mintzberg (1989, pp. 100-103) has identified six:

1. Mutual adjustment through informal communication between parties
2. Direct supervision (one issues orders—others carry them out)
3. Standardization of work processes—specifies work processes of people carrying out interrelated tasks
4. Standardization of outputs—achieves coordination by specifying the results of different work
5. Standardization of skills and knowledge—in which different work is coordinated by virtue of the related training the workers have received
6. Standardization of norms—in which it is the norms infusing the work that are controlled (convent, for example).

As the organization's work becomes more complex, the usual movement seems to shift from mutual adjustment to direct supervision: to standardization, preferably of work processes or norms, of outputs or skills, finally reverting to mutual adjustment (paradoxically also the mechanism best able to deal with the most complex forms of work), according to Mintzberg (1984, p. 102).

Structure in Hospitals

No organization can rely on any single component of the system. Different levels in the systems need different coordination links. Historically, in hospitals and in nursing, direct supervision and standardization of work processes have been the preferred coordination methods. The development and utilization of the nursing policy and procedure manuals is a prime example of that choice. Management also has been the major decision-making entity in the practice of nursing. Management has assumed responsibility and accountability for the practice of nursing. It is only within the past few years that structures have begun to emerge that will carry nursing from the direct supervision/standardization or work coordination mechanisms to more progressive mechanisms to organize and deliver services. Over the past few years as nursing has developed as a recognized profession with its own professional standards, the system has changed toward increased flexibility, as Mintzberg (1989, p. 101) has suggested is the normative progression.

Shared governance currently is the most well-known and concretely organized example of a structure for nursing systems that provides movement away from the more concrete systems of the past toward a more truly flexible, professional practice model. It allows work to be organized so that it reinforces and demands accountability from the professional practitioner for the practice of nursing, and returns to managers the role of managing the environment so that practitioners can focus on the provision of professional care (Porter-O'Grady and Finnigan, 1984, p. xi).

EMERGING PROFESSIONAL PRACTICE ORGANIZATIONAL MODELS
Characteristics of Current Structures

Professional practice organizational models have existed and are constantly evolving in industries throughout the nation. Interestingly, in professional organizations today such as universities, accounting firms, and some hospitals, a certain "core" structure has consistently emerged. It is primarily a bureaucratic structure, yet is decentralized. There are a minimal middle-line management hierarchy (i.e., there are wide spans of control over professionals in the environment) and large, fairly mechanized organized support staffs. In addition, there are somewhat autonomous professional groups functioning primarily under the regulations of their profession rather than the regulations of the institution. Two opposite structures apparently develop within these systems—one for the professionals that is flexible and allows them autonomy for practice; and one for the support structures of the system that is controlled and somewhat centralized. Some level of decentralization has reached the nonprofessional organizational structure but the finite control for decisions clearly still rests with management (Mintzberg, 1984, pp. 174-188).

Approaches to Future Models

In his new book *The Fifth Discipline,* Senge (1990, p. 4) states that the organization that will truly excel in the future will be the organization that discerns how to tap people's commitment and capacity to learn at all levels in the organization. In other words, the capacity *to learn how to learn* may be the key to excellence in future systems. Future professional practice models will need to focus less on structure and more on relationships to meet the newest challenges facing the field. Hierarchy and control issues will be replaced with issues such as professional accountability, professional judgment, and models of integration for professionals. This new system must be an open system capable of intense flexibility.

Today's organizations are full of internal politics and game-playing, widely accepted as the "norm." The professional practice model of the future will address this issue and lead a return to an environment wherein a shared vision between the system and the professionals creates a new level of openness for all (Senge, 1990, p. 274).

In *Megatrends 2000* Naisbitt and Aburdene (1990, p. 298) claim that the great unifying theme at the conclusion of the 20th century is the triumph of the individual. This new focus on the individual is evidenced diversely—from human rights movements to new trends in the management of organizations. Futuristic organizations realize that they are made up of individuals. Organizations do not grow and change—*people* grow and change.

Futuristic organizations also recognize that individual accountability is the foundation of future systems. Individuals provide the service of industries, and individuals provide for the determination and motivation for any changes in those industries. In the health care system, professional practitioners will continue to be the direct link of the organization with its "product." Practitioners will continue to gain visibility and importance in the system.

Individuals will quickly learn that to accomplish the goals of the future system, they will need newer ways to integrate and coordinate with each other. Individuals will learn to work in new types of teams. Senge (1990, p. 10) says that the discipline of team learning starts with "dialogue," the capacity of members of a team to suspend assumptions and enter into a genuine "thinking together." This new art of "dialogue" will be seen in integrative matrixed organizational structures that will link professionals so that they can continue to provide care and learn and grow in the system. Professionals will be the foundation of the future health care system. Management and support staff alike will be the spokes of the wheel, whereas professionals will be the hub. New structures are already emerging that support and validate that premise.

Characteristics of a Profession

Blane (1975, pp. 13-16) identifies six characteristics that are consistent among all professional groups:

1. A defined body of knowledge with specific skills acquired through an educational process
2. An orientation that is service based rather than productivity based or financially based
3. Discipline, peer review, and a code of ethics
4. Autonomy in practice with appropriate legislative and legal sanctions for workers who practice the profession
5. An organized system composed of professionals recognized by society to carry the mandates, roles, and responsibilities of the profession
6. A culture that supports the professional activity

Regardless of the ultimate structural design, the system must allow for all professions to practice and grow. Nursing systems must support the needs of the profession. The developed structure must support and encourage attainment and retention of the attributes listed above. The first of these characteristics regards knowledge and professional education.

Standards of practice and care.   In the last 20 years, the knowledge base of nursing has increased and become more clearly identified. The development of standards of practice and care for specific populations of patients has afforded nursing a clear knowledge base that is recognized as unique to nursing. Those standards are generally developed by professionals independent of the institution and are mandated by the professional organization. Staff nurses need a structure that allows them to determine the system's standard of care (based on the profession's defined standard) for themselves and their peers. Staff nurses need to feel accountability for that activity because of their identification as professionals. For years nursing management has defined the "standard" of care in most institutions. Management wrote the policy and procedure manuals. Management may have asked for staff nurse assistance in some of that activity, but the accountability and responsibility for standards clearly rested with management. New structures that are consistent and that reinforce professional practice environments must be different from current practice.

Nursing as a Service

Nursing is a service profession. The service that is provided is nursing care. Nursing care is delivered to individuals based on assessed needs and modified according to the nurse's evaluation of the effectiveness of that care. A manual or policy book cannot dictate individual patient care. Judgment and knowledge guide nurses in providing care to their patients. Ultimately, the health care system's structure must provide for that element of flexibility that is necessary for professionals to operate. The system must not constrain the professional. It must encourage judgment and its application to meet each patient's needs in the most effective, coordinated, and integrated fashion possible. Finance, productivity, and other similar information should be elements that management monitors and provides to professional practitioners so they can integrate the information into their decision-making cycle. In professional practice systems, management elements must be merged with the practitioner's perspective so that an integrated perspective is available for the final decision maker. Trust that the professional practitioner will make appropriate decisions for the system is also necessary for management to fully understand and appreciate the practitioner's unique role in a professional system.

Autonomy in Nursing

Autonomy in nursing practice is virtually nonexistent in hospitals today. Numerous reasons for this lack of autonomy were suggested earlier, but the absence of accountability by individual practitioners is a primary reason. Nurses desire and need autonomy; however, the system consistently has rejected that opportunity through the controlling structures that have been implemented.

These controlling structures emerged from a traditional hierarchical, bureaucratic structure. They developed from a belief system that management should control all decision making, with little employee participation. It was thought that management should organize, plan, and develop systems so precise that employees merely had to implement the appropriate activities identified by management as appropriate. Management also sought to organize its own field in the same manner. Management created complex systems that encouraged preplanning for all scenarios. These beliefs were incorporated in the systems personnel or supervisory policies, nursing policy and procedure manuals, and other rules and regulations. The intent was to maximize efficiency and effectiveness by providing readily available explicit guidelines for employees and managers alike. The effect may have been consistency in application of like actions by different employees, but these control systems created a loss of individual accountability.

New structures must demand accountability from practitioners. They must establish peer review and disciplinary activities that will require accountability by nurses for all nursing care delivered. They must reinforce the new belief that accountability rests with the individual professional practitioner, rather than with the system.

The Role of Culture

Blane (1975, pp. 13-16) discusses the need for a culture that supports professional activity. Every organization, department, nursing unit, and specialty has a culture. How important is it? Can it shape behavior? What *is* culture? The answer from a typical employee is "It's just the way we do things around here." Culture is the way people act . . . it is the way they are supposed to act. Culture cannot be seen but can be felt. Everyone knows what it is. Culture is one of the most powerful elements in any organization.

Culture can be defined as the summation of socially transmitted behavior patterns, arts, beliefs, institutions, and all other products of human work and thought characteristic of a community or population (Morris, 1971). Culture is derived from the basic belief systems of people. It comes from behaviors generated as a result of those beliefs and values. Those beliefs and values guide individual action and judgment. In creating or restructuring a professional practice environment, it becomes critical that culture be addressed. Hospitals have historically operated like machines or assembly-line bureaucracies. They have created cultures that have reinforced the lack of professional growth and expectations. Nurses have practiced within that culture for a long time. Other professional practice groups have also lived in that culture for a long time. Significant effort is required to change the culture to fully support a professional practice model. Careful planning and persistence are necessary to achieve the right outcome. Careful planning begins with some basic assumptions and beliefs. These basic beliefs that a system must embrace to create the right culture for the support of a new, more professional practice-based system include the following tenets:

1. People are basically good and are motivated to do the right thing when given the opportunity.
2. People want to work and provide services to others.
3. People, when given the right information and perspective, will make meaningful decisions that will be good for themselves and also for others.
4. People have the right and the duty to influence decision making that affects them.
5. Everyone has certain gifts and skills, but we must recognize that not everyone has the same gifts and skills. Everyone must respect diversity — it is the foundation for equality.
6. Everyone has the right to be needed, to be involved, to understand, to affect one's destiny, to be accountable for one's actions, to feel success, to feel meaningful.

These beliefs are the foundation of any professional practice structure. They are beliefs that management and staff alike must integrate into their value system. They are the foundation for decentralization. They are the foundation for organizational change.

PROBLEMS ENCOUNTERED WITH PROFESSIONAL ORGANIZATIONS

Accepting the need for a professional practice approach to restructure the health care system is the first step toward change. Recognizing the need for the expansion of the professional organization to include all professionals in the system—not only the physicians—has entailed new demands. Nurse executives know that the medical model itself is not faultless and thus those issues will also confront the newly formed professional practice groups such as nursing. Increased democracy and autonomy are the gains the professional organization gives to its professionals, but at the same time problems of coordination, innovation, and discretion remain to be resolved (Mintzberg, 1989, pp. 188-192).

Coordination

Problems of coordination involve finding ways to link the more autonomous professionals with the bureaucratically functioning nonprofessional groups. Traditional managers generally control nonprofessional workers and require employees to function and gain direction through the vertical lines of authority. Where does the professional integrate with this approach? The support staff's function is to support the professional practitioners. The need is for a method that enables professionals to clearly articulate their needs to those groups through management. In nursing, many nonprofessionals are delegated direct patient care activities and require the general supervision of the professional for that portion of the job. These same individuals, however, have responsibilities that can and should be supervised through the more traditional routes of the system rather than consuming the time of the professional practitioner. To maximize the time spent by professionals in their practice, the system must provide appropriate support for the professional groups that meet that group's needs. The professionals need to be able to clearly articulate their needs and control who performs certain delegated tasks that, in their view, affect patient care outcomes. Therefore, the resulting system must allow practitioners to make judgments not only about their independent practice decisions but also about some areas of the traditional system that they feel affect their practice. Professionals do this in several ways. First, professionals should coordinate with management to communicate system needs. It is management's responsibility to communicate and mediate the professional and nonprofessional components of the system. Traditionally in nursing, it has been helpful for such mediators to be nurses (nurse managers) who can understand the perspectives and needs of the practitioners and can administer the traditional system through appropriately learned management theories. It is important that a mediator be able to act as a professional practitioner advocate, much as nurses act as patient advocates.

Coordination needs exist between nursing and other professional practitioner groups. Structures are needed that allow practitioners to discuss practice issues and coordinate care in the most effective and efficient manner. Interdependent practitioners must have some mechanism through the formal structure to deal with long-term issues and development and coordination of the standard of care. They also need a culture that supports and encourages informal networking and coordination for day-to-day functions and needs. Collaborative practice committees are becoming more common in hospitals and are meeting the needs for coordination between practitioners. Case management is another example of a coordination link used in some systems (O'Malley, Loveridge, and Cummings, 1989). Innovative systems of the future will continue to create new coordination mechanisms for their practitioner groups.

Innovation

The second problem that professional organizations face is the issue of innovation. As Mintzberg (1989, p. 190) aptly states, "Major innovation depends on cooperation . . . new programs and improvements usually cut across multiple professional lines . . . professional bureaucracies create reluctance of the professionals to cooperate with each other and the collective processes can produce resistance to innovation." Professionals, by their nature, are independent and autonomous. They are familiar with controlling their own decisions. Creating mechanisms to encourage cooperation and thus freeing innovation is a requisite. Professionals must face responsibility for coordination and cooperation. As technology becomes increasingly complex, issues arise that illustrate this point. In the past it was workable to divide the "tasks" along section lines in most medical staff organizations. With the changes in available technology and the current competitive economic environment, traditional section members "cross over" into practice areas. Radiologists, cardiologists, gastroenterologists, and surgeons now all perform the same "tasks." Similarly, in nursing it was formerly easy to compartmentalize patients based on the need of certain skills and knowledge by the nurse caring for the patient. Today it is less clear as nurses find they are asked to care for sicker patients with more complex problems. The need for interdependency and cooperation among nursing specialties is increasing as the system grows more complex. For the system to survive, leaders need to ensure that they address ways to improve the system's viability despite competition among professional practice groups and in spite of the tendency of the professional groups to become rigid, bureaucratic, and independent of others. Freeing professionals to practice more autonomously requires integration of democratic actions. Health care system relationships will not permit these groups to independently become bureaucratic and fail to integrate with the system as a whole. Recognition of that reality is key to the system's viability.

Discretion

According to Mintzberg (1989, p. 190), the third major problem with professional organizations is discretion. Professional organizations force and focus discretion into the hands of individual practitioners, whose skills require the exercise of considerable judgment. The system works well when those professionals are competent and conscientious. Problems arise when they are not. Mintzberg (1989, p. 190) relates this to several factors. One factor is that professionals have been reluctant to counteract their own interests, perhaps because of the intrinsic difficulty of measuring the outputs of the professional's work. Second, professionals have been traditionally loyal to themselves and their professional association and not the system they practice within. Health care executives must ensure that checks and balances are available within the system that require practitioners to address peer incompetence and other relational issues. The Joint Commission on Accreditation of Healthcare Organizations and other accrediting agencies have quality assurance requirements in place because they recognize these natural tendencies of professional groups. There has been considerable publicity about the lack of professional control over peer practitioners in the medical field. This issue led to the establishment of a national data bank for professional practitioner information. Information about all physicians is stored in a computer bank and systems are mandated to access that information before the initial appointment and reappointment of medical staff members to hospital staffs. Nurses and other professional practitioners will soon be mandated to participate in similar activities as a result of consumer demands. Hospitals are the primary locations where these professionals practice, leading consumers to demand access to hospital accreditation information. The trend is clear. Access to such information is being demanded because the system did not implement structures to adequately monitor and police its individual practitioners. Systems of the future will demand that those components be in place. In the future, quality assurance information will need to be collected not only in the aggregate form but also by individual practitioners for every professional in the system.

THE NURSING ENVIRONMENT IN PROFESSIONAL ORGANIZATIONS
Individual Accountability

Individual accountability is the key to effectiveness in professional organizations (Mintzberg, 1989, p. 193). Accountability originates and rests within an individual and creates a sense of ownership for one's actions and their impact on others. With accountability and ownership come obligations for action and followup. As an individual practitioner the professional must be dedicated to working with the client first and foremost: attorney and client, educator and student, nurse and patient. The professional's power base within professional organizations is derived from the working relationship that exists with clients. The structure that exists in professional organizations is primarily built around the needs of the professionals—the need for support and coordination that practitioners have to be able to individually provide service to their patients. The basic relationship remains one-on-one between the professional and the client. Changes within the system must carefully address the need to maintain this relationship of individual accountability between professional and client.

Nursing Groups

Most hospitals are organized by departments or divisions. This practice allows a system to organize delivery of patient care around like-client groups based on the similarity of work processes and equipment required for each group of patients (cardiology, oncology, rehabilitation, etc.). In addition, similar groups of patients are usually cared for by a fairly focused group of professionals who usually serve a specific patient population. This practice encourages the achievement of common standards of care and provides for peer review among like professionals. Well-diversified nursing units allow for increased flexibility and a greater degree of control over individual operations. Unit-based professionals can virtually create their own support structures and build a reasonable, independent, functioning sub-system within the hospital system. Examples of this are seen every day. Diversi-fication of units or divisions within hospitals has only increased in the past few years. As the trend toward more professional practice models increases, so too will the trend toward more independent unit-based systems.

Organization of Professionals

The typical nursing unit is organized around a patient population. There are several groups of professional practitioners who provide care to the patient popu-lation based on their role and responsibilities. Physicians, professional nurses, and professional allied health practitioners all play varied roles in the provision of care to their patients. Each has an individual relationship with the patient for the care directly provided. In addition, each has a responsibility to the other practitioners to participate in coordinating the patients' care. The nurse generally fulfills the co-ordination role. The nurse is usually the professional practitioner who has the most primary relationship with the patient by virtue of the requisites of the work of nursing. The coordination of professionals must be accomplished quickly and be maintained throughout the patient's stay to optimize patient outcomes. However, coordination should not preclude the individual's accountability that must exist and be felt by each practitioner toward the patient. Individual accountability is ac-complished through an understanding and appreciation of each member's unique role.

Facilitation of patient care conferences helps to provide effective coordination of care. It also allows time for education of each discipline to the other's role and the contribution that professional can make to the patient. Most health care disci-plines have become so specialized that most collegial groups do not really know the areas for which specialized practitioners are educated and prepared to assume responsibility. Grand rounds and other educationally focused sessions bring the professional groups together and offer an avenue to increase coordination in the system.

Newer professional practice models also must provide for a structure for the various professional groups to meet as a whole. There are numerous professional issues that should be addressed and organized by like practitioners. Among these issues are development of the professional groups' standards of practice, guide-lines for credentials and privileges, standards of performance, disciplinary proce-dures, quality assurance reviews, educational needs assessments, and establish-ment of research. The system as a whole must address a structure for nurses to organize themselves as a body of professional practitioners to accomplish all ac-tivities that are essential to their practice. In addition, many of these issues must be readdressed at the subunit level or specialty level of organization. Structures must be developed, usually through the use of groups, for the professionals to co-ordinate on a unit level and establish the specialty standards of practice, monitor compliance to those standards, and plan for educational and research needs.

By their nature professional organizations demand the use of groups to coor-dinate the diverse types of practitioners. The key to effective functioning is finding a way to organize the individual professionals so that their individual and interdependent/collegial responsibilities can be accomplished in the system with minimal conflict between professional groups. Each professional has individual accountability to the client. Members also have collective responsibility for control of their profession and their members in the system.

Organization of Support Staff

Nursing units have several groups of support staff available to assist the professional practitioner in the system. The support staff can be divided into two categories: the care support staff and the material support staff. Responsibilities are delegated from the professional practitioners to the care support staff for selected direct or indirect care activities.

Coordination of resources is critical to the delivery of nursing care. The structure in the system must provide for a linkage of the professional practitioner to either directly delegate and control the care support staff, or arrange for management to provide for the delegation and supervision of the support staff through preestablished agreements.

The material support staff generally assists in arranging and providing for the effective organization and efficiency of the environment. Management staff, along with the material support staff in most professional organization models, exists as a support mechanism for the professional practitioner. Management's role is to manage the human, material, and financial elements of the system so that the work of the practitioner can be accomplished. This implies constant communication from practitioners to management as to their needs. Communication is usually accomplished through group meetings established through the development of a management structure. The structure integrates with elements of the practitioner groups as needed so that management receives the information needed to perform well. The practitioner is at the center of the organizational model with management providing a linkage to the rest of the system.

Shared Governance as a Model

Developing and creating a model structure that meets all the critical elements of a professional practice model is a difficult task. It would be difficult enough to create such a structure in a new organization free from any bias or history that may complicate such a task. It is seemingly a monumental task in a system typical of most hospitals. The critical elements are reasonably clear: individual professional accountability by the practitioner, coupled with professional responsibility and accountability for all issues relating to practice. Such issues include standards of practice and care, assurance of the quality of care provided, responsibility for the professional development of the practitioners, and professional review responsibility. The challenge is to create a workable structure that allows all these elements to operate at the same time. Porter-O'Grady and Finnegan (1984, p. xi) are recognized as individuals who initiated the first such structure for nursing in the early '80s. The concept has been called "shared governance."

Shared governance is more accurately described as a set of concepts and beliefs that can emerge from an existing organizational structure but forces significant fluctuation, which brings about changes that are more consistent with behaviors expected in professional organizational models. Shared governance is an accountability-based system. The concept is founded on individual accountability as opposed to individual participation in management. The basic belief system supports the concepts previously discussed in this chapter as well as in Chapters 1 and 2. The actual structure used to facilitate shared governance beliefs varies from organization to organization. Whether a system chooses the councilor or the congressional model of shared governance or others (see Chapter 4) is not as fundamentally critical as ensuring that the structure is sound, complete, and truly integrative of the critical elements arising from the belief system.

PROBLEMS ENCOUNTERED WITH REFORMATTING NURSING WORK GROUPS

Nursing work groups are a significant part of the hospital environment. The grouping of nursing professionals varies from unit to unit, but in most systems, nurses are organized around a particular patient population base. They integrate into their group the full-time unit-based care support staff members and consider the nurse manager the group's leader. This structure is pervasive in most health care settings. Traditionally, the nurses and the support staff report directly to the nurse manager. The professional staff have some degree of autonomy with their practice environment on a one-to-one basis; however, overall the nurse manager is seen as the group leader. In addition, any support staff member who does not report directly to the unit's nurse manager may be viewed as not being within the control of the nursing unit's power base. Such members may be recognized as a necessary part of the team effort, but because of the lack of the direct hierarchical control over them by the group's leader (the nurse manager), they are not recognized as having full membership rights. This is the culture of most units in traditional hospital systems.

For professional practice models to work, there must be some alteration of the basic assumptions surrounding nursing work groups. There must be a way to reorganize the groups along a structure that more appropriately fits and reinforces the professional caregiver's role. The culture of the group must change to accept that new structure and the new relationships that coincide with the new structure. The traditional view of all the team members being the "same" or "equal" needs to be addressed.

Equal but Different

Most professional nurses identify with the support staff. Nurses recognize the value support staff members bring to the system. The professional nurse also recognizes the desire of these individuals to feel needed and valued in the roles that they fulfill. Too often, however, nurses sacrifice their own professional values and fail to act as responsible, accountable professionals to help satisfy the support staff's need to feel "equal" to nurses. The word "equal" is what creates problems. Everyone agrees that all staff members are equal as human beings. Everyone deserves the same respect and treatment. This basic belief is one of the underpinnings necessary for the introduction and maintenance of a truly decentralized professional structure. However, the central point is not "equal"—rather it is "different." That perspective needs to be communicated to the staff nurses frequently so that they understand that being different does not mean that one person is a better human being than another; it merely means that one has a different role and a different set of responsibilities than another. To acknowledge less than that leads to compromise of one's professional responsibilities.

Traditionally, the system has recognized and treated nurse managers differently than staff nurses. There is the perception that staff nurses are not equal to nurse managers. This is reinforced by the historical bureaucratic structures that afford the decision-making authority to management. Society indirectly reinforces these beliefs by perpetuating the concept that the importance of an individual's work and worth within an organization is based solely on a person's salary. That attitude has been a great disservice to all systems.

Nurses must recognize that they are *different* from others, including their fellow support staff members and their nurse managers. Nurses must recognize these differences and accept them without placing a value on the differences. Placing a value, or allowing others or society to place a value, on the differences is the mistake that will lead others to feel they are not being treated equally as human beings. The difference is critical in the implementation of a professional practice model. Management's understanding and integration of this belief into everyday functioning is also critical to success of the transition. The popularity of clinical advancement programs that afford nurses the opportunity to be recognized through the more traditional indicators of success (increased salary and benefits) is a tribute to the nurse executives and nurse managers beginning to respond to the need for permanent changes in traditional attitudes toward the basic "hands-on" care provider. The pyramid that has been the foundation of the traditional health care organizational structure is starting to disappear.

Uses of Licensed Practical Nurses in Hospitals

Prior to strict enforcement of state practice acts and more rigid accreditation standards, licensed practical nurses (LPNs) functioned in expanded capacities beyond their original preparation and education. These support staff members were used to perform advanced procedures and were expected to fill in when registered nurses were not readily available or desired by some systems. Registered nurses sometimes provided supervision for the care given, but overall the LPN was fully responsible for providing the level of care delivered. As the profession of nursing became more organized and nursing started to closely examine the practice of nursing, the differentiation of the practice of "nursing" was questioned. Not only did nursing question the difference in role of the LPN and the RN, but also the difference in role of the RN compared with another RN with different educational levels. Nursing as a profession began to mature and state practice acts followed. Accreditation standards became more rigid and the role of the RN versus another staff member became an issue. For years LPNs had been told, both directly and indirectly through behavior and complacency, that they were prepared to plan and provide the care necessary for the patient. As times changed, nursing began to question whether or not that standard needed to change.

Health systems began to redefine the role of the LPN. LPNs as an organized group have encountered much difficulty and misunderstanding regarding the differentiated practice movement that has entered nursing. It is easy to understand some of the emotional elements experienced by LPNs. The issue at stake, however, is not "equal" but "different." Nursing care systems must stop sending mixed messages to LPNs. The new differentiated roles are clear and understandable. Stability and consistency of application are needed to reinforce the appropriateness and legitimacy of the critical role LPNs play. If inconsistencies exist, there will be continued unhappiness and unrest. The message must be clear and precise—the role is critical as care support staff; however, the final decision making, planning, and evaluation must be provided by the professional practitioners. If that perspective is not accepted and understood by both the professional practitioner and the LPN, then group growth will be inhibited. Reformatting work groups not only involves sometimes redefining who the members are, but also adjusting roles and responsibilities among the members of the groups.

Nursing as a Female Profession

Nurse executives must deal with the issue of nursing as a female profession. Much has been written about the nursing shortage and the predisposing factors that led to the situation regarding the salary compression issue. In fact, many authors attribute the root of the problem to the fact that most nurse are females. Females have a long history of inequality, and it is well documented that long-term oppression can cause behavioral changes in individuals. Beattie (1987, p. 28) defines the condition of "codependency" as "an emotional, psychological, and behavioral condition that develops as a result of an individual's prolonged exposure to, and practice of, a set of oppressive rules—rules which prevent the open expression of feelings as well as the direct discussion of personal and interpersonal problems." As a group, nurses have demonstrated codependent behavior as a result of long-term oppression in health care, coupled with long-term oppression in society by predominant masculine control. Nurses are beginning to recognize the caretaking behaviors that are not appropriate and are beginning to resocialize toward more appropriate acceptance of responsibility. Nurses will continue to be educated and resocialized to envision themselves in a professional context as more professional practice models unfold.

To accomplish this resocialization, consistency and education within a supportive culture are necessary. The change must begin with nurses themselves. Professional nurses must learn to solve problems effectively and to feel comfortable in that role. They must actively listen and communicate clearly and appropriately with their peers, colleagues, and support staff members. Nurses need skills to resolve conflicts constructively. They need to practice assertiveness in regard to their own needs. In short, they need to act and behave as adults in a professional world. They need to accept accountability for their own actions, and expect their peers to do likewise. Nurse executives have a critical role in supporting, encouraging, and rewarding these new behaviors as they occur. Staff nurses must take considerable risks to break out of the old mold and risk new behaviors. Some type of reward or reinforcement must be afforded those who take the risk.

The nurse executive plays a critical role in creating a supportive environment within which nurses will feel more comfortable in taking risks. Traditional management controls create question and doubt regarding the consequences of risk-taking. What will the result be? Ultimately, actions speak louder than words, and nurses will be focused on management's response to the new behaviors. It is imperative that the initial responses be supportive and sincere. Nurse executives and nurse managers alike must portray an accepting attitude for the expression of opinions and ideas. Early in the change process it is important to reinforce the presence of participation and risk-taking as opposed to an in-depth critique of every action and decision. Management must clearly articulate its value for staff members' decision-making responsibility as it pertains to the practice of nursing.

Issues with Staff Relationships

Nursing has always had some type of structure that allowed for the coordination and integration of nurses with other nurses, and nurses with support staff members. Those structures are changing as the environment toward professional practice evolves, but the need has always been addressed in the past. Nursing is comfortable in defining and redesigning its affiliation and linkages within its own "department." The unfamiliarity occurs in reaching out and setting up linkages and networks within the medical staff and other practitioner bureaucracies.

Historically, there has been conflict between physicians and nurses in health care. Some of the conflict is traceable to the history of conflict between men and women. Physicians and hospitals have a unique relationship that is not duplicated in other major industries. Physicians, by virtue of the American health care system, control access to hospitals. Hospitals depend on physician admissions to fill their beds. The critical nature of the relationship is such that the hospital will do whatever is necessary to keep its "customers" happy. Physicians have enjoyed this special treatment for years. Conversely, nurses have been oppressed generally, and have suffered for lack of input and participation in decisions affecting them. They have watched physicians influence decisions for years. Some nurses who have watched this process will even attempt to resolve problems and meet their needs by appealing to the physicians they know who hold power and are listened to by the hospital administration and board. It is natural for nurses to feel angry because of the historical treatment afforded them. However, rather than channel that anger in an appropriate avenue, some nurses direct their anger at the people who benefitted from the system's preferential treatment—physicians. Physicians' long-standing power base in health care systems is diminishing each year; however, it still affords the profession considerable influence beyond that generally afforded nurses and other professionals. Nurses must continually seek ways to resolve their anger and move on to construct better relationships with physicians in the future.

For nurses, physicians, and other allied health practitioners to work collaboratively, they will have to individually accept that their roles and responsibilities are different. "Different" but "equal" is again the key concept in this equation. Nurses and others alike often agree that the primary reason for lack of cooperation among them is that physicians and others are not truly aware of the unique contribution made to patient care by nurses. Hospital units are busy with acutely ill patients. Physicians often visit patients and write orders without seeing the primary nurse. Therapists' schedules are busy and rarely afford them time to discuss their patients' case with the nurse or physician. Physicians and therapists alike do not fully understand the level of education and knowledge needed to provide highly complex nursing care to acutely ill patients. Opportunities for one profession to educate the others regarding their work and its current developments will improve interdisciplinary relationships and levels of understanding. Such interaction will encourage equality as each group realizes the unique contributions of the other. Trust and respect are developed through interaction. The health care system has failed to provide any link for that interaction to consistently occur within health care institutions. As a result, professional groups have grown apart. Quality patient care depends on "fixing" that part of the system.

Shared governance has contributed significantly to the system's ability to bring these practitioner groups together again. Although the initial application of shared governance principles and concepts was to nursing divisions inside hospitals, that has not precluded their natural progression to fields outside of nursing. Nursing recognized the need for the fundamental changes and was willing to take the risk to start the process. However, it is clearly evident that the process need not stop with nursing. The foundation of shared governance needs to be the driving force to accomplish the widespread restructure and redesign of all the professional components of the health care system.

The issues that confront nurses as professionals within hospital structures are the same issues that trouble other practitioners. Autonomy, control, responsibility, accountability, and participation are a few of these common issues. Sharing the experiences of how to address those problems across all professional groups affords an opportunity for all the professionals to realize their similarities. Nursing can help medicine find ways to improve peer review and quality assurance; medicine may help nursing achieve greater accountability for individual practitioner actions; nursing can assist other professional practitioners to find ways to more fully integrate their care with the overall plan of care. All these activities will ultimately bring the practitioner groups closer, improve relationships, and improve the quality of care provided. As the quality of care is improved, the relationships will become further solidified. The vision is clear. Shared governance is purely a catalyst to bring about change.

EMPOWERING NURSES TO PARTICIPATE IN CHANGE
Basic Beliefs

Nurse executives, regardless of their degree of motivation to create a professional practice environment, cannot do it alone. They need their managers' and their staffs' support. They need to create an environment that motivates managers and staff to participate. Empowerment is the goal. One of the basic beliefs needed to support the culture necessary for a professional practice model is that people have the right and the duty to influence decision making that affects them. In professional practice models, affected professionals also assume accountability and responsibility for themselves and their peers. These principles mandate involvement by the practitioner to a degree not previously experienced by most nurses. Participation has always been present in most systems, but participation is different from accountability for practice.

Nurses live out values that are different from those of management. The skills and knowledge needed to manage a group of patients differ significantly from the tools and information needed to manage a practice environment and a group of practitioners. How do systems provide the transition for their staff and empower them to get involved?

Creating a Vision

The first step in reaching empowerment is creating a vision. Nurses and other professionals in hospitals have practiced for a long time in a system whose only vision was to survive financially and provide good care. Such goals are still appropriate, yet coupled with those goals is the need for a new vision of a changed work environment. Nurse executives need to create a vision of a true professional practice environment.

The nurse executive's role in creating and communicating the vision is critical. First, the vision must be a reflection of what the nurse executive thinks and feels. Nurses need to know that the vision is sincere, not just a result of a well-designed recruitment and retention campaign. Sincerity in what is said is as important as constant verbal reinforcement of these beliefs by the nurse executives. Second, the vision must be understood. The nurse executive must describe examples of the vision that reinforce the significance and meaning of the change. Personal commitment to the vision is reinforced when nurses perceive a deep level of understanding of the vision's impact by the nurse executive. Third, periodic implementation of specific actions that support the vision is necessary. General concepts are appropriate ways to focus on change; however, translation of those concepts into specific action steps helps reinforce support for the change over the long term. The nurse executive must be the expert, the cheerleader, and the matriarch of the vision throughout the transition.

Staff members must feel that the culture will be supportive and nourishing of the changes needed. There is no mandate for the final structure of the system to resemble the initial vision—in fact, if it did it might hamper creativity and innovation. The vision needs to be stated in conceptual terms and system beliefs, rather than by articulating structural specifics. Keeping the vision clear and always present will empower nurses and others to act. Their actions will bring the system closer to the goals described in the vision. The clearer the vision, the better the decision-making capability of those working toward the vision. The more people work toward the vision, the more they will identify with it, and thus increase ownership of the goals necessary to attain it.

Decreasing the Fear

As mentioned previously, staff nurses are not familiar with management skills and practices. Historically, managers have taken accountability for all the areas of the practice system, including many of the decisions regarding patient care. For systems to smoothly transfer accountability for certain elements to the practitioners, not only does there need to be a structure in place to organize these new players, but there also must be education for the practitioners about systems and their operation. Most nurse executives would feel personal stress and chaos if asked to manage a full patient load in the intensive care unit because of significant periods of time away from the environment and unfamiliarity with the equipment, new drugs, and practice. The same is true of the staff nurse who is suddenly asked to participate in managing elements of a system with which she is somewhat unfamiliar. In addition to the unfamiliarity with managing groups and systems, the staff nurse has an added element to deal with: fear. Walton (1986, pp. 72-73) refers to Deming's theory in his 14 points to improve organizational efficiency that fear in the average employee is higher in America than anyplace else he has observed. Many employees are afraid to ask questions and take positions. There seems to be an underlying culture that reinforces the fear. It is obvious that fear in a professional system seriously hampers the organization's efforts.

Education of management and staff regarding professional practice systems helps decrease the usual fear associated with change. Information and knowledge are critical elements to address through constant communication. Communication channels that are open and free-flowing will also assist in decreasing fear. The basic premise is that information reduces fear. As more information is available, workers will feel more comfortable in understanding the change, and therefore comfortable in discussing their involvement in the change.

As the professional system's structure matures and responsibility and accountability for the professional practitioner's actions and level of competence are transferred to peer levels, then the traditional management control over compensation and benefits will also be eliminated. Trust must be developed through careful planning and thoughtful collaboration among management and staff members regarding the gradual transition of these economic concerns into the arena of the practitioner. Careful planning itself is educational and greatly improves a person's success rate.

Perhaps staff members' greatest fear is the fear of being fired. Management has traditionally had such power over nurses in hospitals and still retains it in most systems. Physicians are independent practitioners who are not employed by the system and therefore are not concerned about being "fired." They are disciplined through peer review activities. There is generally a higher standard of "proof" associated with that activity than in a normal employee situation. In mature professional practice model systems there has been progress toward the nursing staff's control of entry and exit from the nursing division for professional practitioners. This trend will tend to focus practitioners on peer accountability issues but will also hopefully decrease fear of average staff nurses that the system would choose to fire them without appropriate justification. Professionals need to first feel accountable to themselves and their patients before they can feel accountable to the system that employs them.

Power and the Need for Power Shifts

Power is a complex concept. It extends across all relationships and exists and manifests itself in some form at all levels of an organization. In most organizations, the locus of power still rests primarily with management. Hospitals are no exception. Transition to a professional practice environment will demand a shift in that locus of power and decision-making authority.

Having power implies having control over a situation or person. Generally, people who have power feel "in control," whereas people who do not have power feel "helpless." Helplessness, the belief that one cannot influence the circumstances surrounding one's life, undermines the incentive to learn. It interferes with intrinsic motivation and satisfaction. Professionals are obligated to be accountable and to continue to learn and strive for improved outcomes. They need to feel in control of their practice in order to feel accountable for their practice. The mandate is clear—the focus of power over professional issues in professional organizations must shift to those professionals accountable for the outcomes.

Managers, Challenges, and Changes

Peters (Peters, 1987, p. 345) writes, "I am frustrated to the point of rage—my files bulge with letters about the power of involvement. Sometimes it's planned . . . Sometimes it's inadvertent. But the result is always the same: *Truly involved people can do anything!*" The frustration described by Peters is proof of the power that midlevel management has over any change process. It is imperative that midlevel managers feel ownership in and support the change process.

Restructuring toward a professional practice model entails certain requisites. One is the decentralization of the system, especially the professional arenas. How the majority of nurse managers obtained their current positions is considered below.

Until recently, nursing has not created a clinical track that affords the same salary, benefits, and status as management positions offer. In the past, many nurses, because of internal and external motivators, felt the need to move into management positions to achieve the degree of freedom, flexibility, and participation that management could afford them. The salary and benefits at the management level were also significantly better. No other options for such growth existed. The hospital's most senior nurses frequently moved into management roles as positions became available. In most hospitals, managers continued to fill the clinical expert role in addition to the management role. Then professional practice models emerged. Nurse leaders started to discover that the old ways would not be effective over the long term. They realized that perhaps the system that forced nurses to leave practice and move into management was not the type of system needed for the future.

Today many systems are trying to make the transition to a more logical organizational structure that will enhance long-term survivability. However, through that transition the system is, in effect, "changing the rules" that affect those clinical nurses who moved into management at a time reflective of "older" values. In most hospitals today, these managers are usually the first-line contacts with most professional practitioners; this makes their support even more critical. These managers need the system's support for concentrated education to help them understand their changing role. They will have to understand the need for change and sometimes seek assistance during the transitional process. Finding ways for those who no longer want the management role to return to clinical nursing without economic or status loss will help the nurse executive deal with the frustration that some experience. Those who choose to remain in management instead of clinical nursing should do so because of an independent career choice, not because they are forced to as in the past. Once all the managers realize they have a career choice, and know their role through education and information sharing, they should begin to support the change process and feel ownership for it.

Urgency as Energy

In *Teaching the Elephant to Dance,* Belasco (1990, p. 345) says that a sense of urgency is the source of energy necessary to affect change. Urgency is a good descriptor for health care environments today. Nurse executives would agree that the climate is right, the timing is right, and the motivation is present to move the change through the health system. The urgency comes from the factors demanding the change in the system, including decreasing resources, both human and economic. These decreasing resources are demanding that attention be paid to how the work is currently accomplished and finding avenues to achieve the same results with less use of valuable resources. Numerous examples exist in systems that describe that attempt. Such changes include new nurse assistance positions, increased automation in charting and documentation systems, tighter utilization review programs, and standards based on newer research regarding patient care outcomes. There are also new accounting systems that help quantify the cost of the care provided so it can be coupled with patient care outcome, to bring about desired changes in utilization practices of practitioners. Several research projects have been funded and are ongoing to help clarify the critical factors that cannot be compromised without an undesired change in patient outcome. The urgency will continue as the population of America ages. Predictions are dramatic as to the impact this single demographic phenomenon will have on the health care system (Rubin and others, 1988).

The nursing shortage has had a dramatic impact on hospitals throughout the United States. It also clearly has increased the focus on nursing's problems with the current structure and systems, and has created a sense of urgency toward the resolution of those problems. Timing is a critical element in any change process. It is clear that timing is now prime for nurses and other professionals alike to be energized by the urgency of the situation and work toward change. Nurse executives need to appreciate the sense of urgency and understand it for what it is— energy moving toward action.

OBSTACLES TO EXPECT
Expect Change to Be Slow

No matter how well planned the restructure and change, problems will be encountered. The ability to anticipate some of the obstacles to be encountered helps maintain focus and momentum. Knowing that certain behaviors and situations are likely to occur provides the opportunity to plan to handle those problems even before they occur. Older organizations tend to have more formalized behaviors (Mintzberg, 1989, p. 106).

Change occurs slowly. Well-established systems have developed and formalized approaches to problem resolution. Historically, those approaches have not included employee participation to the degree that is necessary today. Changing the basic concepts of operation of any complex system, especially one as complex as a hospital, requires extensive time and energy.

Emphasize the Long Term

Managers and nurses alike will occasionally exhibit short-term memories. Frustration will be a nurse executive's companion. It will be challenging to remind people to think ahead and keep the vision clear. One way to sustain motivation over the long term is by setting short-term goals and short-term successes. Developing a timeline maps the change process. Periodic success—points that can be publicly acknowledged—should be included in that timeline. Staff and managers alike need to be reinforced; all influence the achievement of long-term success. Once achieved, everyone should hear about the success. Spreading the word spreads enthusiasm.

Remind People the System is in Transition

Because change itself is a long-term venture, the change facilitator will encounter problems regarding expectations and timing. Even if the long-term vision is clear, it still takes years to complete and stabilize any new system. In the interim, people will be confused between the vision and the reality. It is important to inform people of the change process and the expected levels of compliance with the new system. The system will be in transition and, therefore, people need to be tolerant of the inconsistencies in the short run. To be tolerant, there must be understanding. Leaders must encourage everyone to take responsibility for the vision and begin to understand and appreciate the current position on the continuum of change. Formal and informal channels of communication are critical in keeping people informed. The change agent should stress that situations may seem to be in conflict with the long-range plan. Examples of successful systems help to remind people that the change is possible and working in other settings.

Expect Critics and Skeptics

Staff members need their questions and remarks answered directly and should be encouraged to participate in analyzing the issues they present. Respect for staff members permits them to voice their concerns. Hospital systems are complex. Managers use a vocabulary that is foreign to most staff nurses. Unfamiliarity usually creates caution. Unfamiliarity with a management change that could affect a worker can create fear and distrust. If the system does not keep nurses informed and up-to-date, critics and skeptics will increase. Free-flowing information and participation will alleviate unfamiliarity and thus decrease criticism. Talking directly with the critics is helpful. Determining what their issues are, if legitimate, facilitates some resolution. Another strategy is to enlist the help and support of critics. Finding a role for them to play creates a sense of ownership in the process. People usually want to do the right thing.

Confront Procrastination

With today's dynamically mobile health care environment, when is there time to bring about large-scale change? Most days can easily be filled with "firefighting" rather than determining long-term strategy. Most chief executive officers, nurse executives, and staff leaders find it difficult to maintain focus on long-term change amid chaos. Thinking about the world of the average staff nurse can be even more perplexing.

Staffing shortages are universal, as are cost constraints. Patients are more acutely ill. Patients and families are more informed and thus have greater expectations regarding nursing care. Doctors feel controlled from all sources and probably attempt to control whatever elements they feel they still can influence. Most nurses are female, wives, and mothers with increasingly complex role demands. Within such an environment, there is there room for nurses and time to participate in creating change? Convincing nurses that change is needed is not always necessary, but helping them find the time is vital.

Procrastination is a major problem for both the executive and the staff nurse. Procrastination is worsened by the fact that the change is long term. The strategies to deal with procrastination are similar to other strategies previously discussed. People need to be informed. Projects should be broken down so that small successes can be achieved. Successes should be visible so some outcome is recognized. Success encourages motivation and participation. Participation and success by some staff nurses in the change process will generate participation and eventual success by others.

Exhibit the Right Attitude

A project of any length will naturally involve some mistakes. Mistakes are not a problem—negative reaction to mistakes is more generally a problem. Any negative circumstance can be viewed with a positive perspective: if nothing else, at least a lesson may be learned. The entire incident can become an opportunity for motivation. Staff nurses may fear participating in real change and risk-taking if they do not know their leaders' probable reaction to failure or mistakes. Attitude is important. Even leaders make mistakes. The organization can recover.

Change is inherently difficult. It brings joy and some pain and hardship. It causes people to question basic beliefs and challenge the past. It forces people to reexamine and question everything they do. Change forces people to become self-reflective and question their motivation and creativity. It creates uncertainty and confusion.

Change also brings revitalization and rejuvenation to the workplace. It allows people to relieve boredom and daily routine. It cleanses and challenges. Change brings opportunity and growth. Change challenges those affected by it to view it in the most positive light, and believe that chaos and creativity are positive experiences, exhilarating and finitely necessary for growth.

SUMMARY

Today's health care system demands a new perspective from nurse executives. That perspective needs to be adaptive, responsive, facilitative, and supportive of change. Organizational structures of the past need to be reevaluated in light of this new perspective. Professional practice models such as shared governance are emerging as concrete examples of ways that hospitals can address these new demands.

The foundation for professional practice models is accountability. Nurses must be accountable for the delivery of nursing care and have an obligation to fulfill the mandates of the system to achieve that end. The system reciprocates by offering appropriate levels of support to those professionals through human, material, and fiscal resource allocation and coordination. The relationship must be one of mutual respect and commitment to the goals determined by both parties. Problems occur in any system and will occur with professional practice models. Through a shared commitment, problem resolution becomes more effective and efficient. Systems for dealing with common problems related to professional practice models can be discussed and resolved early in the structure's development.

Hospital nursing divisions have historically been complex organizations. They have a history of reinforcing dependency-type behaviors in nurses and other professionals through complex controlling structures. Requisites for change include a firm, consistent set of values, long-term commitment by the nurse executive and others, constant evaluation and reevaluation of each element of the system, and education of all parties to keep the vision alive. Keeping the vision alive is the primary goal of the nurse executive. Other steps will follow more easily if the vision remains clear and understandable. Obstacles are to be expected during the redesigning of a nursing organization. Nurse executives should expect obstacles and view potential roadblocks as opportunities and validation that the change process is effective and the goals are attainable. The vision of change is not without problems or possibilities.

REFERENCES

Aiken, L. (1990). Charting the Future of Hospital Nursing. *Image,* 22(2), 72-77.

Beattie, M. (1987). *Codependent No More: How to Stop Controlling Others and Starting Caring for Yourself.* New York: Harper & Row, p. 28.

Belasco, J.A. (1990). *Teaching the Elephant to Dance: Empowering Change in Your Organization.* New York: Crown Publishers, p. 345.

Blane, G. (1975). The Hospital as a Professional Bureaucracy, *Trustee,* 28(10).

Holling, C.S. (1976). Resilience and Stability of Ecosystems. In E. Jantsch and C.H. Waddington (Eds.), *Evolution and Consciousness: Human Systems in Transition.* Reading, Mass.: Addison-Wesley.

Mintzberg, H. (1989). *Mintzberg on Management: Inside Our Strange World of Organizations.* New York: Free Press.

Morris, W. (Ed.). (1971). *The American Heritage Dictionary of the English Language.* Boston: American Heritage.

Naisbitt, J. and Aburdene, P. (1990). *Megatrends 2000: Ten New Directions for the 1990's.* New York: William Morrow, p. 298.

O'Malley, J., Loveridge, C.E., and Cummings, S.H. (1989) The New Nursing Organization. *Nursing Management,* 20(2), 29-32.

Peters, T. (1987). *Thriving on Chaos: Handbook for a Management Revolution.* New York: Harper & Row.

Porter-O'Grady, T. and Finnigan, S. (1984). *Shared Governance for Nursing.* Rockville, Md.: Aspen Publications.

Rubin, R.J., and others. (1988). *Critical Condition: America's Health Care in Jeopardy.* Washington, D.C.: National Committee for Quality Health Care.

Senge, P.M. (1990). *The Fifth Discipline: The Art and Practice of The Learning Organization.* New York: Doubleday.

Smith, KK. (1984). Rabbits, Lynxes, and Organizational Transitions. In JR Kimberly and RE Quinn (Eds.), *Managing Organizational Transitions*. Homewood, Ill.: Irwin.
Walton, M. (1986). *The Deming Management Method*. New York: Putnam, pp. 72-73.

BIBLIOGRAPHY

Aiken, L. (1990). Charting the Future of Hospital Nursing. *Image,* 22(2), 72-78.
Beattie, M. (1989). *Beyond Codependency and Getting Better All the Time*. San Francisco: Harper & Row.
Beattie, M. (1987). *Codependent No More: How to Stop Controlling Others and Starting Caring for Yourself*. New York: Harper & Row.
Belasco, J. (1990). *Teaching the Elephant to Dance: Empowering Change in Your Organization*. New York: Crown Publishers.
Blane, G. (1975). The Hospital as a Professional Bureaucracy. *Trustee,* 28(10), 13-16.
DePree, M. (1989). *Leadership Is an Art*. New York: Doubleday.
Holling, D.S. (1976). Resilience and Stability of Ecosystems. In E. Jantsch and C.H. Waddington (Eds.), *Evolution and Consciousness: Human Systems in Transitions*. Reading, Mass: Addison-Wesley.
Morris, W. (Ed.). (1971). *The American Heritage Dictionary of the English Language*. Boston: American Heritage.
Mintzberg, H. (1989). *Mintzberg on Management: Inside Our Strange World of Organizations*. New York: Free Press.
Naisbitt, J. (1984). *Megatrends: Ten New Directions Transforming Our Lives*. New York: Warner Books.
Naisbitt, J. and Aburdene, P. (1990). *Megatrends 2000: Ten New Directions for the 1990's*. New York: William Morrow.
O'Malley, J., Loveridge, C.E., and Cummings, S.H. (1989). The New Nursing Organization. *Nursing Management,* 20(2), 29-32.
Peters, T. (1987). *Thriving on Chaos: Handbook for a Management Revolution*. New York: Harper & Row.
Peters, T.J. and Waterman, Jr., R.H. (1982). *In Search of Excellence Lessons from American's Best Run Companies*. New York: Warner Books.
Porter-O'Grady, T. (1986). *Creative Nursing Administration: Participative Management into the 21st Century*. Rockville, Md.: Aspen Publication.
Porter-O'Grady, T. and Finnigan, S. (1984) *Shared Governance for Nursing: A Creative Approach to Professional Accountability*. Rockville, Md.: Aspen Publication.
Rubin, R.J. and others. (1988). *Critical Condition: America's Health Care In Jeopardy*. Washington, D.C.: National Committee for Quality Health Care.
Senge, P.M. (1990). *The Fifth Discipline: The Art and Practice of the Learning Organization*. 1990, New York: Doubleday.
Smith, K.K. (1984). Rabbits, Lynxes, and Organizational Transitions. In JR Kimberly and RE Quinn (Eds.), *Managing Organizational Transitions* (pp. 267-294). Homewood, Ill.: Irwin.
Walton, M. (1986). *The Deming Management Method*. New York: Putnam.
Woititz, J.G. and Garner, A. (1990). *Lifeskills for Adult Children*. Deerfield Beach, Fla.: Health Communications.

4   *Models of Shared Governance: Design and Implementation*

Beth E. Foster

This chapter focuses primarily on the forces driving nursing toward new management models, specifically shared governance, and the mechanisms necessary to establish and maintain these models. Included in the discussion are the environment from which shared governance has emerged and the primary models extant today.

It is important to remember there is no one "right" way to structure a shared governance model. Each organization has unique issues. The important factor is that the design be consistent with the purpose.

FORCES DRIVING CHANGE

The changes in today's society in general, particularly in health care, are propelling nursing to move in new directions. Social upheaval related to the women's movement has had a profound effect on nursing's struggle to create a meaningful place in health care. Institutions within the health care system have long been replicas of traditional male-oriented systems. As members of a predominantly female profession, until recently nurses have been socialized to accommodate the male-oriented system. They have learned to play the games necessary to survive by developing unspoken tactics (Stein, Howell, and Watts, 1990).

Because nursing education developed in hospitals and was financially supported by them, its structure and function became institutionalized in a form that still exists in many organizations. Hospital-based nursing schools existed to provide services that supported the values of the hospitals and to provide an unchanging supply of new nurses (Porter-O'Grady and Finnigan, 1984). The step from hospital-based nursing school to the hospital's nursing service, both often controlled by the same nursing director, was an easy one for new graduates. The familiarity of expectations between the two removed much of the anxiety ordinarily experienced in transitions and perpetuated the role of nursing as a source of service to the hospital.

The movement of nursing education from hospitals to institutions of higher learning was a major step in establishing an academic base for nursing practice. This triggered the beginning development of nursing as a profession (McNichols and Miller, 1988; Porter-O'Grady and Finnigan, 1984).

In addition to the women's movement and professionalization of nursing, other societal changes affect organizations. As job security has decreased in economically uncertain times, so has organizational loyalty. In addition, widespread skepticism of government, institutions, and industry has developed because of a loss of confidence in both organizations and their leaders. These changes are challenging the traditional bureaucratic organization that has been prevalent in industry (Heller, 1984; Peterson and Allen, 1986). Employees desire more control over the work environment. Participative management models have been successful in improving employee morale and perceptions. As Peterson and Allen point out, to view the need for change in management structure as limited only to enhancing professional practice in nursing does not fully appreciate the same need for change occurring in the rest of the industrial world. The control and decision-making issues related to these changes, however, have helped to shape the models of shared governance in nursing.

During this time of change, both managers and staff are experiencing dissonance in their work. The work is more complex, workers are better educated, and no single person can be relied on to provide all the information and answers.

Bureaucracy is defined as "government characterized by specialization of functions, adherence to fixed rules and a hierarchy of authority" (Webster, 1988). Most large organizations today would be referred to as bureaucratic in structure. The common perception is that little work is accomplished in a bureaucracy, al-

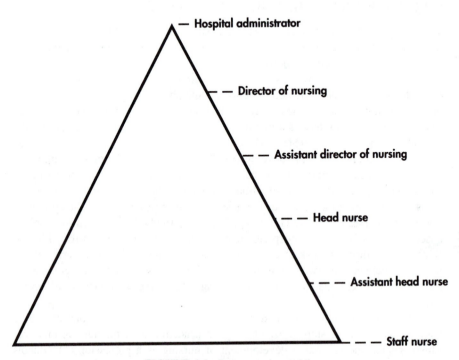

FIGURE 4-1. Bureaucratic model.

though this structure was designed to create efficiency and centralize control. The many hierarchical levels and an expanded scope of accountability as employees moved up in the organization resulted in layers of personnel between the staff and the highest level of management. Top-down communication and tight control characterize this model as shown in Figure 4-1.

Placement within the structure and reporting relationships become critical status issues. Decision making and policy development are kept at the highest levels and communicated down the line. The result of such structured systems is that managers at the top levels make decisions and are held accountable, while the work of the organization is performed by those who have had no input into the decisions. Although this may have addressed the need for improved production, little attention was paid to the higher-level human needs of the workers.

NURSING IN A BUREAUCRATIC STRUCTURE

The majority of nurses identify with the bureaucratic type of structure common in hospital settings. Most have become familiar with its workings. Unfortunately, this format often conflicts with the current roles for which professional nurses are educated (Ketefian, 1985).

Fiscal constraints have become a major concern of the health care community within the past 5 to 7 years. As an increasing percentage of the gross national product is consumed for health care (12% and increasing), the need for creative leadership to confront the problems of health care delivery in a cost-efficient manner was one of the findings of the Commission on Nursing (Lynaugh, 1989). Coupled with massive fiscal constraints is a demand-driven shortage of professional nurses. This supports the need for new methods of organizing nursing departments to enhance the professional component of the practice arena to recruit and retain nurses in the profession.

System structure reflects the values of the organization. When bureaucracy takes precedence over professional practice issues, care will be compromised and staff will be frustrated and unable to fully participate in the activities associated with their practice. Conflict between the profession and the institution results (Porter-O'Grady, 1985).

One approach that has been used to avoid this conflict is decentralization, a format frequently found in hospitals and other professional organizations. This approach maintains a hierarchical structure and thus may be referred to as a professional bureaucracy. It does decrease the layers of management by moving the authority for decisions to a lower level of the hierarchy, but accountability for decisions is retained at the management level. For example, in a decentralized structure, the nurse manager, rather than the director or administrator, has the responsibility for decisions regarding the practice environment on the unit, although it is not her role as a manager to perform those clinical activities. This places both the staff and manager in an untenable situation.

Because this structure does not effectively transfer accountability to the practicing clinician, it is not equal to the decentralized decision making required in promoting professional accountability. Only when both the authority and accountability for an activity rest with the individual or group performing the function is true decentralization in place.

An organization's commitment to true decentralization is no stronger than its faith in the individual worker. Leaders in such organizations are responsible for sustaining this vision of the individual as professional and evolving policy and structure to support that vision.

Rather than attempting to control the organization, leaders serve as teachers by articulating these values and fostering the climate that develops and unites the individuals in the organization into a common purpose.

PRINCIPLES OF SHARED GOVERNANCE

It is important to remember that there is no one "right" way to structure a shared governance model and that the system and the work it facilitates are more important than the creation of a structure. However, the following basic principles and structures to support them will be present in a shared governance model:

1. Staff are elected by their peers to the positions they hold in the shared governance structure.
2. Clinical nursing staff are given accountability for all issues relating to nursing practice. This includes standards, quality assurance activities, and peer processes associated with clinical practice. Throughout the organization clinical nurses rather than managers are represented on all committees that affect nursing practice. Conversely, nursing management, rather than making clinical decisions, is accountable for the provision of necessary financial, human, and material resources for the nursing staff to do its work. Nurse managers are responsible for managing the budget, ensuring that adequate numbers of staff are hired, and ensuring that the interface between nursing and the departments that support nursing functions appropriately.
3. An acknowledgment of the role of the clinical nurse as central to the hospital's mission of patient care exists. The nurse executive no longer sees herself as the sole representative of the nursing department, and supports the representation of a clinical nurse at the highest level of the organization. A key difference between a bureaucratic organization and shared governance is that the potential exists for a staff nurse to represent nursing staff on the board of directors of the hospital. If the nurse executive is not a board member, other ways may need to be found to acknowledge the staff nurse in the organization's power structure.
4. Staff has a shared role with management in the issues of salary, budgeting, staffing, and working conditions. Such involvement may take various forms, but adequate information on these topics must be provided to staff for their input to be meaningful. Management no longer has absolute control of these processes.
5. Bylaws or rules define the operations and structure of the nursing organization. These provide a clear definition of roles and accountabilities within the department of nursing. To ensure that the processes undertaken cannot be

changed casually by present or new management, the bylaws or rules should be approved by the board of trustees.

6. Clinical staff are represented at the executive level of the department of nursing. The structure selected to accomplish this is often a coordinating or executive group composed of staff and management. This executive group would generally address those issues affecting the entire department (for example, approving the departmental budget or developing the bylaws). They may also assume a role in determining or assigning accountabilities to appropriate groups within the structure.

7. There is a well-defined process for all members of the department to meet to review pertinent issues and the work of the department. Minimally, an annual meeting should occur at which the leadership may be elected.

INITIATING THE MODEL

Considerable work and creativity are involved in establishing an organization that supports shared governance. The implementation process involves a period of at least 3 to 5 years. It is a lengthy process because of the extended preparation period necessary for both management and staff as each phase of the new model is unfolded.

The change from a bureaucratic structure to shared governance is not a matter of rearranging a few structures and lines. As the underlying principles are examined, it becomes clear that it is a systemwide shift not only in organizational structure but in basic beliefs (Krejci and Malin, 1989). The clinical nurse, rather than the nursing administrator, has the pivotal and critical role in the department. Ferguson (1980) describes a distinctly new way of thinking about old issues as a paradigm shift. When the practice of nursing in a bureaucratic structure is compared with the practice of nursing in a shared governance structure, the concept of paradigm shift is helpful in analyzing the process.

Elements of a new paradigm must grow in a culture that will support them. Determining the cultural norms of an organization helps ensure selecting a program that can succeed over time. Allen and Kraft (1984) describe the organizational culture as containing "two organizations—one with visible, articulated, expressed, and stated goals, policy statements, and procedure manuals; the other invisible and unconscious, lying quietly under the surface, but actually determining what will happen in the long run." It is critical that both "organizations" be assessed.

When the decision has been made to redesign an organization, a number of questions must be asked. Among the first are "What is the work of the organization?" and "What structure would facilitate the accomplishment of this work?" These are critical questions that cannot be answered in isolation from the current organizational culture.

The structure that is created is not simply a mechanical drawing with labeled positions but the framework that will integrate the functions and work. It will necessarily be open to communication and information flow required to facilitate decision making and timely activity. Mechanisms must be present to respond not only to the work of the department but also to the needs of the employees as human beings and as a professional staff.

The cardinal rule is that shared governance cannot be implemented by management fiat. However, nursing leadership often will begin the process by informally exploring with individuals and groups their concerns, thoughts, and beliefs of how nursing is and could be practiced at their institution. In some instances the impetus to change occurs because of overt staff dissatisfaction and in others because of the desire of the nurse executive to develop a more professional model of practice.

Regardless of the primary impetus to change the nursing organization, changes so profound necessarily must be led by the nurse executive. The concept of leadership in shared governance is changed dramatically, so the nurse executive must be comfortable with the relocation of much decision making. This needs to be carefully considered because shared governance will not succeed without this support. The current bureaucratic structure has been supported through design of the nursing organization (role descriptions, rules and regulations, reporting relationships) and nursing also has the power to redesign it. However, no one functions in a vacuum. The interrelationships between departments also need to be considered in the design. Naisbitt (1982) states that change occurs when changing values and economic necessity meet. This is clearly the situation in nursing and health care today.

To assist in the necessary redesign, Porter-O'Grady and Finnigan (1984) suggest a series of questions that should be asked relating to the role and work of nursing as a service, how nursing's work is viewed and valued within the institution. The fact that the structure must include the functional aspect of practice makes this task more complex.

1. What are the essential activities of nursing that require organizational and structural support?
2. What role does nursing currently play in the organization and does this meet the organization's expectations?
3. What are the goals of nursing and what roadblocks must be overcome to accomplish them?
4. What linkages will coordinate activities within the department and in the hospital as a whole?
5. How can a professional practice model for nursing best "fit" the current structure and culture of the institution?
6. How can nursing most effectively support the vision and goals of the organization?

Why is the change to shared governance so difficult? Shared governance is not an easy concept to understand, and developing departmental consensus on its meaning is more difficult. This is especially true when the required changes in behaviors are not fully understood by the individuals involved. In addition, breaking away from traditional roles that have provided meaning and status will be resisted.

STRATEGIZING THE MOVE TO SHARED GOVERNANCE

Both nursing and general administrative leadership must be committed to the changes that must occur. The concept of shared governance will not be totally understood by the Chief Executive Officer (CEO). However, the CEO must agree to generally support the necessary process required to implement shared governance.

The CEO/COO's beliefs about nursing and how he or she interacts with the nursing department will be key factors in the nurse executive's approach to shared governance with him or her. It is important to remember that the hospital administrator will probably come from the traditional management background found in most hospitals today. The process and effects of shared governance will be viewed in that context. Nevertheless, the executive or operating officer may come from a broad spectrum of styles within the traditional framework, from autocratic to participatory. Knowing this style will guide the nurse executive in presenting the issue.

The hospital administrator regards his or her leadership as institutional but recognizes nursing as a large and important part of the system. Particularly in today's health care environment, the CEO will try to balance clinical and budgetary concerns. Most administrators are concerned about quality patient care but must approach it from a nonclinical point of view. The administrator is therefore dependent on the nursing executive's interpretation of how any changes in the department will affect quality of care. Because quality is primarily a matter of individual perception, the response that quality of care will be affected can be unsettling by its lack of definition. The ability of the nurse executive and hospital administrator to communicate with confidence on issues such as this when the administrator is essentially dependent on the nurse executive's clinical interpretation, in combination with the CEO's experience with nursing, will be important factors in assessing how this history will facilitate or constrain the introduction and acceptance of shared governance.

Knowing the administrator's preferred style and value system will be important in planning the strategy to move to an open and participatory system. Developing the plan with emphasis on those aspects that will best reflect the values of the administrator and working to enhance the institution's goals will facilitate acceptance and support.

Because the outcome unfolds over time, apprising the administrator of the early phases is appropriate, emphasizing areas that may be of particular interest that the nurse administrator can support. Regular follow-up, as successes occur, or when noise in the system is expected, should maintain confidence and support. As changes occur that are important to the administrator's value system, they can be emphasized (Porter-O'Grady and Finnigan, 1984).

Other officers of the corporation, especially in the human resources department, will need to be informed of activities. Because the vice president for human resources is concerned about all employees and their working situation, the changes that occur in the nursing department will be of great interest. Because nursing is a large department and affects nearly every department in the hospital, the human resource officer's views of nursing as a department and its role within the institution will be factors to consider in presenting shared governance as a concept. Nursing has not always felt understood by human resources personnel; thus it is not uncommon that animosity or a certain level of wariness exists between these two departments. As recruitment and retention issues have become more critical in nursing, a general appreciation of human resources in making changes in the work environment has occurred. This should help to facilitate the integration of new concepts related to shared governance.

Activities traditionally considered as the human resources department's responsibilities (developing job descriptions and evaluations) will eventually become part of the new governance process; therefore collaboration with the human resources officer will be an important strategy. Inability to complete the process once implementation has begun will create a feeling of betrayal in the nursing organization with long-term effects on morale.

Having the knowledge and skills of the experienced human resource expert who understands and supports the needs of the professional can be valuable to the nurse executive. Because resources from management, education, and development are often within the domain of the human resources department, implementing strategy to meet the developmental needs of the nursing department in the transition to a new form of governance can be a joint collaboration. If this project is undertaken without adequate support, the changes that occur will be limited.

Peer leadership in the institution also should be informed of the changes and strategies that will be undertaken. Time demands to implement and sustain the program will be substantial, and the nurse executive's role will change. As accountabilities are transferred, the executive will be less involved with traditional day-to-day activities related to nursing practice. This will decrease the level of detail to which she ordinarily has ready access because many decisions will be moved to other members of the department. Other administrators will need to be informed of progress, although the difficulties encountered in departmental activities related to the changes that are occurring will not be easy for them to appreciate.

MOVING AHEAD

When support for change has been determined, the next step is to explore with nursing management and staff how the process should unfold. Literature review, attendance at presentations, use of consultants, and, when possible, site visits of models of interest have been used to discover usable models.

The particular model selected is not as critical as how well it fits the organization. This fact will be emphasized by any nursing leader who has implemented shared governance. No process of this magnitude should be introduced without an assessment of the organization and a plan for preparing individuals and groups for the change ahead. Much will be learned in the process of development. The reasons for shared governance become clearer for staff and management as the concepts and models are explored.

In discussing early implementation, Wilson (1989) points out the need for consensus regarding what shared governance means since each position in the organization will experience a different role change. For example, the role changes of the manager will be expressed differently from those of the staff nurse. In addition, there are varying levels of skill and maturity as well as trust issues and personal agendas within the nursing department.

STEERING FUNCTION

A steering committee is helpful to oversee the shared governance process. The committee should be limited to 10 or 12 members and be composed of staff and management. The exact number of each is not critical, but it must be understood that the process is a collaborative effort between staff and management. Two satisfactory approaches are: (1) an equal number of staff and management; (2) a proportional number, with more staff representation because the major focus will be in the area of staff expertise, patient care. In this early phase of development, a mix of half staff and half management is probably appropriate. The group will often be selected rather than elected, with elections subsequently occurring as the new structure begins to function. The level of sophistication and professional maturity in the group will influence its progress and format. An additional administrative representative who is not associated with nursing can lend credibility to the necessary activities.

The same questions related to changes necessary to move to a professional practice model asked during the nursing administrator's assessment should be asked of this group. The questions provide a focus to the discussions that have the potential to move the group from individual and unit-based issues to a broader outlook of the department and institution.

This larger view is important because nurses tend to view their work environment in terms of the interaction between themselves and their patients and the units on which they work. One strength of group work is uniting nurses from various areas of the hospital whose perspectives may differ significantly.

The structure is the framework through which the department will perform its work. How this occurs may be easier to visualize when the models are reviewed. The values and beliefs of both the organization and department will be demonstrated as the roles of staff and management are described.

Because this group will help the nursing administrator lead the department through the change associated with shared governance, it is of primary importance to support an education process for them. Shared governance will require a systemwide effort to reach a mutual understanding of the term *shared governance;* thus the steering committee will need to attain some level of comfort with the concept. This process will not be easy because it will represent a reversal of many well-established patterns of thinking and behavior.

A good starting point is a discussion of nursing's place in the current health care field and how it was reached. Information on the health care setting and the continued expected changes will help to clarify why the bureaucratic structures under which most nurses function are no longer appropriate. A focused review of nursing as practiced at the institution will help put the current organizational structures in perspective.

Information on shared governance in nursing and similar structures in the business world is readily available. Videos, educational programs, use of consultants, and site visits offer additional opportunities to understand the concept. Unfortunately, there is little information on the actual implementation available in print. Most hospitals that have implemented, or are in the process of implementing, shared governance have personnel who are eager to discuss their work over the telephone.

Group discussion about the information within the committee will be necessary for continued development of a shared meaning of the concept. Because each role will be affected differently, the interface of the various perceptions is important (Wilson, 1989). The first obligation will be to select the model that most closely fits the needs of the organization and establish a timetable for implementation. The model may be altered as necessary, provided the basic criteria for shared governance are met. Until members of the steering committee are fairly comfortable with the newly acquired information, they will be understandably reluctant to try to explain it to others. Skepticism both within and outside the group is to be expected. Animosity by peers may occur because of the time required away from the unit for such a poorly understood concept.

Assistance in supporting the steering committee members in their communication efforts is warranted because this is generally a new role for them. This is especially true for staff members who may be uncomfortable with the prospect of giving information when they still lack confidence in its content. Because the management role will change significantly, committee members who are managers may find themselves in a position of relaying information that will not be well received.

Opportunities to discuss anticipated questions and explore responses to these questions can decrease some of the associated anxiety. In addition, managing information can be facilitated by structuring the process and monitoring information flow so that clear expectations are established. For example, it should be determined who will have basic responsibility to communicate information about the steering council activities to the staff on each patient care unit. During the early phases, complaints regarding lack of general institutional knowledge about the process are not uncommon.

INITIAL ACTIVITIES

Part of the educational process will evolve from the primary activities of the group. As beliefs about and hopes for nursing are examined, the philosophy and purpose of the nursing organization will need to be reviewed. It is unlikely that these two documents will reflect the new thinking about nursing and its role in the institution. Many philosophies are sufficiently vague that almost any concept will fit in them. In such cases, a more specific definition should be written. Developing a clear statement of beliefs is a challenge for most nursing departments. It will be necessary, however, if it is to be translated into meaningful objectives. It should provide a framework for later development of bylaws.

The purpose of the nursing department should also be developed by this group.

Identifying and validating the nursing department's reason for being will continue to clarify the new role for nursing. Necessary elements to address will include services provided to the organization and the authority for such services, the organization's commitment to education and research, and how it will be utilized in patient care, as well as how the environment will be structured to support nursing's growth and continued development (Porter-O'Grady and Finnigan, 1984, p. 171).

After the philosophy and purpose are determined, the critical objectives of the department will be developed. These objectives should be quite specific but applicable to the department at large. Department objectives should include the development of the patient-nurse relationship, nursing's participation in supporting the departmental and institutional goals, how work will be organized to support the practice environment, and standards for assessing results. Specific examples of objectives can be found in the appendix of Porter-O'Grady and Finnigan's book on shared governance (1984, Appendix A). A time frame of 4 to 6 months will be needed to complete this beginning work.

As staff and management personnel are informed of progress, anger may be expressed that only a few people are involved in the decisions. Even when groups have elected their representatives, nonparticipants may not have fully understood what responsibilities would be assigned to the steering group. This will be especially true when long-held values are threatened.

For managers, anxiety related to role change can be expected. Because power and authority are vested in management in bureaucratic systems, the change to a shared governance structure can be expected to evoke feelings of uncertainty and resistance. Staff may feel uncomfortable as they realize the security of bureaucracy, wherein someone else had the final accountability and responsibility for decision making, is being changed. There may have been significant effort to communicate, but the concept was not clearly understood (Gramenz and Jameson, 1982).

The work of the group continues to clarify the process for members. When the core functions have been completed, a mechanism to develop councils or other working groups will be needed.

At this point the group should be functioning well together. The initial lack of trust between management and staff will have been overcome generally, although it may resurface in times of stress. During such times it will be important to remind the group to view the broader professional issues common to all members and that roles, although different, will be structured to support each other. The initial activities will have clarified many of the early uncertainties. Several members will likely develop a leadership role in the organization. Members volunteer to attend staff meetings when issues needing clarification surface, or they plan educational forums to keep enthusiasm and interest high.

THE ROLE OF MANAGEMENT IN THE EARLY PHASE

In most hospitals nursing management has one or more meeting forums. Because the magnitude of change in the organization required for shared governance cannot occur without management support, the group already in place should begin to work on the management role early in the implementation process. Generally, this will be the first council or forum functioning. The management members of the steering committee will be able to communicate with the council on their activities, which can facilitate movement. Because many managers may perceive negative consequences in this new governance process, management steering group members will need support (Eckes, Marcoullier, and McNicholas, 1989; Wilson, 1989).

COUNCILS

In this chapter the term "council" denotes a decision-making group. Regardless of the exact group structure, existing committees that generally fit the identified areas of accountability should be used. This creates less turmoil and gives value to the previous work of the committee. The leadership, title, and responsibilities can be changed through designation by the steering committee (Porter-O'Grady and Finnigan, 1984). If no such committees exist, then the role of the steering group is to create the format and design a process for selection of members. In the latter case, as long as 12 to 18 months may be necessary to establish the groups. This will depend largely on the level of maturity and sophistication of both the steering committee and the nursing staff.

SELECTION OF CHAIRPERSONS

Chairpersons serve a highly visible and important role in the councils. Most chairpersons have had no preparation for this activity and need support to learn the new skills required. Craig's (1989) study indicated that the staff involved wanted help to learn the new role and more formal training about shared governance as a model. Providing educational opportunities on group process and decision making yields benefits, enhancing the speed and effectiveness of council activities.

One effective way to select leaders of the forming governance groups is to select a staff member from the steering committee to be chairperson. This allows the forming group to have a leader who understands the fundamental process. If the steering committee does not have appropriate or available staff members for the chairperson position for all newly forming groups, a management or administrative member can be selected from the steering committee to serve as a representative in his or her capacity as manager or administrative representative. In this fashion, the steering committee, as it coordinates and controls the process, can become the executive or coordinating council or forum. Any additional members will gradually be replaced as chairpersons are chosen. Throughout the duration of the steering committee stage, the ratio of management to staff should generally remain constant.

Because council members are also inexperienced, they may not always choose effective chairpersons. If reasonable opportunities for education and counseling do not effect change that permits the council to function effectively, the chairperson will need to be replaced. This can occur through counseling and resignation or the executive committee can act to remove the chairperson. The structure of the group should require a chair-elect to serve as an understudy for the year before assuming the chair position. Thus role rehearsal occurs as an ongoing process and prepares the chair-elect for the chairperson's activities.

ESTABLISHING A TIMETABLE

Some members of the steering committee may find themselves unable to continue to serve. If the group is well underway, it may choose not to replace members because of the time required for a new person to "catch up" to the other members. Throughout the process the steering committee works on the timetable established at its outset. This helps the group recognize success when projects are completed and to know when deadlines are not being met. Because projects such as developing philosophies and a statement of purpose are less concrete than the usual nursing activity, it is easy for work to fall behind schedule. Monitoring progress becomes critical because the implementation timetable will depend on regular movement.

As each council or forum is formed, activity related to its accountabilities should be communicated to the steering group. How the accountabilities are addressed will not be prescribed—that is the work of the council or forum. When the guidelines have been established, they are submitted to the steering committee for review and approval or clarification if necessary. This ensures the appropriate framework is being followed in the transfer of decision making. The major projects for the coming year should be identified and a timetable established.

All forms of shared governance will address in some fashion five major areas of emphasis: practice, quality, education, peer relations, and governance.

How will the five areas of accountability be supported? In bureaucratic structures, management assumes accountability for all the nursing activity and the staff does not actually assume accountability for their work. Outcomes of care, therefore, become the responsibility of someone other than the caregiver. In shared governance models, assignment of accountability for patient care is to the staff nurse, and the integrating structures to support this change must be in place.

A strong value statement about the clinical nurse is made in allocating accountabilities. The message is clear that clinical nurses have accountability and authority for clinical practice in the institution. Because this role has usually been assigned to management, the structure must be designed to avoid this. The activities of practice and quality groups are at the core of professional practice. Work in these areas convinces others of the seriousness with which nurses view their practice and professional responsibilities (Knowlton, 1982). This is an example of structure supporting the desired process and outcome.

IMPLEMENTING A STRUCTURE FOR PROFESSIONAL PRACTICE

Nurses in bureaucratic structures have been alienated from the type of supportive network that moves them beyond focusing on tasks to a focus on nursing as a whole. In a bureaucracy, the roles of management and staff are essentially isolated and decisions are made for staff by managers who have been granted that authority by the position they hold. The design of shared governance creates the necessary linkage for networking and integration of all elements of nursing practice. This is done by establishing mechanisms that ensure that professional nursing staff are accountable for the practice of nursing and managers are accountable for appropriate support of the practicing nurse. The allocation of accountability for various work roles is established in the mandates of the various councils or forums.

No "required" format exists for shared governance, but the underlying principles must be reflected in the structure design. A design to support principles may be difficult to visualize. It is helpful to organize the structure around the five major areas of accountability, indicating the mechanisms of support. The general controls to monitor the work of the group are common to all five areas and include keeping minutes of all meetings, setting group expectations for individual participation and the specific work of the group, and establishing guidelines to monitor progress.

PRACTICE STRUCTURE

Nursing practice is at the center of any shared governance system and will generally be the first structure formed in relation to staff accountability. Whereas other councils will address issues vital to practice, this group will establish the authority of the staff nurse in all areas of clinical practice. Because of the accountabilities addressed, the composition of this body should be primarily staff nurses, a manager and a nursing administrator for input to staff on their areas of expertise, and any additional information that will assist the staff in decision making. A clinical nurse specialist should be also be a voting member of the council in organizations with this role.

The following list of key elements to be addressed may be used to begin the determination of nursing accountabilities:

1. Develop standards of practice
2. Establish job descriptions for all clinical nurses
3. Review and reaffirm the nursing care delivery system or select and implement a new system
4. Appoint nursing representatives on all hospitalwide committees and task forces affecting patient care
5. Establish criteria for unit-based shared governance committees

QUALITY STRUCTURE

The focus of work in this body is the quality-control aspect of nursing practice. Often this function has been performed by nursing management even though the measurement is usually related to staff practice. In the shared governance format, staff nurses not only identify the appropriate monitors and criteria, they also determine the need for corrective action or opportunity for improvement. Finally, as a quality issue, the credentialing of nursing staff must be established to help ensure nurses are qualified to practice. This council will have a similar composition as the practice council. The program will need to be integrated with the hospital quality assurance plan. The person responsible for the overall hospital plan should sit as a nonvoting member of the council to facilitate this process.

The following key activities should be undertaken to fulfill the quality obligation of the department:

1. Assess and review data sources, and establish department priorities
2. Develop measurable monitoring criteria and instruments
3. Assess standards on a regular basis to ensure they are current and being met
4. Evaluate deficiencies and recommend action to eliminate the deficiencies
5. Establish credentialing mechanisms and a peer review format for all clinical nurses
6. Approve all nursing research activities

EDUCATION STRUCTURE

The education program for the department is designed and initiated by this council or forum. Education is the cornerstone of keeping the practicing nurse informed and able to meet the standards established by the practice and quality councils. Because of the diverse needs that will probably be presented, there should be a staff representative from each unit as well as a nurse manger, nurse administrator, and clinical nurse specialist. This may cause some difficulty with group dynamics because of the number of people involved. The council will essentially provide overall direction of the resources, both human (through the nursing education division) and financial (through education funds available) for the department to meet its educational requirements. Primary accountabilities will include:

1. Identification of short- and long-term educational needs of nurses within the department
2. Ensuring that a program with adequate flexibility to meet the learning needs of experienced and beginning practitioners is available
3. Incorporation of new standards and nursing research
4. Development of specific and consistent evaluation processes for nursing education programs
5. Review and approval of the budget for nursing education activities

NURSING MANAGEMENT STRUCTURE

Nursing management is often the first active council group because it generally already exists in some form, and initiation of shared governance cannot begin at the unit level without the support of the managers. As noted earlier, the narrowing of focus in the management role will be a major change. The role of the manager moves from controlling and directing to facilitating and integrating the functions of the unit. This council will address the accountabilities of management in shared governance through the following activities:

1. Allocation of resources for staff, budgeting, and supplies. Staff input is sought in determining these allocations

2. Provision of support in clerical and other nonnursing areas so nursing care can be delivered appropriately
3. Implementation of the decisions of the nursing councils on the nursing unit
4. Facilitation of interdepartmental problem solving
5. Establishment of mechanisms to develop skills necessary for problem solving, decision making, and patient care management
6. Creation of consistent methods to monitor the level of staff accountability. Council activities are structured to enhance leadership skills appropriate to the manager in a shared governance setting
7. Shift in clinical decision making to staff personnel.

EXECUTIVE OR COORDINATING GROUP

Regardless of format, the work of the members is to ensure that there is overall coordination of activities and that departmentwide decisions are made in a timely fashion. The coordinating group is composed of the chairpersons of each council or committee and the nurse executive. Through this format staff nurses develop a role at the executive level and a forum for the nurse executive is provided directly to the leadership of the governance system. The group functions as the central point for the coordination of the activities of the individual councils and is accountable for decisions that affect the entire nursing department.

1. Mechanisms for communication related to decisions of the councils, resolution of conflict, and facilitation of decision making between councils are established. For example, is an issue being addressed in the appropriate council? Has a decision been made that will negate the outcomes of another? This becomes important as decision making becomes spread over a wider base than in the traditional model.
2. Decisions that affect the entire department are implemented. An example is final approval of the department's annual budget.
3. The work of all the governing groups is reviewed and the efficiency of the overall nursing department is evaluated.
4. Bylaws for governing the established groups and all members of the department of nursing are developed and revised as necessary.
5. General guidance to the nurse executive on issues of concern to the department is provided.

CORPORATE BODY

Another aspect of governance is the work of the corporate body of nursing. All nonprovisional members of the professional nursing staff make up this body. At intervals specified in the bylaws, the members meet to ensure that the business of the department is being appropriately enacted. In this manner, members of the nursing staff retain the overall final authority for departmental activities even though the majority of the work is done in nursing councils or forums.

Participating in the collective body of nursing to approve actions affecting all professional nurses helps establish a strong foundation that integrates beliefs and activities. A forum for discussion and decision making affirms the role and accountability of each member of the professional nursing staff for the way nursing is practiced. These activities are a demonstration of the department's commitment to participation and collaboration.

At least annually, officers of the body should be elected, bylaws reviewed, and reports on the activities and issues of the nursing body given. Although the specific purpose of the meeting is to provide opportunities to enact the business of the department, the opportunity for social interaction and education is also valuable.

CHECKS AND BALANCES

Although the emphasis is on transferring legitimate authority for decision making to nursing staff, checks and balances for the overall system do exist. This important issue may be lost on the participants as the program unfolds. Three basic controls exist:

1. Nurses at the administrative level are advisory members of councils to ensure decisions are consistent with overall organizational goals and objectives.
2. Rules, regulations, and bylaws that direct the work of each committee, council, or other formal group are clearly delineated.
3. A mechanism for resolution of differences between groups or between groups and the administrative role in the nursing organization exists.

Boyle (1984) provides valuable insights into the need for checks and balances that provide structure and coordinates activities in instituting participatory management in a large industry.

SHARED GOVERNANCE ACTIVITIES

The council accountable for nursing practice should establish the necessary criteria and accountabilities for each unit to establish a unit-based shared governance committee. These committees, which can be used with any shared governance model, are an extension of the system at the unit level. Those who are not participants in departmental governance activities will have an opportunity to see and participate in the principles of shared governance in their day-to-day work in a more visible fashion. These groups function as subsets of the practice council/committee and make decisions on practice issues at the unit level. If committees already exist on the unit, they may be able to continue functioning within the new guidelines.

The precise structure of the unit council is not critical provided the basic principles required to support its work are in place. The composition of the group is an issue that requires some insight. Some unit councils are composed of all professional staff members; some include nonvoting members who are not professional nurses (i.e., LPNs), and others include all members of the unit with a variety of categories of staff.

Care must be taken that registered nurses make decisions on issues pertaining to their professional accountabilities, and that they do not isolate themselves from other members of the staff who also work as part of the unit team. The skill with which this is accomplished, regardless of the final format, will affect how professional nurses and shared governance are perceived by others. As a subset of the departmentwide practice group, how practice is managed on the unit will reflect already established standards.

When shared governance moves to the unit, the need for new skills in learning expected roles should be anticipated. Decision making and the use of power may be problematic, and conflicts can emerge. Craig (1989) mentions these two themes in her study of implementation and outcomes of shared governance. The interface between management and staff may not be well understood by the participants. Staff personnel may feel all decisions are theirs, or they may feel frustrated because the manager does not make the decisions and allows the group to flounder. The manager will have had experience in her new role in the management forum, but she may not feel comfortable or secure. The management group has the most difficult role change, and challenges to the nurse manager's authority by the staff may occur. If a mature steering committee exists, they can be helpful in guiding the unit-based committee. The need for a supporting relationship between management and staff and the role each plays as presented jointly by a staff nurse and a manager can enlighten groups struggling with the realities of implementation. Boyle (1984) describes the stabilizing role of the steering committee in implementing participative management in a non–health care setting.

Throughout the process, it will be important for the nurse executive to divest herself or himself of roles that belong to staff and managers. This will be difficult during the formation period because the functions and structure will not yet be developed and coordinated. In addition, the remainder of the institution is still functioning in a bureaucracy. The councils or forums that are actively forming will need much information from management and administration so they can understand why certain movements or decisions may be required. Collaboration with steering committee or council members will be critical. Otherwise, the fragile trust that exists will not be sustained.

BYLAWS

Bylaws to govern the department are important because they not only provide a framework for the work of the nursing organization, but they will also serve as a "snapshot" to describe the values and associated processes that can be expected to occur. It may be tempting to develop bylaws early in the process of shared governance to provide some structure. Organizations who have done this successfully have found that it takes 12 to 18 months of work. It is difficult to develop bylaws at the beginning because a clear picture of shared governance has not emerged, and the structure as viewed at the start may require a number of revisions. Otherwise, individual councils would not be able to make adjustments as the structure develops. Regardless of when the bylaws are developed, the professional nursing organization will need to approve them by at least a majority vote. It will be difficult for nurses to do this with clear understanding before the councils and forums have begun to function. Porter-O'Grady and Finnigan (1984) provide a detailed discussion and specific examples of bylaws.

THE ISSUE OF VETO

In some organizations the nurse executive may retain veto power over decisions. Veto power in any form of shared governance organization has major implications. Because the basis of the organization is shifting accountability from management to staff, this cannot be fully achieved if veto power is retained, which sends a message that a lack of confidence exists in the system itself or the professional staff cannot be fully trusted (Porter-O'Grady and Finnigan, 1984).

Conversely, because of the nurse executive's accountability to the board of trustees and the chief executive officer to support organizational initiatives and priorities, what type of interface should exist when conflict does occur? An important control mechanism in each decision-making group is the information and interpretation of the administrative representative. If this proves inadequate because of a rapidly changing situation or other gap in information, the nurse executive will generally meet with the group making the decision and provide the necessary additional information or interpretation. When resolution cannot be accomplished, the executive group, which includes staff nurses and a manager who are chairpersons of the councils, will take action on the issue. The leadership role of the nurse executive is critical in establishing credibility throughout the unfolding of the shared governance process, and the work that has been done before such conflicts arise will be realized here. Bylaws must fully address the process of conflict resolution.

MODELS

To provide a clearer visualization of the relationship of structure to process, the most common models of shared governance with a centralized coordinating function will be briefly described followed by shared governance as a unit-specific model. It should be understood that a model is simply *one* prototype that can be studied and modified to meet the needs of the organization. As many models exist as do institutions with shared governance.

COUNCILOR MODEL

The councilor model is structured to involve staff nurses in the widest possible range of activities related to clinical practice. Decision-making councils are established based on the functional areas of professional practice (see Fig. 4-2). Approval of staff council decisions by administration or other management groups is not required. All nursing managers and administrators will be involved in activities that support, facilitate, or integrate functions necessary to implement decisions made by clinical nurses in councils representative of the areas of practice. Except

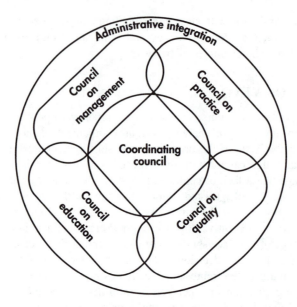

FIGURE 4-2. Councilor model. (From Porter-O'Grady, and Finnigan, S. Shared governance for nursing: a creative approach to professional accountability. With permission of Aspen Publishers, Inc., 1984, p. 105.)

for the management council, councils will be primarily composed of staff nurses. If the organization has clinical nurse specialists, one should be included in each clinical group. A single nurse manager will have the only nonclinical vote in each staff council. The nurse manager's role is to advise the council on management implications as issues are discussed. One administrative-level nurse without a vote advises each staff council regarding how various issues affect the goals and objectives of the department and institution at large. Effective communication of this information will assist the council to make appropriate decisions.

The size of the hospital may affect the actual number of staff members involved in any council, but no single area should dominate. Generally, all clinical areas should be represented. Large councils (more than 15 members) may become cumbersome to manage because effective decision making is difficult in larger groups.

The management council will include all nurse managers, directors, and the nurse executive. The council's primary shared governance functions are to manage the fiscal, human, and material resources for the institution in concert with decisions made in the clinical councils. The management team becomes the agent to ensure that decisions of the councils are implemented on the units, within the available resources. Because this role is much different than the role previously assigned to the management team, the council provides an opportunity, through its work as a group, to identify needed developmental activities. The management council provides a forum for discussing and assigning management accountabilities and roles. For example, when a department project or incident is identified, management accountabilities can be assigned based on the role developed by the council members.

The coordinating or executive council is composed of the chairs of each council and the nurse executive. As noted earlier, this council presents the staff nurse with the opportunity for a significant role at the executive level. The primary purposes of this council are to coordinate the activities of all the councils and, as necessary, to make decisions that affect all areas of the nursing department. The coordinating function is vital because decision making is now spread throughout the organization rather than solely at the management level. There will be debate throughout the implementation process regarding who should make certain decisions. Often, involvement by more than one council is necessary. For example, when unit-based shared governance committees are established, they will deal with practice, quality, and education issues. Decisions involving more than one council will be reviewed to be certain they are congruent and have been addressed by the appropriate groups. It is expected that ambiguity will continue in any shared governance organization, but comfort should develop with experience.

The role of the council chairpersons is important because their position affords them an opportunity to expand their view of the nursing organization within the institution. This expanded knowledge base should enhance their decision-making skills. Conversely, the nurse executive has direct access to the leadership of the governance representatives on a regular basis, which expands her knowledge of current staff concerns. The resulting collaborative relationship will serve the department and institution well. With only five members, this group can be convened, should it become necessary, to make critical decisions that cannot wait for regularly scheduled meetings. Communication is integrated and decisions are made in a timely fashion.

Constraints of this model are its complexity, particularly when moving issues through the system. As noted earlier, there is a broad decision-making base, and the ability to integrate activities becomes a crucial factor. Cost and time involvement also need to be considered. It will be necessary to build the cost of staff participation into the nursing budget. Small groups, few in number, with clear accountabilities and goals will minimize confusion and help to focus governance activities. As previously noted, the coordinating council plays a key role in integrating department activities.

CONGRESSIONAL MODEL

In the congressional model, all members of the nursing department (RNs, LPNs, nurses' aides) belong to the nursing congress. The overall structure is similar in format to the federal government with elected representatives, a cabinet or executive council, and committees. Figure 4-3 depicts the structure of the congressional model.

The president and a cabinet of officers are elected by the congress from a slate of nominees. Nominees may be both staff members and managers, but at least

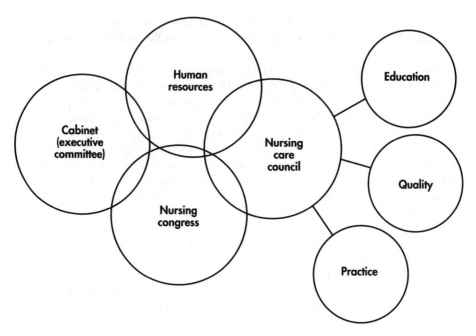

FIGURE 4-3. Congressional model. (Adapted from Rose Medical Center, Nursing Congress Bylaws, 1983. Used with permission.)

50% are staff. Committees or councils are formed to represent the five areas of nursing accountability and are responsible for specific activities that are defined in rules or bylaws. As committee work is completed, it is presented to the cabinet for action. The cabinet becomes the coordinator of shared governance activities, monitoring the effectiveness with which committees perform their work, and advising the nurse executive on matters of concern to the nursing congress.

The nursing care council monitors and coordinates the activities that relate to the practice of nursing, including all functional areas of clinical practice in the general categories of practice, education, and quality assurance. Subcommittees are formed to provide direction in all areas of practice, and these subcommittees present reports and recommendations to the council for action.

If issues require further consideration or intervention after review by the council, they may be referred by this council to the cabinet. The nurse executive and the chairpersons or a representative of each subcommittee form the nursing care council.

A unique characteristic of this model is that a council dealing with human resources is created. It is composed of representatives from all clinical areas and an administrative human resources representative. The council advises hospital administration on issues of concern to the nursing department such as staffing, recruitment and retention, and other employment-related activities. Participation in institutional planning and development around human resources activities may be offered.

In a general sense, a parallel organization is formed by nursing within the institution at large. This is a constraint that needs to be considered before implementation of a congressional model. The ability for the format to be replicated in other parts of the organization should be assessed. In addition, opportunities to create linkages with other hospital departments such as establishing a professional relationship committee to enhance collaboration between nursing staff and other personnel who work with patients can help to decrease the isolation of nursing from its support areas.

ADMINISTRATIVE MODEL

The administrative model follows more traditional lines of separation between management and practice. A practice structure and a management structure are established. Management and staff have separate groups that focus on their specific functions and accountabilities. The areas of accountability for staff may be defined in various ways but should address the categories defined earlier—practice, quality, education and development, peer relations, and governance. Figure 4-4 depicts the structure of the administrative model.

In this structure, the clinical group work is done by staff committees. All practice issue recommendations from the various staff committees are referred to an umbrella group or council composed of both managers and staff. This group makes decisions on the recommendations it receives. In some models a separate integrating forum for all clinical issues and all management issues may exist between the committees and the executive group because many concerns may relate to more than one committee. This format can streamline the work of the executive committee to some extent since it may prevent the need to refer the work to another committee that will need input. The group composition may vary but will be most representative if a majority are staff nurses. The nurse executive role, whether through the vice president or director level, is represented in the clinical forum to provide a departmental and institutional view of the issues brought before it. It is also a source of important information for administrative nurses to learn staff concerns. When there is a management component, the issue will be referred to the appropriate management structure. In all shared governance models, there will be many instances when decisions between management and the clinical staff will overlap. This will not change as the model matures, but the comfort level of those involved should increase. Each committee should have a specific purpose with developed goals and objectives, and the bylaws should reflect the membership, responsibilities, and roles of all groups established as part of the system.

A key characteristic of the administrative model is the structural familiarity in discussing, recommending, and moving decisions upward. The decision-making body, however, will be composed of both staff and management. This group should be composed of at least 50% staff or a representative proportion in the institution of staff to management. It can be assumed that the decision on composition will reflect the degree of commitment to staff nurse participation within the nursing organization.

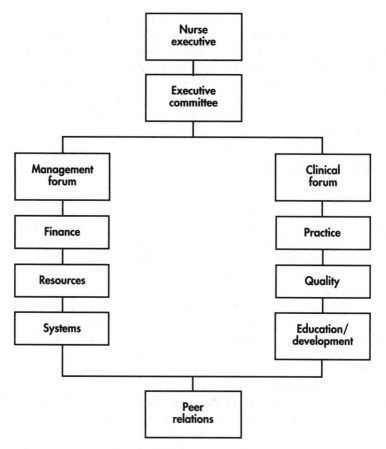

FIGURE 4-4. Administrative model. (From Porter-O'Grady, T: Shared governance and new organizational models. Nursing Economics 5[6]:286, 1987.)

As noted earlier, this model is familiar in format and may be the model of choice in organizations that are more traditional. It may also be practical in the use of existing committees, because less reorganization may be necessary.

However, the potential exists in this traditional format to revert to old management-centered processes. This is especially true when the staff is not proportionately represented on staff and management committees. When there is equal representation between the two groups, it may be expeditious for the nurse executive to assume the role of tiebreaker. To prevent this situation, staff representation should be greater than 50%. Clear mechanisms for resolution of conflicts involving staff decisions and nursing administration should be developed. Most organizations now use the councilor, congressional, or unit-based structure. Pinkerton and Schroeder (1989) provide in-depth information of the administrative model.

UNIT-BASED MODELS

Several institutions have established models that are unique to each nursing unit. Unit-based models, as depicted in Figure 4-5, differ from the more traditional format because there is no central integrating function with staff input at the executive and coordinating levels. Each unit is authorized to establish its own governance system. There is considerable latitude so that each unit can establish a format that seems to best meet its needs. The functional areas of accountability are addressed on a unit-by-unit level. Some institutions have one or more units that have chosen to eliminate established managers, dividing the management function among the group's members.

In providing control, each unit submits its plan to the nurse executive to ensure there is no conflict with other policies and standards in the department. Generally, the members of the administrative team with overall responsibility for the unit will have advised unit staff of possible conflicts while developing their model. Regardless of the flexibility of the nurse executive and administrative staff, administration still approves decisions related to practice in this format. This remains a central issue even if *all* plans are approved as submitted.

Perceived benefits of this approach are that the process is faster than waiting for the entire department to organize itself, and units can form groups at their own

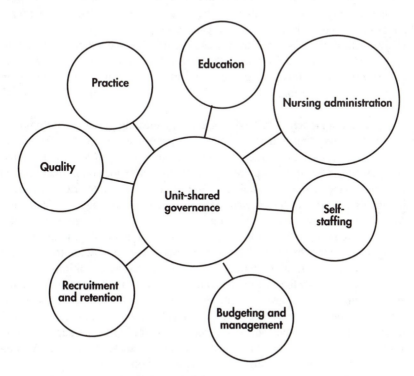

FIGURE 4-5. Unit-based model.

pace. Innovation can be encouraged and groups learn from each other. Conversely, no unit would be required to form a shared governance model. A high value in this format is given to recognizing the individuality of groups.

One of the constraints of unit-based models are that the coordinating function and a role at the executive level for staff nurses are not part of the design. Therefore, there must be executive approval for the format that defines the practice of nursing on any particular unit. Rather than staff nurses making decisions with the nurse executive on departmentwide decisions and integrating issues relating to accountability, nursing administration fulfills this function.

Some organizations have started with the unit-based model and later developed a departmental integrating and control function that gives staff full decision-making authority over practice issues. Until central integration and control are present, shared governance cannot be said to be fully implemented.

COLLECTIVE BARGAINING

Establishing effective shared governance models in unionized hospitals has begun. Several unionized hospitals are currently in that process of adopting shared governance models. The challenge of integrating the contract and the governance structure in a fashion that continues to promote decision making at the staff level is a major undertaking. Obviously this can be accomplished only in an environment where change beneficial to all involved can occur.

Unfortunately, there is a dearth of literature on implementation of shared governance within a union environment. In general, those issues that exist when trust is lacking will exist in this setting. Active effort to keep communication open will be critical because relationships, especially in the beginning, are likely to be tenuous.

A suggested approach is to begin exploratory meetings jointly with union and management negotiating teams so that all members feel invested in the process. During the early phase the participants must agree to be open to all conditions of change that may need to be explored. This presents a major commitment for both union and management and is likely to cause some anxiety. Because it is uncertain which issues will arise, concerns are apt to surface surrounding long-standing issues or areas of current stress. The union wants to protect the contract, and the process may be seen as "caving in" to management, undermining union authority, or trying to eliminate the union. Management may expect the union to not be fully cooperative to maintain their control or to place bargaining conditions in the contract that interfere with the full implementation of shared governance. Some management members of the group might also be concerned about giving staff, who are union members, so much decision-making authority. In addition, there may be concern about giving management information to the union or appearing to be supportive of the union. The concerns of both parties are quite similar. Acknowledging these concerns can be helpful if it is understood these issues will only be resolved over time as the working relationship develops. If it is possible to involve a consultant, it will generally be easier to be more objective and to defuse difficult situations.

If both parties agree to proceed with the project, specific mechanisms must be in place to ensure ongoing involvement of the negotiating teams, staff, and corporate officers of both the union and the hospital. Although the corporate officers are less directly involved, lack of their support at critical junctures can make the task more arduous. If they are regularly informed of issues and progress, difficulties are less likely to arise. To bring them to the table to resolve an impasse or inform them of a major change they did not anticipate disadvantages the process.

A suggested format will provide support at several levels. In addition to meetings with the negotiating teams, the union negotiator and selected officers of the bargaining unit should meet with nursing administration, preferably the nurse executive and one or two other nurse directors. Meetings should occur at least monthly to review progress, discuss changes, and begin to study contract content and language once the process is underway. Items of conflict or concern that have surfaced between meetings should be discussed so they can be referred for resolution to the appropriate individuals or put on the agenda for further discussion. The work of this group is excellent preparation for negotiations because members will have discovered that even the most difficult issues can be discussed without animosity. Successes develop trust and a willingness to continue the commitment.

An additional informal meeting with union officers and nursing administration should also include a manager and two or three staff members from the same unit. If there is tension regarding an issue on a particular unit, it is good to invite the manager and staff from that area. These meetings allow discussion and clarification of information related to the concern. A monthly luncheon or other regularly scheduled meeting in a relaxed setting works well. This provides an opportunity for members of the nursing staff to observe union and management leaders solving problems together and to be comfortable participating in that activity. This is an important factor in the overall process, since trust issues will surface often. This is especially true during times of stress.

The number of meetings may seem complicated and cumbersome, but the various groups provide a solid foundation for problem solving and enhance the possibility of success in this sometimes arduous undertaking.

The need for a steering committee is not eliminated by the work of the groups described above. These groups support the work of the steering committee. Staff nurses on the steering committee are union members. They should be given the opportunity to choose whether they are to be elected by bargaining unit members or appointed by union officers. Satisfaction of the membership with the choice of their representatives may become an issue, and it is important that members feel comfortable with how their representatives were selected. The steering committee will be more focused on how practice should be structured to accomplish the goals of shared governance, and the negotiating team will need to discuss broader issues related to collective bargaining and how the contract may be affected. There is an opportunity for the negotiating team to deal with current health care issues and the concept of shared governance in the early phases while the steering committee undergoes its own educational process. Once the program is underway, quarterly meetings of the negotiating teams are probably adequate, whereas the steering committee should meet at least monthly.

The question of whether shared governance should be included in the contract will arise. Because most contracts are of shorter duration than the implementation of shared governance, the concern is almost certain to occur. Two factors are of particular importance: Professional practice cannot be negotiated and contract language, by intent, tends to be restrictive. Contracts are usually negotiated for 1- to 3-year periods, and it is important that items not preclude activity of the councils that are forming. Careful review will be necessary so these activities are not defined by the contract rather than by council members. Sensitivity should be exercised so that the language of the contract and the ongoing shared governance process are not in conflict. The effort is not to unduly restrict the work of the staff in developing their model.

It is helpful to acknowledge in the contract the work being undertaken and language indicating the mechanism to be used when changes are needed in the contract. A single article in one major hospital contract recognizes that shared governance is being implemented and indicates how contract changes will occur, the role of the contract during the interim phase, and what mechanism intervenes should the process cease to exist. No further mention of shared governance appears in the contract. The article was written by the steering committee and submitted to the negotiating teams before the start of negotiations.

Development of an article in the contract is an initial process. Meetings between union and management leadership should help to prepare for negotiations in which contract language will be changed. Meeting and identifying specific areas for cooperative change present a challenge. Conversely, the opportunity to jointly work out language without the added pressure to complete negotiations is beneficial. Some of the concerns surrounding traditional areas of confrontation such as grievance and disciplinary action can be defused if a trusting relationship was developed during the implementation phase. Nevertheless, language that is mutually satisfactory will be needed. It should be as nonrestrictive as possible so the need of staff to develop formats and structures that promote professional practice is not impaired. For example, by limiting language to phraseology such as . . . "mechanisms shall exist for settlement of disagreements" . . . rather than a detailed procedure to be followed for specific grievances allows the appropriate councils to determine how these issues will be handled. In this manner an activity such as peer review is not precluded. It is also important to acknowledge that under this format management will also relinquish its traditional role in the grievance procedure.

Just as using the bureaucratic structure to begin implementation of shared governance seems incongruent, so does the resistance of the union in giving their members decision-making authority in the workplace. However, the historical perspective of each must be considered, with sensitivity shown as concern is expressed and resistance encountered. Because neither party will be experienced in addressing contract issues in the context of shared governance, a sense of perspective in working through the difficulties of doing what has not been done before can add some excitement and perhaps a sense of humor to the challenge.

Steering committee members will be important leaders in establishing shared governance. Because of the work in which they have been involved, they will be more knowledgeable and informed than their peers. Major changes in established relationships between management and staff are needed, and committee members will require support to deal with reactions of their peers to these changes. Reactions will be related to both staff nurse accountability and a lack of understanding of the need for controls and a defined management role. As previously noted, staff may resist accepting accountability because an activity has always "belonged" to management. Conversely, they may feel they no longer need any management input and can make rules as the need arises. This can be resolved effectively in the steering committee because the knowledge base has been expanded during the preparation phase. A staff nurse and manager from the steering committee are an excellent team to work with groups experiencing difficulty in adjusting to the changes.

TRENDS IN SHARED GOVERNANCE MODELS

It is difficult to describe shared governance models because many modifications have been made. It is unclear how to categorize some models. As a result, the concept remains somewhat hazy. Because no single model exists, it is difficult to envision it precisely. The principles on which it should be based are much easier to state.

Some institutions have developed models in which other members of the organization join with nursing in an integrated or collaborative model. In some cases, this emerged as an accommodation to particular circumstances in the institution. For example, some unions have claimed the model represented a collective bargaining unit for nursing so other staff were integrated. Finding ways to integrate others into shared governance is of interest because of nursing's tendency to become isolated from the rest of the organization. In Mershon's interview with Bocchino (1990) the tendency of nurses to isolate themselves from the larger health care system is discussed. Pinkerton and others (1989) also address this issue in relation to the difficulty of having a progressive group working with personnel in other departments who have not developed as fully. As noted earlier, the literature of other disciplines indicates employee needs of more responsive and humanistic work environments. Finding organizationwide models that help members work more effectively together may be the next step in shared governance.

SUMMARY

The selection of a professional practice model that meets institutional and departmental needs requires careful analysis. In addition, knowledge that adequate support within the institution exists is a prerequisite to begin the process.

There are as many models for shared governance as there are hospitals where it has been implemented. The models described in this chapter should serve only as guides in the development of structures most appropriate to the culture and work of an organization.

Because uncertainty is a normal part of change, anxiety and even some chaos are to be expected in a project of this magnitude. Providing adequate information about the project and fully involving both staff and management are critical to success. This is especially true as traditional roles change and old identities are challenged.

A formal group of staff and management should be established to oversee the project and help the nurse executive lead the department through the necessary changes. Establishing clear goals and timetables will prevent a loss of momentum, especially when broader issues such as philosophy, purpose, and mission are being defined.

The steering committee plays an important role in integrating the work of various forums and councils. Throughout the process communication is a key factor in decreasing resistance to change. There will be a knowledge gap between council members, who are formally involved, and other unit staff. When unit governance committees are established the staff members who are not involved with council work will have an opportunity to apply the principles of shared governance to their day-to-day activities. The need for new skills in learning expected roles should be anticipated because conflicts can be expected, particularly in the area of interface between staff and management.

Union and management are beginning to find ways to integrate professional practice models with collective bargaining agreements. Although the issues are complex, full participation between the two groups and an openness of all parties involved will be necessary to succeed.

New management structures that challenge the traditional bureaucratic organization have evolved throughout the work force. This has been the result of employee dissatisfaction with models that fail to recognize basic human needs and an increasingly complex and changing work environment. Nowhere has this been more true than in health care. New models of shared governance will continue to evolve, such as organizationwide models that facilitate cooperation. Shared governance is the process that moves nursing to the future and should not serve as an end point or constraint to resolving new challenges that will inevitably develop.

REFERENCES

Agreement Between Borgess Medical Center and Michigan Nurses Association (1990). Article VI— Professional Nursing Coordination Council, 8.

Allen, R. and Kraft, C. (1984). Transformations That Last: A Cultural Approach. In J.D. Adams (Ed.), Transforming Work (pp. 36-37). Alexandria, Va.: Miles River Press.

Bocchino, C. (1990). An Interview With Kathryn M. Mershom. *Nursing Economics*, 8(2), 19-28.

Boyle, R.J. (1984). Wrestling With Jellyfish. *Harvard Business Review*, 84(1), 74-83.

Craig, C. (1989). Shared Governance [Consider This]. *Journal of Nursing Administration*, 19(11), 15, 41.

Eckes, A., Marcouiller, M., and McNichols, M. (1989). Growth of the Shared Governance Model. *Nursing Administration Quarterly*, 13(4), 35-47.

Ferguson, M. (1980). *The Aquarian Conspiracy* (p. 26). Los Angeles: J.P. Tharcher.

Gramenz, N. and Jameson, P. (1982). Pitfalls and Possibilities: Staff Nurses' View of Shared Governance. In On the Scene: St. Joseph's Hospital, *Nursing Administration Quarterly,* 7(1), 39-41.

Heller, T. (1984). Authority: Changing Patterns Changing Times. In J.D. Adams (Ed.), *Transforming Work* (pp. 88-95). Alexandria, Va., Miles River Press.

Ketefian, S. (1985). Professional and Bureaucratic Role Conceptions and Moral Behaviors. *Nursing Research,* 34(4), 248-253.

Knowlton, G. (1982). A View of Shared Governance From the Medical Staff. In On the Scene: St. Joseph's Hospital, *Nursing Administration Quarterly,* 7(1), 46-47.

Krejci, J. and Malin, S. (1989). A Paradigm Shift to the New Age of Nursing in St. Michael's Hospital: A Shared Governance Model. *Nursing Administration Quarterly,* 13(4), 41.

Lynaugh, J. (1989). *Twice as Many: And, Still Not Enough.* Secretary's Commission on Nursing (Vol. II). Department of Health and Human Services, Office of the Secretary, Washington, D.C., pp. VII. 1-3.

Merriam, Webster, Inc. (1980). *Ninth Collegiate Dictionary* (p. 146). Springfield, Mass., G & C Merriam.

McNichols, M. and Miller, J. (1988). Control over Practice. In Pinkerton, S. and Schroeder, P. (eds.). Commitment to Excellence (pp. 168-169). Rockwille, Md., Aspen Publishers.

Naisbitt, J. (1984). *Megatrends* (p. 208). New York, Warner Books.

Peterson, M.E. and Allen, D. (1986). Shared Governance: A Strategy for Transforming Organizations. *Journal of Nursing Administration,* 16(2), 11-16.

Pinkerton, S. and others. (1989). St. Michaels Hospital: A Shared Governance Model. *Nursing Administration Quarterly,* 13(4), 35-47.

Pinkerton, S. and Schroeder, P. (1988). *Commitment to Excellence.* Rockville, Md., Aspen.

Porter-O'Grady, T. (1985). Credentialling, Privileging, and Nursing By-Laws. *Journal of Nursing Administration,* 15(12), 23-27.

Porter-O'Grady, T. (1986). *Creative Nursing Administration, Participative Management into the 21st Century* (pp. 83-85). Rockville, Md., Aspen.

Porter-O'Grady, T. and Finnigan, S. (1982). Shared governance at St. Joseph's Hospital: St. Joseph's Hospital. In On the Scene: St. Joseph's Hospital. *Nursing Administration Quarterly,* (Fall), 27-59.

Porter-O'Grady, T. and Finnigan, S. (1984). *Shared Governance for Nursing: A Creative Approach to Professional Accountability* (pp. 4, 31-32, 45-46, 105, 124-125, 165-186). Rockville, Md., Aspen.

Stein, L., Watts, D., and Howell, L. (1990). The Doctor-Nurse Game Revisited. *New England Journal of Medicine,* 322(8), 546-549.

Wilson, C. (1989). Shared Governance: The Challenge of Change in the Early Phases of Implementation. *Nursing Administration Quarterly,* 13(4), 29-33.

BIBLIOGRAPHY

Aiken, L. (1987). The Nurse Shortage: Myth or Reality? *New England Journal of Medicine,* 17(10), 641-645.

Barbis, M. (1990). Shared Governance Begins at the Unit Level. *Innovator,* (Spring), 8.

Barry, C.T. and Gibbons, L.K. (1990). DHHS Nursing Roundtable: Redesigning Patient Care Delivery. *Nursing Management,* 21(9), 64-66.

Boyadjis, F. (1990). Empowerment Managers Promote Employee Growth. *Healthcare Financial Management,* 44(3), 58-62.

Howard, D. (1987). Outcomes of Shared Governance on Staff Nurses. *Journal of Nursing Administration,* 17(12), 9.

Johnson, L. and others. (1983). A Model of Participatory Management With Decentralized Authority. *Nursing Administration Quarterly,* 8(1), 30-46.

Jones, L. and Ortiz, M. (1989). Increasing Nursing Autonomy and Recognition Through Shared Governance. *Nursing Administration Quarterly,* 13(4), 11-16.

Kotter, J.P. (1990). What Leaders Really Do. *Harvard Business Review,* 68(May-June), 103-111.

Kramer, M. (1990). Trends to Watch at the Magnet Hospitals. *Nursing '90,* 20(6), 67-68, 70-74.

Luderman, R. and Brown, C. (1989). Staff Perceptions of Shared Governance. *Nursing Administration Quarterly,* 13(4), 49-56.

McDonagh, K. (Ed.) (1991). *Nursing Shared Governance: Restructuring for the Future*. Atlanta: K.J. McDonagh & Associates.

Neis, M. and Kingdon, R. (1990). *Leadership in Transition*. Shaumburg, Ill., Nova I.

Ortiz, M., Gehring, P., and Sovie, M. (1987). Moving to Shared Governance. *American Journal of Nursing*, 87(7), 923-926.

Peterson, M. and Allen, D. (1986). Shared Governance: A Strategy for Transforming Organizations. *Journal of Nursing Administration*, 16(2), 11-16.

Taylor, C.M. (1990). Shared Governance: A Three-Year Perspective. *Aspen's Advisor for Nurse Executives*, 5(5), 4-6.

CHAPTER

5 Nursing Staff Roles in Unfolding Shared Governance

Sheila Smith

One of the hallmarks of a profession is control over its practice. To create an accountability-based professional practice model, a different environment and structure are required in the workplace. Nurses must be able to assert their place within the organization. They must be viewed as interdependent, not dependent, health care providers with equality of status, who are responsible for their practice and those areas that affect their practice. The practice of nursing encompasses a unique body of knowledge and a broad scope. The professional nurse is the only one capable of making decisions about the practice and the areas that affect it.

A systems approach must be used in the development of an accountability-based professional practice model. The model must address the needs of the professional nurse. It must provide support for the clinical practice and care delivery. A structure must be implemented that supports the role of the nurse and guarantees her the ability to make the decisions that affect her practice. Shared governance is a professional practice model that places accountability and authority for practice decisions at the level of the clinical nurse. Shared governance is a framework of concepts applied through a structure that ensures the application of the principles. The structure itself is not shared governance. Rather, the structure supports the application of the concepts.

The shared governance model will be unique in each institution, dependent on its culture, needs, and unique characteristics. Shared governance is an evolving model. The significance of the change requires careful planning and implementation. It is sometimes difficult to determine where to begin such a complex and dramatic change process.

"Would you please tell me, which way I ought to go from here?" (Alice)
"That depends a good deal on where you want to get to." (Cheshire Cat)
Alice's Adventures in Wonderland by Lewis Carroll

An understanding of the ultimate destination is basic to the change process. It assists in the development of the plan. It provides the direction. After the target or goal has been set, knowledge of the present state and the past will aid in the development of strategies. Evaluation and continuous assessment are necessary to ensure continuous progress to goal attainment. Therefore it is necessary to know

111

where you are going, where you are, and where you've been to determine the best way to attain your goals. Finally, you must be able to ascertain when you've arrived.

KNOWING WHERE YOU ARE AND WHERE YOU'VE BEEN

Before embarking on the implementation of a shared governance model, it is imperative that an in-depth assessment and analysis of the division of nursing and the organization be conducted. This part of the change process is too frequently minimized. The assessment and analysis provide valuable information to guide the planning and implementation process, as well as the development of strategies to ease the transition.

There are three possible targets of change: knowledge, attitude, and behavior. Hersey and Blanchard (1977) developed a model that conceptualized the type of change required and the length of time for the change to occur. Their model illustrates that change in knowledge may take a relatively short period for an individual and slightly longer for a group, whereas changes in attitude and behavior are respectively longer for the individual and longer still for a group. Identification of the target of the change will provide directions with regard to the areas of the change and the length of time required.

The movement to a shared governance model involves a change in all three areas. New knowledge will be needed concerning the concepts of shared governance. The staff and managers will need to acquire new knowledge and skills to successfully function in their changing roles. The requisite attitudes or values differ from those in a traditional model. Behaviors must be altered as the roles are transformed.

Examination of the key areas from both a historical and a current perspective will assist in the identification of potential areas of strengths and deficiencies within an organization. The historical perspective may indicate the reactions that may occur and the rationale for these reactions or perceptions. It may aid in the identification of potential areas of conflict. The appraisal of the current status of key areas will substantiate the areas of potential strength for continued development and support through the change process. It provides the foundation on which to build and support the system (Kanter, 1983).

The division of nursing is a dynamic system that operates within the larger hospital system. A change in one area affects the whole. As the assessment is made, the areas should be examined within the context of the system in its entirety. The areas of assessment should include not only the division of nursing but also the hospital at large.

ASSESSMENT AREAS
Culture

The norms and rules within any organization are indicators of the values and the beliefs held by that organization. An accountability-based professional practice model requires basic assumptions regarding the belief and value of the nurse as a professional and her ability and right to exercise control over her environment and practice. The values and beliefs necessary in a shared governance model include concepts that relate to the professional nurse's commitment, ability, value of contributions, collaboration, and equality of status with other health care professionals (Peterson and Allen, 1986; Porter-O'Grady and Allen, 1986).

How is the division of nursing viewed within the organization?
How are employees viewed?
What value is placed on employee contributions?

Structure

Structure is the composition of the organization. It refers to the arrangement of the system. It includes not only the reporting relationships but also the committee and meeting structure. The transition process of the structure will be affected by the current organization. The new structure will be based on the requirements and needs of the organization.

What are the formal and informal lines of power and authority?
To what degree is the organization decentralized?
What is the level of staff participation in decision making?
Define the purpose, membership, and responsibilities of all committees, task forces, and groups within the division.
Define the purpose, membership, and responsibility of other hospital committees in which nursing is involved.

Knowledge and Skill Level

Knowledge is a structure of ideas, facts, and concepts used in a particular endeavor. Skill is the functional ability to perform a set of characteristics or actions required for an activity. To produce a specific outcome, the ability to combine knowledge and skill in an effective manner must exist. To make the role transition and successfully function in a shared governance model, special knowledge and skills are required of the staff nurse and the manager. Although it is true that the implementation process of shared governance does assist in the development of staff and management, a basic level of competency is required in certain areas for success of the change process. These areas include, but are not limited to, assertiveness, change process, group decision making, team building, conflict management, leadership, communication, group process, facilitating, and interpersonal skills.

What are the developmental levels of the staff and unit managers?
What are their strengths and areas for further development?
What are the assets of each group?
Who are the key leaders of change within each group?

Intergroup and Intragroup Relationships

The movement to a shared governance model affects all members of the nursing division. As the structure unfolds, the expectations, relationships, and roles change. It is a difficult period characterized with fear, uncertainty, and conflict. A basis of trust and team cohesiveness is an important foundation. Role clarity is essential. An understanding of the current roles helps in the transition. Some role uncertainty is unavoidable during the implementation process, which may be heightened with greater conflict if there are preexisting role ambiguity, role conflict, and territory issues. These areas also need to be evaluated in the context of the whole organization.

How would you characterize the relationship of nursing with other departments?

Does a collaborative relationship exist with other members of the health care team?

Are there unresolved territory issues?

Who and where are your supports?

What is the level of trust within the division (between and among levels)?

Are roles clearly understood and valued?

Resources

A change of this magnitude requires a sizable commitment of resources. The highest resource usage will occur during the planning and implementation phase. Resource utilization will be ongoing and requires planning and budgeting. Resources include people, time, money, energy, and expertise. Early in the process much time will be devoted to planning. After the initial planning, resources will be spent on participation and learning of skills and concepts. These two areas will be greatest during the implementation phase, but they will be a constant requirement for system maintenance caused by turnover.

What are the available resources?

How can you maximize the resources?

Do you require external resources?

Communication

Communication is vital in the change process and key to the attainment of a shared governance model. In a traditional model, poor communication has a negative impact on the effectiveness of the organization but does not prevent its functioning. In a shared governance model, an ineffective communication system interferes with the ability of the structure to function. The communication system will evolve as the structure unfolds. The structure will drive the needs of the communication system. However, open, multidirectional communication lines are needed during the development of the shared governance system to decrease confusion, conflict, and to provide feedback so that the system can be modified.

What are the formal and informal lines of communication?

How efficient, effective, and accurate is the current system?

Is information freely shared?

Is there free communication across departments?

Response to Change

Many factors influence an individual's response to change. Previous experience with change can positively or negatively affect feelings regarding change. Knowledge of the organization's previous response and experiences with change can provide information that may be useful in predicting future responses. Individuals' perception of the effect of the change on them or misperceptions regarding the change may cause some fears. Lack of knowledge about the change may lead to confusion and misinterpretation.

Does the organization promote risk taking and change?

What are the past experiences with change?

Review past successes and failures in implementation of change. What were the influencing factors?

Analysis

All hospitals are unique and each implementation plan must be individualized. As the assessment areas are reviewed, and analysis of the strengths, deficiencies, and their importance and effect in the change process must be examined. The identified strengths can be further developed and capitalized. A plan for development of the problem areas and a time frame for resolution can be generated. Areas of deficiency must be viewed in terms of their degree and level of importance. Depending on the area and the degree of deficiency, it may be necessary to develop the area before initiating the planning process for the structural changes. Thus the beginning of the change process may start before introduction of the shared governance concepts and theoretical framework.

It is important to conduct an analysis that encompasses the "total picture." The overall stability of the division and the organization is an important factor. Because of the magnitude of the change and the length of time required for implementation, a stable environment is required. This type of change will cause conflict and some instability. The organization must be able to withstand the process. After a certain point is reached, it will be impossible to return to the previous structure without serious consequences. Although it has been reported that a shared governance model is an effective deterrent to unionization, it should not be undertaken during a time of union threat because this is usually a time of great and long-standing instability. The shared governance model may an effective deterrent to unionization, but it should be instituted only as a proactive strategy.

With a thorough analysis, some responses, behaviors, and areas of conflict can be predicted, which assists in the development of strategies and a phased planning process.

HOW TO GET THERE
The Evolving Model

The shared governance model is an evolving model. As the structure evolves, so to do the roles, skills, educational needs, and problems.

After an initial planning phase, the implementation and the transition of the structure occur. This phase is marked by chaos, confusion, and uncertainty. The next phase is one of development, regrouping, and clarification. The final phase is the refinement phase of integration. These phases should be viewed as a continuum. Overlapping areas and blurring between phases will occur.

Before developing the plan for implementation it is important to first determine the destination. A vision must be developed; without knowing the destination, it is impossible to develop the route.

VISION

A vision is an ideal, unique image of the future (Kouzes and Posner, 1987). A vision sets the direction for development and change. It provides the standard to which to aspire. The vision must first be defined, and then be shared, marketed, and sold.

The vision should be broadly communicated. The nursing staff of the division as a whole needs to know the direction that is being set. They need to understand what to expect and what is expected of them.

Marketing the vision involves relaying the positive impact that this change will have on individuals, helping them to view the change as necessary and desirable.

Selling the individuals means that they accept and support the vision. The vision becomes their vision. They accept the responsibility for the attainment of the vision.

The idea for pursuing the implementation of the shared governance model may come from several sources. For it to be developed into a vision, however, requires the senior nurse executive's support and commitment to its development. She must be willing to accept the key leadership role in the process. Change cannot occur without this commitment or involvement. The senior nurse administrator is the only one who has the authority and power to restructure the organization. She is the one who will pass the authority to the staff. The nurse executive is charged with creating an environment that fosters staff nurse accountability. She assists in the development of structures, systems, and expectations that promote the development of staff accountability. She must model the management role changes.

PHASE I—PLAN DEVELOPMENT

As the vision takes shape, a planning group should be formed that is representative of the division. Staff members should be included early and in the process be well represented. Small representation from the other categories should be included. The group should contain approximately eight members who form a broad representation. They may be selected or volunteer. They are usually considered the leaders and innovators within their peer group. The planning process should be led by a change agent who possesses an overall understanding of the theoretical framework of the model. This person must be highly skilled in the change process and should be at the administrative level in the nursing organization. The planning group will develop the initial implementation plan. This group should be viewed as a task force with a defined goal. Its only purpose should be the development of the initial implementation plan. After this has been accomplished, the group should be disbanded. The continued implementation and developmental process should be facilitated by the change agent in conjunction with multiple key staff and managers. As the process unfolds, more individuals become involved with the implementation and development. Over time, the role of the change agent is phased out as the shared governance structure and participants assume its continued refinement and development.

Before members of the group begin their work, it is important that they process a solid foundation of knowledge about shared governance. Educational resources and programs should be made available to the members. The plan will focus on three major categories: education, structure, and support programs.

Education

Education is an ongoing, continuous process. It is required before, during, and after implementation. There are two major areas of education. One area involves the knowledge of the concepts of shared governance. The other concerns the skill and knowledge necessary for the staff and management to function in the shared governance organization.

The plan for education of the concepts of shared governance should develop strategies to address four needs. One is the basic knowledge of concepts for all members of the nursing division. Second is a more in-depth knowledge base for the members who are involved in the implementation. A third area is a method for orientation of new employees. The fourth area is an ongoing re-education, a clarification of concepts, and a more in-depth knowledge of concepts for staff that will be necessary throughout the process.

Shared governance is a complex conceptual model. A full understanding of the concepts and principles will initially be difficult to grasp. It will be helpful to simplify the terms, concepts, and principles. Concrete examples assist in the comprehension. Resources such as articles, books, and video tapes should be made available. Conferences and networking with other institutions are useful. Education of shared governance should be made available to all personnel. Requiring some mandatory education concerning the concepts may be desirable. It gives a message of the importance of the model. More extensive education should be targeted at those most involved in the change process. As the model develops and the system changes, it will create a new level and need for knowledge concerning shared governance. A re-education may be requested and will be required; during employees' first exposure, a frame of reference for the information did not exist. New questions will arise, and there will be a need for more specific and detailed information. As they begin to work in the system they are better able to understand the concepts, the effects, and the application. There may also have been an initial lack of interest or resistance to the subject. It is impossible to teach someone who does not want to learn. Whereas formal and informal education provides a basis or background of knowledge, true understanding occurs only with involvement in the development of, or participation in, the shared governance structure. As new people enter the system, it is necessary to provide education. It may be helpful to initiate shared governance education into the orientation program early in the implementation process.

In addition to educating the members of the division of nursing concerning the concepts of shared governance, there is a need to provide information to others in the organization. When the decision is being made to implement a model, the senior nurse administrator should begin discussions with her superior and peers. It is important for them to understand what is being undertaken and why. Senior management support will assist in dealing with the negative reactions that may occur within the hospital. Periodic updates and more in-depth information should be shared throughout the process. When the implementation begins, a brief description of shared governance should be shared with the rest of the organization. It will be too early in development to provide many specific details of the model. It would be confusing to explain the structure because it will be evolving and changing throughout the implementation. There will be fears from other departments within the organization. Some will be expressed, others will not. Most concerns will be in regard to the effect of the change on them. They may fear loss of control or that nursing is isolating itself and will not make collaborative decisions. It is best to address these concerns as they are expressed. Reassurance will be needed, with emphasis that they should continue their interactions with nursing as before. As the structure changes, management will be responsible for assisting them through the shared governance system. Other departments should use the same contacts as before the shared governance structure was initiated. This contact is generally from management. The nursing manager is responsible for introducing and assisting other department managers through the new process of the shared governance model. This decreases the likelihood of a negative first experience for nonnursing departments. It prevents confusion and frustration, particularly early in the model development when it is changing and evolving. The manager can facilitate smooth interaction and follow-through. After the structure is fully developed, staff will learn over time how and whom to access in the structure. A common reaction to the concept of shared governance is that it is, or will lead to, a union. Clarifying the concept and sharing the literature can alleviate this concern.

The largest need for education exists in the area of the skills and knowledge required by the staff and management to make the role transition and to function successfully in the new system. Both formal and informal education and development are required. The assessment and analysis will provide the information regarding focus areas. As previously mentioned, some skill development may be necessary before the process is started. Other skills will need refinement as implementation occurs. The informal and formal education should coincide with the developing model. As the various changes occur in the structure and the roles change, different educational needs will surface. An understanding of the role transition and the model's development will provide direction to the educational plan. The education should initially be targeted at the individuals who are actively involved. Continuous education will be essential because of turnover and increased participation will create an ongoing need.

Role Transition

Staff. The authority and responsibility for the professional practice of nursing are invested at the staff nurse level in a shared governance model. By definition responsibility is the obligation to perform an assigned task to the best of one's ability. Authority is the right of decision concerning the responsibility. Accountability is answering to someone for what has been done. Responsibility cannot be delegated. Only an individual can be accountable. In a traditional model, there was incongruence in assignment of accountability, responsibility, and authority. The staff nurse was given responsibility for her practice but lacked the authority. This made it impossible to fulfill the expectation of accountability. As the staff role develops and expands, the staff members become responsible and accountable for their own practice. The organizational structure supports this movement and is developed so that failure to function in a responsible and accountable manner is not rewarded. The initial role transition begins with the acceptance of responsibility by the professional nurse for her practice. It then moves to involve the areas that affect that practice. The final expansion is the acceptance of responsibility and accountability for the entire nursing professional practice at the organization. Thus the staff nurse is not only responsible for her own practice delivery, but also that of her peers and the division of nursing at large. This requires a change in the perception of the work from a job to a profession. Some may view this change with fear and resistance. It does place greater requirements on the staff nurse. These requirements include time, skill, knowledge, commitment, and effort. Personal obligations increase. Staff members become responsible not only for their direct care delivery but for all things that relate to that care. They also have an obligation to the care delivered by their peers. They are responsible not only for the positive outcomes, but also the negative outcomes. They must rectify the problems that relate to practice issues.

The role transition of the staff occurs over time as the organization changes. At any given time, the staff will be at varying levels of development. The effect of the organizational changes will be seen in the behavior and personal growth of the staff. Argyris (1962) contends that in the traditional organization the workers are kept in a state of immaturity because they lack control of their work and their environment. This encourages behavior that is passive, dependent, and submissive. Argyris identifies seven stages or changes that take place as an individual moves from immaturity to maturity. Each change is viewed on a continuum within each stage.

The first stage is the passive state, characterized by little involvement in activities that affect the individual, the organization, or the profession. Feelings of powerlessness and a victim mentality may exist; these yield to increasingly greater involvement in activities and decisions. Support and reassurance are important at this stage. Expectations should be set and role modeling should occur.

Second is the highly dependent stage. In this stage staff members may be uncertain of their capabilities. They may lack self-confidence and fear errors or mistakes. They may not trust that they actually have the authority to make decisions or control their practice. They seek support and reassurance. They may wait to voice ideas and opinions until those of the manager are known. There may be a tendency to rely on or refer to the manager. As the individuals gain more confidence, they will move toward progressively higher levels of independence. The need for the manager's assistance, although always necessary, will diminish. The manager needs to be attuned to these feelings. A safe environment that fosters acceptance for errors and mistakes is important. Acknowledging past mistakes of managers may decrease anxiety. Positive reinforcement and development of skills should be the focus. The manager must avoid the temptation to rescue the staff and should moderate their participation in decision making.

In the third stage, staff members are capable of behaving in only a few ways. The staff will be involved in many issues and situations to which they have not been previously exposed. They will vary from the simple to the complex and will require a variety of responses. In the beginning the staff will draw on a limited pool of skill, knowledge, experience, and expertise. Their ability to match the approach required in a given situation may be limited. As they acquire new skills and knowledge, they will be better able to function in many complex situations by use of a variety of approaches. In addition to acquiring new interactive skills, the staff will need to gain an understanding of the politics and complex structure of the hospital. Information and an understanding of a broader prospective should be provided. They will need an understanding of the integration within the division and within the hospital.

During the fourth stage, there is a tendency for the staff to have shallow, casual interests. When staff involvement begins, it may be on a superficial level. Members may tend to focus on the things that directly affect them. Their understanding of the extent of the new organization and the responsibility and impact may not be recognized. Their understanding will increase as they become more involved and as the model continues to unfold and develop. The feeling that this is only a temporary fad that will eventually disappear and that its impact on them is minimal, particularly if ignored, will change. A new level of interest will emerge as they begin to feel the effects of the changes. A deeper interest and a stronger commitment will grow.

In the fifth stage, the time perspective is short and narrowly focused, encompassing only the present. Tunnel vision may be evident, with a lack of understanding of the system as a whole and integration required. Staff members may only be aware of their own perspective. As the implementation process begins, there will be a tendency to deal with issues in the context of the present; the focus of the various groups will be in the "here and now." The ability to solve problems may be limited. They will require assistance in assessment of the problem and the analysis of solutions. Initial problem solving may deal only with the surface issues. The issue may not be viewed in its entirety or in regard to the impact of the decision on others. The need for others to be involved in the decision may not be considered. This is partially because of the lack of knowledge and understanding of the intricacies and complexity of the division and the organization. As the groups begin to understand their roles, define their work, and comprehend the complexity and integration within the division and the hospital, there will be a shift to more in-depth problem-solving abilities. The need for long-range planning and integration will be apparent. The focus will shift to viewing the picture in its entirety. Active involvement in development and direction of the goals will occur. There will be a realization of the need to consider all the factors: financial, regulatory agencies, hospital goals, etc.

The sixth change that occurs is in the concept that the employee is subordinate to others. In nursing, because of the position of the profession and the effects of the women's movement, staff members may exhibit suppressed group behaviors. They may not view themselves as equal to others within the organization. They may exhibit behaviors of horizontal violence. They may be reluctant to assertively interact with other professional members of the health care team. Until nurses view themselves as equal to others and assert control over their own practice, they cannot expect to receive respect or acceptance of authority for making practice decisions.

Finally, there is a lack of awareness of self that moves toward awareness of and control of the "self." Staff members initially may not have the ability to view themselves objectively. They may be unable to identify areas of strength and areas that require assistance or development. Understanding the concept of interdependence with others may be difficult. They may shy away from objectively viewing themselves and their peers. A strong sense of self-identity must develop. Nurses should become aware of the perceptions of others but learn not to build their self-concept totally on those perceptions. As a greater understanding of themselves and others emerge, their ability to function within the structure will be enhanced.

Management. The unit manager's role is the position that is most profoundly affected by the move to a shared governance model. It is also the key to the successful implementation and the position that exhibits the most resistance to the changes. This unique set of circumstances creates a challenge to the move to a professional accountability-based practice model. Those experiencing the greatest impact and who are the most resistive are the ones who can influence the success of the outcome.

Unit managers may fear that their positions are in jeopardy because of the implementation of a shared governance model. There is no easy response to this fear. Most institutions that have implemented a shared governance model have not eliminated management levels but may have been able to reduce the number of positions within a management category. The purpose of shared governance is to implement an accountability-based professional practice model that places control over practice at the clinical nurse level. The ability to decrease the number of managers should be viewed in the context of the economic health care climate and the recent management literature on organizational structures and layers. It has been suggested that there should be a maximum of five levels within an organization and that three levels should be adequate for most (Peters, 1987). The decision to decrease or eliminate management levels should be made during the assessment phase and will be institution-specific, depending on the needs, complexity, and size of the organization. A change in the maintenance organization or a decision to change should be made before implementation of the shared governance structure is begun. If the intent is to remove levels or decrease the number of managers, it should be made clear how, when, and why. Hidden agendas and plans will only interfere with the change process.

The traditional role of the unit manager has been that of controller, director, supervisor, and decision maker (Porter-O'Grady, 1986). The unit manager was responsible and accountable for the activities of the department. Even if she was highly participatory, the final responsibility, decision, and outcome rested with her. As the authority for professional practice and those areas that affect it is shifted to the staff, and the staff become accountable, the unit manager's role must change to that of facilitator, coordinator, integrator, and supporter (Porter-O'Grady, 1986).

The new environment requires different management skills. The unit manager not only must be proficient in the traditional management skills but also must possess leadership abilities. Leadership and management are distinct, complementary, and necessary (Kotter, 1990). Management is systems, control, order, quality effectiveness, and productivity. Leadership is the facilitating of change. Management plans and budgets; it is the process of tasks. Leadership sets a direction and the strategies to achieve the vision. Management achieves the plan by organizing and staffing. Leadership unites people and creates commitment and understanding of the vision. Management attains the outcome by controlling and problem solving. Leadership achieves through inspiring, motivating, and maintaining the movement toward the vision.

In traditional models, a strong manager could successfully function and achieve the outcomes because it was possible to rely on the authority of the position. In a shared governance model, the authority has been shifted to the staff. Strong management skills are still required, but they are focused on systems management and fiscal, material, and staff resources. Strong leadership skills are necessary to assist the staff in the change process, the development of the skills and the model. Management in a shared governance model focuses on systems support and resources—to ensure that staff nurses have the necessary resources to perform their work. The clinical nurse should not waste time dealing with inadequate systems or resources. Staff nurse hours should not be spent on securing resources (equipment or supplies) or in dealing with inadequate systems. Inefficient systems will devour nursing time that is taken from direct patient care. Management's role is to assist the caregiver to deliver quality care.

Leadership of change is an active, demanding, and continuous role. It involves five practices: (1) challenging the process, (2) inspiring a shared vision, (3) enabling others to act, (4) modeling the way, and (5) encouraging the heart (Kouzes and Posner, 1987). A leader challenges the status quo and seeks ways to continually improve. Leadership requires the ability to take risks and an openness to mistakes. Inspiring a shared vision is accomplished by helping others envision the future, by encouraging them to become enthusiastic and committed, and by assisting in seeing the value and the benefits of the vision. Leaders must be able to enlist involvement and ownership in that future. A leader enables others to act by support and collaboration. They form a team. Leadership must have the ability to access the strengths and areas of development of the staff, to find the unique areas of interest and motivation for individual staff members. The leader strengthens the team with skills, knowledge, communication, and information.

The manager must model the pathway for change by setting the example and living the value and the belief. Managers set high standards and expectations and must meet them and expect others to do the same. It is important to make the vision concrete and a reality. One way is to start with small achievable wins that can be built upon—encourage the heart. A change of such magnitude is draining. Frequent encouragement is necessary. Accomplishments should be recognized, and everyone must feel part of the success. Positive behaviors must be rewarded. Those who are not contributing should be neither punished nor rewarded.

Structure

Before the structure changes are implemented, careful consideration should be given to the type of model to be used. There are three basic types of models: the councilor, the administrative, and the congressional models. The models should be fully investigated and matched to the organizational culture, environment, and needs. Although there are three basic types, no model is developed exactly the same in every organization. Although it is helpful to study other models in other institutions, they should be used as a guide only. The model should be adapted to the particular institution and meet the unique needs of that system.

After the model type has been chosen, a vision of the model should be developed. The vision of the model will be modified as the model unfolds, but it will provide direction to the change process. The structure should be loosely defined, followed by definition of the groups and broad outlining of accountabilities. These will become more specific, detailed, and refined as the process evolves. Minimally, the structure should provide forums to deal with issues that relate to practice, education, quality assurance, and management. Other areas may be defined, for example, research, personnel, or recruitment. The current structure should be reviewed next, with a list of the committees, task forces, and meetings that currently exist. Their purpose, work, and membership should be defined and compared to the future structure. The steps to transform the groups should be determined. It is desirable to limit the disruption of the various groups' work. In some instances there may be a need to make dramatic changes. Others will make a slow transformation. Each group's accountability in the new structure must be ascertained. Can its work be included at this time? If not, the group's work and a timeline to incorporate it should be determined and reported to the group responsible. Some groups may need to be disbanded; others may not be part of the shared governance structure but may be part of the management structure. However, their purpose and function may need to be redefined. The transformation or disbanding of groups will be resisted. It is important to objectively review the purpose and justify its continued existence.

The current groups' membership and chair positions should be compared with the new structure. If they contain predominantly management personnel, it may ease the transition to slowly replace the membership with staff. Co-chairing a manager and a staff nurse briefly will allow for some skill development, ease the transition, and prevent disruption of the group's work.

At the divisional level, the council or forum that should be first initiated will depend on the current structure. It may be possible to use an existing group structure and, with modification, easily make the transition. The strengths and developmental level of the groups should be assessed. Although the development of the councils or forums will not occur simultaneously, there should not be a lengthy time lag until group development. It is important that the groups be developed in a relatively similar time period. The shared governance model is a systems model and the councils or forums are interdependent. Integration will be difficult and may ultimately affect the success of the new structure.

The level of the development of the structure requires consideration. There are three possible approaches. One is to begin development at the unit level on some trial areas. This approach may be perceived as "safer" because it allows those who have concerns or fears regarding the changes to test the system. Unit-based structures also allow more participation. Staff members have the opportunity to be exposed earlier and more directly to the shared governance system. Skill development will begin and be better developed for the divisional council. A drawback to initiating change at the unit level is that the units who have begun may be perceived as elite or privileged. Isolation from the division and hospital, particularly in terms of goals and direction, is a danger. As the unit structure develops it will quickly reach a point beyond which it will not be able to progress. It requires a divisional structure for guidance, support, and direction. Frustration over the inability to influence practice decisions at the divisional level may emerge.

Development at the divisional level also has some benefits and some negative aspects. The initiation at the divisional level can aid in the development of the unit-based structure. It can serve as a model and assist in coordination and sharing between the units. Beginning at the divisional level may also give more credibility, legitimacy, and momentum to the change process. One problem with only divisionwide councils is that the new structure becomes just another hierarchy. There is too much centralization with little opportunity or few forums for unit-based decisions.

Simultaneous or closely developed systems may be the best alternative. This approach to change has the benefits of the other two approaches and minimizes the drawbacks. Skills are developed at both levels. There is better understanding of the model because of increased participation and more exposure. Improved integration between the unit and divisional structure can occur. Staff members have forums at the unit and divisional level in which to assume accountability for their practice.

Regardless of the level of the approach of the structure, the unit-based structure is vital. There must be a structure that allows unit-specific decisions.

One of the requirements of a shared governance model is the need for centralization and decentralization. The system needs to be centralized in its goals and directions. There is a need for some unity and overall standardization and guidance. The divisional councils provide that unifying focus and direction. The service delivery is decentralized. It is important to maintain a degree of decentralization so the unique needs of the departments can be met. Practice, education, and quality assurance issues arise on a unit that are individualized to that area. To address these needs, a structure must also exist at the unit level that empowers the staff to assume responsibility and accountability. Without a structure in place, the previous incongruence exists and management maintains authority and control. It also sends a confusing message in terms of commitment to the concepts of shared governance. In some systems, elaborate decision trees have been developed that outline the route to be taken when a decision is required. Essentially, this process assigns urgent practice decisions to the manager with confirmation by staff at a later time. It assigns nonurgent practice decisions to staff groups. This can be a dangerous practice: it suggests that only a manager is capable of urgent, and therefore important, decisions. The need for a decision tree can be eliminated by empowering staff chairs and co-chairs to act in lieu of the staff groups.

There is a delicate balance between too much centralization, in which the divisional decision-making forums become another hierarchy, and too much decentralization, when there is lack of integration and each department becomes isolated and out-of-step with the needs, direction, vision, and goals of the institution.

In many instances there will be decisions or policies that only outline the direction. The specifics and the implementation may vary among units, thus requiring the units to further define the policy as it uniquely relates to them. The development of a unit structure also assists in the integration of the model between the division and the various departments. There is a system by which needs, issues, policies, and information can flow and be addressed at the appropriate level. Multidirectional communication is aided. The unit structure supports the premise that a shared governance model is a "bottom-to-top" structure for information, communication, and decisions, as compared with a traditional hierarchy where all decisions flow down from management to the staff.

The unit structure need not exactly mirror the divisional structure. The unit structure should be developed to meet the unique needs of the unit. The structure should allow responsibility and accountability for issues that relate to practice, education, and quality assurance. This can be accomplished in a variety of structures. Some units have developed multiple groups to accomplish these areas, whereas other units use one group for all. The possible types of structures may be as varied as the number of units.

Support Programs

As the plan is developed, it is important to examine the programs that support and facilitate staff nurse accountability for nursing practice. In addition to the structure, these support programs assist in creating an environment that fosters accountability. Although these are not essential in implementing the structure, they are important to the development of a professional practice model.

Primary nursing or case management.   The delivery of nursing care model is the foundation for control of practice. A model should exist that provides a vehicle for individual accountability for patient care delivered and its outcome. It allows decentralized decision making and invests responsibility in an individual. The professional nurse has autonomy for her practice delivered to her clients. It is the first level of practice accountability. It is incongruent to have a shared governance model in place without a delivery of care model that is also accountability based.

Peer review/peer input.   As professionals, the assessment of the quality of care delivered by peers further demonstrates control over all aspects of practice. It allows the professional group to evaluate care, thus assigning members a role accountability beyond their own practice. The evaluation of peers is a component of professionals. Accountability to society by professionals can be accomplished through a peer review process (Passos, 1973).

Job description and performance appraisals.   As the roles begin to evolve, the job descriptions and performance tools should be revised. They should reflect the changing roles, responsibilities, values, and expectations. Professional accountability and responsibility should be clearly delineated.

Clinical advancement.   This program should also reflect the accountability regarding practice. It should emphasize the accountability for one's own practice, the practice of peers, the nursing division, and the profession at large. A clinical advancement program is a professional advancement program. It acknowledges the professional nurse for advanced professional skills. It provides a method for advancement within the clinical practice setting. Increased autonomy and accountability are provided by a clinical advancement program. It also impacts patient care through improvement of quality outcomes, and promotes retention through job satisfaction, recognition of advanced clinical skills, and expanded clinical roles.

Competency-based orientation.   A competency-based orientation ensures attainment of a minimal standard of skill and knowledge level of the clinical practice nurse. It provides for quality care delivery. This method promotes professional accountability for the quality of the education. It further demonstrates autonomy of the profession.

Standards of practice.   Standards provide a basis for measurement; they are a model by which to judge. They provide a direction and a foundation for quality care. A hallmark of a profession is its ability to define its own practice and standards. All professionals possess a unique body of knowledge and work within a conceptual framework.

Conceptual model.   A conceptual model offers a unifying focus for practice decisions. A consistent approach is ensured. It serves as a tool that promotes holistic, in-depth patient care and practice decisions. A common reference point exists.

PHASE II—CHAOS, CONFUSION, AND UNCERTAINTY

This phase is the period of most resistance and conflict. "Noise" within the system may be present in varying degrees throughout the 3- to 5-year implementation process. This period will be the most difficult. There will be a struggle between the previous structure, roles, and expectations and the new emerging ones required by the shared governance model.

Opposition may be negligible at first but will become more noticeable as the structure and changes begin to unfold. Resistance will be seen at all levels. There are four reactions or behaviors that might be seen (Pinkerton and Schroeder, 1988): frustration and aggression, passive resistance, indifference, and acceptance. Conflict also frequently occurs.

Frustration and aggression.   This active resistance may be overt at first but will later become covert. Deliberate sabotage and manipulation may occur. Accusation and projection onto other groups is common in the unit manager group.

Passive resistance.   Individuals may unite to resist the changes. They may be responding to real or perceived threats, and use information as their ammunition. Withholding and distortion of information, as well as covering of mistakes, may be seen. Opponents will actually contribute to errors to prove their points, and to make a case for not embracing the change.

Indifference.   Individuals may ignore the situation by not taking part in the activities. They may attempt to divert the attention. They may rationalize why they are unable to get involved or implement the model on their unit at this time. Withholding resources of time and information may be evident in managers, as well as staff. Managers may also withhold assistance to staff for the development of the model or skills or may manipulate the staff to fail.

Participation of the staff can be frustrating in the implementation. As with any change, a small, committed group will be the high participators. Initially, it may be necessary to convince people that they want to be involved. As effects of the system become apparent, a new level of interest will develop. Choosing topics of significant importance to the staff can stimulate interest and involvement. In most cases, there will always be those who choose not to participate. It is important to design the structure so that expectations of involvement are evident. The structure should not reward nonparticipation; only participative behavior is to be rewarded. This may include peer pressure, evaluation standards, career ladder moves, etc.

Acceptance.   There may be the appearance of acceptance, but this may not represent genuine acceptance. Only over time will the outcome of the acceptance and the level of participation be known.

Acceptance of change may be affected by many factors. As mentioned, previous experience with change will influence the response to new changes. Fears of perceived loss of control, power, or authority may be present. Fear of the unknown, an inability to conceptualize the change and new role, or fear regarding the ability to successfully function in the new system may constrain the acceptance of change. Lack of knowledge, understanding, or skills may also hinder acceptance. The inability to perceive the need or value of the change may exist. Philosophical differences should be examined. Change is difficult even for those who philosophically agree with the change. A sense of comfort with the familiar is replaced with a sense of loss and the uncertainty of the unknown.

A safe, supportive environment is necessary to facilitate acceptance. Opportunities to openly verbalize fears, concerns, and uncertainty should be provided. Educational resources and opportunities for skill development should be available. The ability to participate in the implementation of the change is helpful. The benefits derived from the change should be communicated. Information sharing concerning the change, as well as clarification of new roles and expectations, is necessary throughout the process. The hindrance to acceptance will vary with each individual. Multiple strategies to assist with acceptance will be needed.

Conflict.   Problems and conflicts are a part of implementing any change. They should not be viewed negatively but should rather be seen as an inevitable part of the process. Not all conflicts or problems are bad. They can often assist in the further refinement or clarification of the system. It is important, however, to view these conflicts objectively. The cause should be examined to determine a strategy to address them. It is important to analyze the conflict and address it but do not allow the conflicts to change the course or the direction of the change. There are many possible responses to objections within the system. The response depends on the type of objections, the severity, and amount, the impact on the change, and the timing. There are several types of responses to objections to change.

No response.   At times simply allowing the objection to be voiced so that it can be resolved is all that is necessary. This response shows trust and that it is acceptable to question and challenge. Overreacting or reacting to an objection may cause it to escalate; it may be best to wait and ignore it.

Cooperation.   Enlisting the involvement of the resisters gives them an opportunity to be involved and make choices. In this way, it becomes their change process.

Diplomacy.   Individuals whom the resisters trust and respect can help persuade, sell, and convince.

Decrease the rate of change.   It is important to moderate the change with the group's ability to absorb it and adjust to it. It may be necessary to decrease the rate of change to allow a deescalation of conflict. However, a forward momentum should be maintained. If objections completely halt the movement, a powerful reward for continued resistance is created.

Hold the line.   This approach emphasizes reasserting the expectations, clarifying roles, and reviewing the vision.

Warning.   The direction should be clearly set, and those who are unable to support the change must examine the appropriateness of their continued place within the organization.

Not all members of management or nursing staff will wish to or be able to effectively function in a shared governance system. However, it is important to assess the individual in-depth and allow ample time for acceptance and participation. Every effort should be made to ensure ample opportunity and resources for skill development.

Display support from upper level and other levels.   Support of the changes can be displayed in a variety of ways. Verbal confirmation, as well as public positive praise for those who are involved and supportive of the change process, is important. Role modeling of the expected new behaviors can be influential.

As the structural changes begin, chaos, confusion, and uncertainty will occur. For a period of time, the organization will have portions of two systems, the old traditional structure and the new developing shared governance structure.

The system will experience some degree of chaos as everyone struggles with working within two systems. The transition process of the structure change cannot be instantaneous, but a short transition is desirable. As issues arise, particularly early in this period, it may be difficult to determine which process should be used. The groups' progress and exact stage in the change process will be unclear. In addition, the newly formed groups may not yet be ready developmentally to handle all issues. The nurse administrator's role at this time should be to assist in this assessment. She should direct and moderate the systems. Delay in resolution of the problem and delayed decisions should be expected.

In the initial planning process, the council structure and areas of responsibility are loosely defined. As the groups begin to meet, there will be confusion regarding the structure, systems, and process. Role confusion will also be evident. Managers and staff will grapple with changing roles and new expectations. During the first 1 to 2 years, the structure will be undergoing continuous and dramatic change. The councils should begin by more clearly defining their work. They need to begin to develop their accountabilities.

There will be a lack of understanding regarding the shared governance system. Initially, the groups will be internally focused. They are interested only in what relates to their particular group. At this time, many misconceptions may emerge, which may hinder movement. Managers and staff may see no difference between a participatory structure and shared governance. Shared governance is *not* participatory management. In participatory management the manager invites staff involvement in decisions. The manager is not obligated to use the staff input. In addition, the manager retains the final authority and accountability of the outcome of the decision. By contrast, in a shared governance model the involvement in decisions is a right, a defined role in specified areas. Accountability and the authority rest with the staff.

Staff members will experience uncertainty regarding themselves and others; there will be a time of testing. They are unsure whether they will actually be allowed to make decisions instead of management. They may not yet trust management or the system. Skepticism will be projected. Reassurance and support will be necessary. As decisions perceived as important by the staff are made by the staff, the distrust should begin to dissipate.

Mistakes are unavoidable as the decisions are being made. An atmosphere that accepts errors must be created (Peters, 1987). Management must allow mistakes. They must help staff learn from mistakes, view them openly, and be able to talk about them without fear of punishment. Unit managers may find it difficult to allow staff members to make mistakes, or they may actually contribute to mistakes by not sharing information or assisting staff in the development of skills. The manager should not allow the staff to make blatant errors, but should assist them in examining the cause of the issues, developing alternatives, and evaluating the outcomes of the alternative. This is accomplished not by dictating answers, but by asking appropriate questions, thus allowing the staff to choose the answer.

Early in the decision-making stages, a reluctance to make difficult decisions may be noted. This may occur among both staff members and management and usually involves making decisions that will be unpopular with both peer groups. There is fear of rejection and anger. The groups may need to be challenged to make the difficult decisions. They will need support through the process. In the past it may have been easier to pass the difficult decisions to someone else. Assisting the staff through this stage will be aided by building their self-confidence. Talking through issues can be helpful. Those involved in the decisions need to support each other. Often having the opportunity to express the negative reactions aimed at them is helpful in dealing with the stress. After staff members have experienced this in a few situations, they are better able to handle the negative reactions of their peers and have the self-confidence to deal with the situation without personalizing it. Through the process they gain insight into the difficulty of decision making and acquire new understanding and respect for other decision makers.

Issues of nonsupport are evident in staff as well as management. There may be a lack of trust within the groups. Communication and information are important. Explaining the system and how it works may be helpful. An open invitation to observe the decision-making forums gives staff members who are not involved the opportunity to see the process firsthand. It also gives the message that the system is open and that there are no secrets.

It is expected that the major changes will be championed by a few leading innovators. They will be the change agents. As they lead their peers through the change process, they will experience conflict resistance and lack of understanding and support. Breaking new ground is never easy; they are paving the way for their successors. No one will be able to understand what they have had to accomplish. It is important not only that they receive support from their superiors but that there be opportunities for them to interact and set up supports among themselves.

The overall concept that staff make decisions that relate to practice and management makes decisions that relate to business issues and resources may sound clear, but it is not. There are many issues that seem to have components of both. It may not always be clear who should make what decision. As these issues arise it may be necessary to use the guideline that whoever is responsible for the outcome should have the accountability of the decision. In some instances it may be necessary to divide the decision into parts for different groups. If this is not possible because of the nature of the decision, one group may need to seek input from the other. Only one group can make the decision. When it is unclear who should make a decision, the executive council does not make the decision but rather decides who makes the decision.

In the beginning there is a lack of boundaries as the groups struggle for their identity. They are rapidly assuming responsibilities. They are initially timid but move quickly to challenge any boundaries. Boundaries must be placed; there needs to be clear definition or chaos will result. The resultant structure will become as unwieldy as the previous one with confusion of roles and overlapping responsibility. Reeducation of the principles and clarification of the direction will be needed. It will take time for the staff to understand the structures and the interrelationships within the hospital and the division.

Time is an important issue throughout the process of shared governance. Staff members need time to participate in the decision-making process. They may feel pulled between the needs of their patients and their commitment to the duties on the forums. Other staff members may resent the time away from patient care and the extra burden it places on them. Managers feel the pressure to provide the resources to support both activities. This is clearly a challenge for the unit manager. There must be a balance between the direct patient care activities and the non-direct patient care activities. Both are important to quality care. Sufficient resources must be available to meet the patient care requirements so that quality is not affected. If time is not spent on development of the practice and the things that affect it, the quality of patient care will be negatively affected. The divisional budgets and staffing must be designed to include adequate time for both activities. It may be necessary to prioritize the goals and projects of the division. Attempting to accomplish too many things at once may overextend the resources (energy, time, money). The resource of time is primarily the responsibility of the unit manager, but staff members have responsibility to negotiate their time needs with and for their peers.

The principal educational needs in this phase concern the concepts, principles, structure, and systems of shared governance. Skill development should focus on assertiveness, decision making, and consensus building. Support and much guidance and direction are essential.

PHASE III—DEVELOPMENT, REGROUPING, AND CLARIFICATION

The most skill development and process development occurs in the third phase. This phase can begin anywhere from month 6 to month 12. It lasts approximately 1 to 2 years. As the councils begin to more clearly define their work, guidelines for each council should be developed. The guidelines should define the accountabilities, the membership, the roles, the operating procedures, and the election process. These will take several months to generate. The council members will spend these first several months struggling to define their work and developing a process to accomplish it.

One area that affects group process is the size of its membership. The ideal group size for effective interactions is approximately eight to twelve members. Although this size may not be possible within every institution, a concerted effort should be made to limit the size to the minimum required. Some may argue that full representation is required initially. This should be avoided because the transition will be difficult and an effective group process cannot occur with large numbers. It will delay group development. The group should contain a representative number that adequately reflects the various types of areas. Initially, there will be much controversy over this issue. Many will think that every area should be represented. The responsibilities of the representatives are critical. Their role may need clarification, and problems with accountability for their role must be handled.

The membership is responsible for representing the interest, concerns, and ideas of the groups that they represent. A formal communication system between the representatives and the units should be established. There may be confusion regarding the decision process of shared governance. Representative decision making in shared governance is frequently confused with democratic rule.

Democratic rule is not used in a shared governance structure. The disadvantages of democratic rule include special interest groups, narrow focus of problem outcomes and decisions, and unequal representation of groups. A representative model is used in the decision-making forums of a shared governance model. This is often confused with democratic rule. The role of the representative in the decision-making forums is to represent the interest, ideas, and concerns of the staff who have chosen them. However, they are not there to represent only the majority opinions or a special interest group. The representatives participate with an open mind to weigh all the available information and ideas and to make the best decision possible for the patient, the entire staff, and the hospital. They have an obligation to elicit input and to relay rationales for appropriate decisions. The staff members have the responsibility to keep informed and to give input when requested. In addition, they must support the decisions of the group regardless of their agreement or disagreement. The staff may need to be reminded that they were not present to hear all of the information and the discussion that may have influenced a decision. They must trust and support their peers that if they had been in similar circumstances with the same information, they would have made the same decision. The circumstances and information will vary at different times.

Although it is important to allow access to and involvement in the process, it is unrealistic to try to design the system so that no decisions are made without input. Some issues require a broad perspective. However, if there is proper representation, there are adequate and diverse viewpoints for most decisions. The groups need to be able to make decisions without surveying the staff. This is a "judgment call"; however, with advance circulation of the agenda, individuals will have the opportunity to provide input. As the trust level increases, the staff are supportive of the decisions made without their input. The representatives are able to determine the appropriate times when input is critical.

Group dynamics may cause problems with group interactions, group process, or decision-making abilities. Many members may have had limited experience in group problem solving. Some of the problem areas that may develop include "group think," inequality of membership, and lack of consensus.

Facilitating an atmosphere that promotes open disagreement and values individual diversity decreases the likelihood of "group think." Initially, some members may not be vocal or may shy away from disagreeing with a peer. The chair must foster an environment that promotes critical thinking. Group process must be structured to seek outside information and innovative ideas. Discussions and decision making should explore all alternatives. All members should be encouraged to actively participate.

Inequality of membership will surface early in the group's development. Managers, educators, and clinical nurse specialists who may be members of these groups will be initially influential. Staff members may tend to defer to the other members. Managers and specialists must be aware of their own influence. Staff should be allowed to present their opinions first. It may be necessary to preface their input with the statement that it is opinion and should not be regarded as the better approach. The non-staff members should use strategies that assist in the development of in-depth problem solving by questioning and allowing staff to examine all factors and components. In addition, chairpersons must be cognizant of their potential influence within the group. The staff may view such individuals as leaders and may also acquiesce to their ideas. Each chairperson's responsibility is to ensure and facilitate group process. The chair facilitates the discussion and decision making. Chairpersons need to resist setting their own agenda and control of the decisions. The chair should consider similar strategies as the non-staff member such as giving opinions last, giving no opinion in some instances, and encouraging other members' participation.

Decision by consensus implies open communication. Everyone has had the opportunity to state an opinion and influence the opinion of others. Members do not feel that they were not heard and understood (Arndt, 1988). They should not feel that if only they were understood, the group would not have made that decision. The environment is one of support. The decision chosen is the one that the most people support and those who oppose it are willing to support it because they were heard.

As in any group, it takes time for the group to develop a relationship and a team approach. The staff members and the staff chairpersons may be inexperienced in their new roles. They will need assistance from the facilitator in conducting an efficient meeting. The facilitator role is generally filled by a nurse administrator. The purpose of the role is to assist the chair and chair-elect in skill development. By meeting with the chair, the facilitator can assist in development and coordination of the council. Reviewing the group process and dynamics, the facilitator can assist in the development of strategies to improve group effectiveness and efficiency. The facilitator also serves as a resource on hospital, division, and regulatory policies and requirements. She provides a broad divisional and hospital perspective. It is important that chairpersons acquire an understanding of the politics and the structure of the other systems within the hospital. The interest, decisions, and concerns of the council are represented by the facilitator in other hospital forums.

The skill acquisition by staff members and the chairs will require both informal and formal education. Educational needs will include agenda development, minute writing, memo writing, conflict resolution, group leadership and facilitating skills, group problem-solving skills, and effective leadership of meetings.

When the councils first begin to meet, there will be a tendency to process work at the meetings. Items will be placed on the agenda and it will be apparent that insufficient information concerning the problem is available. Even when the problem is well described, additional gathering of information is required. Another problem that may arise is that actual program development may occur in the meetings. These problems will initially hinder the work and cause gross inefficiency and ineffectiveness at the meetings. Most work and the gathering of data should occur before these items are placed on the agenda. Issues should be fully investigated with some alternative solutions prepared before being discussed. New programs and policies should be presented in a final draft form. Thus meetings can be used for final decisions and approval with a decreased need for drastic development or revision. As the skills of the chairpersons and members increase, the frequency of issues that require more than one meeting for resolution will decrease.

After meeting efficiency and effectiveness improve, the shared governance structure may still delay the time it takes to make a decision. The overall process, however, remains efficient because those responsible for implementing decisions are also those who make them. Implementation time is shortened. However, in any organization, there must be an established, accepted, and understood method for making quick decisions when they are required. This method should include staff members. This is usually accomplished by empowering the chairperson to make decisions in lieu of the group. The chair, then, must report to the group the decision and rationale for review and critique. There may be a tendency to revert to the previous manager decision process, but this approach should be avoided.

As decisions are made and policies and programs generated, the operations may become difficult and may warrant attention. The major responsibility for putting the decisions into operation lies with the staff. However, the manager also has a role. Managers may perceive that these issues no longer concern them and attempt to shirk this role. Clarification of both the manager's and the staff's role in this area may be necessary.

As the group gains skill and confidence, other issues may surface. In the early phases, some timid and reluctant behaviors may have been exhibited. With the newfound confidence, this may have yielded to the other extremes of wanting to make all decisions and a challenging of self-governance.

Early in the process it is not unusual for the staff to challenge management that all decisions should be made by them. This is an expected developmental reaction caused by lack of sophistication, maturity, and understanding. Not all decisions within the division should be made by the shared governance structure. The system is an evolving system. As it is developed and refined, more of the decisions may become the responsibility of the shared governance model. It is the responsibility of the nursing administrator to evaluate the staff and system readiness and appropriateness of the decisions. Initially it will be important to start in the more simple and concrete areas of practice and to expand the areas as the staff members develop the skills and an understanding of the structure and its relationship to the division and the interrelationship with the rest of the hospital. Determining when and which issues are appropriate will require staff insight. Allowing certain areas to assume responsibility before they are ready may prove troublesome, yet it is important not to withhold them.

Some may misinterpret that *all* activities and responsibilities within the division are determined with the shared governance structure; literally, this would be management by committee. Kanter (1983) identifies the need for parallel organizations. Two parallel organizations should exist. One is the traditional management or maintenance organization that is defined by lines, job descriptions, and reporting relationships. The other is a highly participatory structure like the shared governance structure that is defined by bylaws. It is the means by which the division manages change and attains its goals. It allows staff members to determine their practice and the areas that affect care delivery. These two structures need to be integrated within the system. There are a complementary relationship and a flow of information, decisions, and programs between the two structures. Participation should be balanced. It is not a replacement of leadership or the management structure. It is the method by which the division chooses to accomplish its work.

In some literature reports, the terms *shared governance* and *self-governance* are used interchangeably. There is an important distinction between these two terms. *Shared* refers to an equality of positions. It is a requirement of all of the professionals in the division. It sets a tone of collegiality and collaboration. In a shared governance model the staff members have control over practice decisions, but management also is involved and has a perspective and an expertise. Similarly, the management decisions are made by the managers, but staff involvement is also sought. There are a sharing of authority and accountability and a collaboration on the development and attainment of goals. *Self-governance* implies a total separation of areas of responsibility. It may establish a "we-they" atmosphere. There needs to be a close collaborative relationship and atmosphere. They are interrelated and cannot properly be developed separately. Synergism is vital. Synergism is the combination of the parts greater than the sum of the individual pieces.

Early in the development of the groups there will be confusion and a lack of cohesiveness and integration among the decision-making forums. Each group will struggle to define its work and its accountabilities. There may be group conflict. Challenging of each other's decisions or their right to make the decision may exist. Communication among the chairpersons is critical. The nursing administrator also must assist the staff in understanding the process, as well as integrating the groups. As the accountabilities become more well defined and as the relationships are developed, a more cohesive approach should emerge.

As the system changes, the need for accurate, timely, and efficient communication grows. This need is more complex in a shared governance model because the number of participants and the amount of information are significantly higher. The system needs to be multidirectional.

One of the accountabilities of the councils is the development of a comprehensive communication system. This is generally assigned to the education council. It will become apparent early in the implementation that the previous communication system is woefully inadequate for the shared governance structure. Constant monitoring and refinement of the communication system are necessary. There can never be too much communication. The goal should be to make being knowledgeable and informed inevitable.

PHASE IV—INTEGRATION, REFINEMENT, AND CONTINUED EVOLUTION

Toward the end of the final phase, the council chairpersons have initiated the movement toward coordination and integration. That step involves the negotiation and synthesizing of the guidelines of all the councils. The accountabilities must not be in conflict and the operating procedures must be consistent. Election processes, membership, roles, and so on should be similar. These guidelines will form the basis of the bylaws. The formal development of the bylaws should not be undertaken until the second or third year of the implementation process. During the first 2 years, the structure will undergo continuous and dramatic change.

The members of the executive group (vice president, staff council chairs) should evolve into a cohesive leadership team for the division. They are responsible for the integration and interdependence of the divisional councils. In the beginning, their group process was comprised predominately of communication and information with little understanding of the executive council role. At this point in the process, the group dynamics and skill ability should be emerging to facilitate the continued development of the model.

Staff members may have also processed little understanding of the purpose of the executive council. There may be fear of too much power being placed with too few people. Reassurance that the executive council does not overrule the other councils may be required. Reeducation concerning the function and purpose will be necessary.

Integration of the shared governance model is important in three areas. First, there must be integration among the division councils. As previously stated, the councils are interdependent. The direction and the goals must be coordinated. Initially, there is a lack of understanding of how the councils' work is interrelated. Issues and new programs will frequently affect more than one council. The groups initially will work in isolation. When the accountabilities and the intergroup process have been developed, intragroup process should formulate. The shared governance structure has a unit component and a divisional component. Integration of the unit-based shared governance structure and the divisional structure is the second level of integration. These two components are interrelated. The divisional council sets the broad standards and guidelines, and the unit council determines the implementation plan and the program specifics. Issues, problems, and decisions need to flow between the division and the unit. The third level of integration occurs at the hospital level. The shared governance structure is a systems model that must fit within the larger hospital system. Ultimately the values, goals, and direction for the division of nursing flow from that of the hospital.

All members of the nursing division are responsible for integration. The staff members are responsible for the integration between the unit councils and divisional councils. At the unit level the unit manager should assist with the department's integration with other hospital departments. The nursing administrators should focus on ensuring integration of the divisional councils with the hospital management, committees, and systems.

KNOWING WHEN YOU'VE ARRIVED

The planning process should include the development of an evaluation plan. The implementation process occurs over a 3- to 5-year period. It is an evolving systems model that is affected by the environment. Periodic evaluation assists in refinement of the model as it evolves and adjusts to the changing needs of the organization. Development of pretesting of selected areas before the implementation process begins may be desirable for a comparison study on the effects of the model.

The evaluation of the shared governance model should focus on the intended purpose of the change. What was the reason for the reorganization of the structure? What were the problems with the previous structure that the shared governance structure will improve? From these questions, the objectives of the model can be determined. The objectives of the implementation should be formalized. The objectives then serve as the basis of the evaluation from which criteria can be developed. The evaluation system is designed by the objectives. Well-delineated objectives and criteria direct the selection methods and the development of the evaluation system. The evaluation system must coordinate and integrate the several kinds of objectives. A summary evaluation should be conducted while evaluating the component parts. The evaluation must draw conclusions and make recommendations.

There will most likely be several reasons for implementing the model. The program evaluation criteria may focus on several areas. The components of program evaluation should include structure, process, and outcome. The relationships of the components should be explored (Clemenhagen and Champagne, 1986).

Structure criteria relate to the organization of the system and the resources that are necessary for that system to function. The resources used include human, time, equipment, training, and education. All have an impact on finances. The quality of the resources should also be assessed. Although some of these costs relate to the start-up of the process, there are ongoing maintenance costs that should be quantified. The financial impact should be compared to the previous organizational structure. It is important, therefore, to quantify the resources of the existing structure before the changes begin. This may include quantifying the current committee and meeting structures in which all nursing staff are involved within the division and the hospital. This includes the number of hours and dollars for these activities. This area may require close monitoring throughout the implementation process. Careful resource assessment is necessary so that needs can be budgeted and allocated. In addition, periodic assessment is helpful so that adjustment and streamlining of the structure occur. In many institutions a cost reduction has been realized after the full implementation of the model.

Process criteria focus on how the system functions to accomplish its work. They assess the interactions within the system itself and among other systems. The efficiency and the effectiveness of the system are evaluated. Decision making, communication, integration of divisional councils, integration with the unit councils, and integration with the rest of the hospital systems are a few of the possible areas for evaluation.

Outcome criteria evaluate the effect of the system. The effects are examined as they relate to the program objectives. The objectives may describe characteristics, behaviors, or the state of the nursing organization. Examples of effects include improved nurse satisfaction, staff accountability and control of practice, increased staff professional development, and improved trust and teamwork.

The evaluation of the components must include the examination of the integration and relationship among them. The analysis provides information that examines the program design, the resource utilization, and the achievement of the program objectives (Clemenhagen and Champagne, 1986). Analysis of the relationships of the components is the only way to evaluate the overall efficiency and effectiveness of the system. It guides and directs the complex decisions for the system's evolution and refinement.

The methodology for evaluation can be determined after the objectives and criteria have been established. Several approaches may be necessary. Prioritizing the essential versus the desirable outcomes may be necessary (Rezler and Stevens, 1978). Also, unexpected outcomes may occur that may need evaluation.

Assessment and measurement are used in the evaluation process. Assessment is the collection of quantitative and qualitative data to define behavior. Measurement assigns numeric values to objects and observations (Rezler and Stevens, 1978). There are a variety of types and numbers of tools that can be used to evaluate the shared governance model. The formats may include observations, surveys, and questionnaires.

The evaluation tool chosen will partially depend on the criteria being evaluated. However, there may be a range of choices for any given criteria. An established tool may be used for evaluation. Another alternative is the construction of a tool.

An established tool has the advantage of providing well-established reliability and validity indexes. For example, there are a variety of tools that evaluate nurse satisfaction, effectiveness of communication, or decision making. There are also tools specifically designed to evaluate a shared governance model. Although these tools have not yet been fully developed or established, they may provide valuable data and the opportunity to compare results with other institutions. A disadvantage may be that the tool does not fully meet the criteria. However, an alternative of adapting the model to the needs should be considered.

The construction of an evaluation tool offers the appeal of tailoring the tool to the unique needs of the institution. One disadvantage is the time and complexity of the undertaking. The feasibility and usefulness of utilizing an existing tool or the adaptation of a tool must be weighed against the time and expense required in the development of a new tool.

The evaluation system itself must be reviewed and revised throughout the process. The quality assurance group should assist in the development of the plan. The overall responsibility for the efficiency and effectiveness of the shared governance system rests with the coordinating or executive group. They define the objectives and use the evaluation results in the refinement, growth, and the development of the model.

SUMMARY

The implementation of shared governance is a significant undertaking in any organization. The change in structure involves a change in the culture of the organization. The culture is defined by values. The values are expressed in how members interact to accomplish the work. Structures and systems within an organization support and influence behaviors and values. Figure 5-1 depicts this interaction.

As an accountability-based professional practice model, shared governance is based on concepts and principles that promote a new set of values. With changing values, behaviors must also undergo transformation.

Behaviors are the expression of the values held. They are also influenced by life experiences, experience in the organization with others, as well as observation of behaviors within the workplace (norms, rules, rituals, etc.). Role expectations also impact behavior. However, the formal written or spoken expectation may be different from those encouraged or implied. Skill and knowledge affect behavior. Increasing knowledge and skill to impact changing values and behavior is helpful. It may be an unsuccessful strategy if the role expectations and the behavior experiences of others, particularly of management, continue unchanged or incongruent.

The organization systems and structures assist in supporting the values and be-

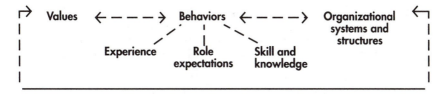

FIGURE 5-1. Culture.

haviors. Concurrently, structure and systems development are shaped by values and behaviors. As the organization moves toward changing values, the structure and support systems must be redesigned to meet the values. For example, the system and structures include committee structure, organizational chart, communication system, performance appraisals, job description, etc.

Transformation of the culture involves diligence, careful planning, and time. The following steps summarizes this complex process:

1. Confirm and commit to the new values.
2. Create a vision and enlist others.
3. Role model management changes first.
4. Promote and set expectations.
5. Build skill along the way.
6. Change structure and systems to support the new values.

REFERENCES

Argyris, C. (1964). *Integrating the Individual and the Organization.* New York: John Wiley & Sons, Inc.

Argyris, C. (1962). *Interpersonal Competence and Organizational Effectiveness.* Homewood, Ill.: Dorsey Press.

Argyris, C. (1957). *Personality and Organization.* New York: Harper & Brothers Publishers, Inc.

Arndt, C. and Huckaboy, Z. *Nursing Administration: Theory for Practice with a System Approach.* 1988, St. Louis: C.V. Mosby Co.

Bennis, W. *The Planning of Change.* 1977, New York: Holt, Rinehart & Winston.

Boyle, E.M. (1984). Wrestling with Jellyfish. *Harvard Business Review,* January/February, 74-83.

Clemenhagen, C. and Champagne, F. (1986). Quality Assurance as Part of Program Evaluation. *QRB,* November, 383-387.

Hersey, P. and Blanchard, K. (1977). *Management of Organizational Behavior Utilizing Resources.* Englewood Cliffs, N.J.: Prentice-Hall.

Kanter, R.M. (1989). *When Grants Learn to Dance.* New York: Simon & Schuster.

Kanter, R.M. (1983). *The Change Masters.* New York: Simon & Schuster.

Kotter, J. (1990). What Leaders Really Do. *Harvard Business Review,* May/June 103-111.

Kouzes, J. and Posner, B. (1987). *The Leadership Challenge.* San Francisco: Jossey Bass Publishers.

Krejci, J.W. and Malin, S. (1989). A Paradigm Shift to the New Age of Nursing. *Nursing Administrative Quarterly,* 13(4).

Marchette, L. and Holloman, F. (1987). The Research Quality Assessment Connection. *JQA,* Fall, 16-19.

Martinko, M.J. and Gardner, W.L.(1982). Learned Helplessness: An Alternative Explanation for Performance Deficits. *Academy of Management Review,* 7, 195-204.

McDonagh, K. and others. (1989). Shared Governance at St. Joseph's Hospital of Atlanta. *Nursing Administrative Quarterly,* 13(4), 17-28.

Passos, J.Y. (1973). Accountability: Myth or Mandate? *Journal of Nursing Administration,* 3, 17-22.

Peters, T. (1987). *Thriving on Chaos*. New York: Harper & Row.

Peters, T. and Outen, N. (1985). *A Passion for Excellence*. New York: Random House.

Peterson, M.E. and Allen, D.G. Shared Governance: A Strategy for Transforming Organizations, Part Two. *Journal of Nursing Administration,* Vol. 16, No. 2 (February, 1986).

Peterson, M.E. and Allen, D.G. Shared Governance: A Strategy for Transforming Organizations, Part One. *Journal of Nursing Administration,* Vol. 16, No. 1 (January), 9-12, 1986.

Peterson, M.E. (1983). Motivating Staff to Participate in Decision-Making. *Nursing Administration Quarterly,* 7, 2 (Winter), 63-68.

Pinkerton, S.E. and Schroeder, P. (1988). *Commitment to Excellence: Developing a Professional Nursing Staff,* Rockville, Md.: Aspen Publishers.

Porter-O'Grady, T. (1989). Shared Governance Reality or Shame? *American Journal of Nursing,* March, 350-351.

Porter-O'Grady, T. (1987). Shared Governance and New Organizational Models. *Nursing Economics,* 5, 6 (November-December), 281-286.

Porter-O'Grady, T. (1986). *Creative Nursing Administration: Participatory Management Into the Twenty-First Century*. Rockville, Md.: Aspen Publishers.

Porter-O'Grady, T. and Finnigan, S. (1984). *Shared Governance for Nursing: A Creative Approach to Professional Accountability*. Rockville, Md.: Aspen Publishers.

Rezler, A.G. and Stevens, B.J. (1978). *The Nurse Evaluator in Education and Service*. New York: McGraw Hill Book Co., 228-238.

Roberts, S. (1983). Oppressed Group Behavior: Implications for Nursing. *Advances in Nursing Science,* 5(4), 21-30.

Smith, S. Evaluating a Shared Governance Model. *Aspen Advisor for Nurse Executives.* 5, 9, (June).

Vlcak, D. Decentralization: What Works and What Doesn't. *Journal of Nursing Strategy,* 8(2), 71-74.

6 Change Strategies for Moving to Shared Governance

Vicki D. Lachman

PLANNED PROCESS OF CHANGE

Coping with change has led nursing departments to use "band-aid" solutions that do nothing substantive for nursing. Changing to shared governance is a long-term strategy. It is a transformation rather than a simple change because of the paradigm shift. Shared governance shifts the authority and accountability to individuals and groups most capable of dealing with a constant need to manage change.

Why is there so much discussion about change? Change is occurring faster, it is more complex, and it reaches deeper into the fabric of our lives. It has an impact on all aspects of an individual's personal and professional life. This rapid rate of change will continue; therefore organizations need to plan for and to implement change at the same time. Shared governance provides a model for this continuous management of change.

Identifying the process and principles of planned change is important to individuals implementing shared governance. As a model, shared governance provides the change agent with a structure for implementing change. Shared governance as a process provides the nursing department with guidelines for empowerment of staff.

The concept of planned change is founded on the principle that people have a right to determine their own future and have the capacity to do so. This concept assumes that human beings have an innate drive toward self-development. The chapter focuses on the process, principles, and problems related to planned change.

Lewin (1947) clearly articulated elements of the change process in his simple unfreezing, change, and refreezing theory. The component of unfreezing is the most difficult step for all involved. A preformed plan for enacting shared governance cannot be bought; in fact, the process of developing such a plan plays a key role in the creation and modeling of empowerment.

The process of unfreezing involves a design for an action plan based on the vision of the nursing department. This plan is not intended to limit or restrict. It is meant to guide and facilitate the actions of all individuals involved in the change.

As part of this decision process, the "where and how" elements begin to emerge. Creative ways to detour around identified roadblocks and types of interventions that will be needed become clearer. The types of support needed will vary but usually include financial and clerical, and the use of experts. Contingency plans are explored as the design team examines potential resistance. Part of this design process is determining the degree of commitment and ways to increase it.

During this period of unfreezing, the current state of the organization is examined. It is important to assess the present culture of the organization, its managerial styles, and its reward systems in order to determine the readiness of the organization for the empowerment of its staff.

A culture that bases promotions on longevity, "contacts," or both is not using empowering behaviors. A nursing department that promotes on the basis of competencies agreed on and compliance with standards of practice is a department of nursing in transition to empowerment. A final part of the plan for change involves ensuring that a structure is in place for continuous evaluation of the change process.

For example, as a ripple of change begins to affect other departments, a format for problem solving, without which the change might falter, will necessarily emerge. As a format for conflict resolution evolves, roles are clarified, cooperation improves, and individuals increasingly support the change. Ongoing, continuous information exchange and conflict resolution among the groups responsible for decisions become critical.

In the transition process, balancing a nursing department's equilibrium is necessary for organization stability. Below are four factors to consider for achieving equilibrium:

1. Enough stability to facilitate the achievement of current goals
2. Enough continuity to ensure orderly changes in both the ends and the means
3. Enough adaptability to react appropriately to external opportunities and demands and to changing internal conditions
4. Enough innovativeness to allow the organization to be proactive (to initiate changes) when conditions warrant (Kast and Rosenweig, 1974)

Unfreezing for a change is an involved process that requires creativity and, ultimately, a dynamic plan of action. Planned change is evolutionary for shared governance. In shared governance, no one remains unaffected by change. Planning for changes involves application of certain principles.

Principles of Change

Having a set of general principles rather than a rigid blueprint helps nursing departments maintain a focus on empowering human beings. Below are eight principles of change to use for implementation of shared governance (Funches, 1990; Vogt and Murrell, 1990).

1. **Homeostasis.** Change can potentially upset an individual's or an organization's stability. The subsequent resistance is the result of the organism's attempt to automatically compensate for the changes. Therefore the change must be reinforced or the organism will return to old patterns. A nurse manager is the key

reinforcer of change in coaching staff members to take charge of changes in their unit.

The most powerful source of resistance to change deserves special attention, because all organizational cultures have at least one source. When change involves something or someone considered sacred, change will cause considerable upheaval or stress. Examples include a dress code policy or a well-connected employee who should be removed or rigid adherence to a certain model of nursing care delivery.

Other common sources of resistance are listed below; all must be examined in the design and implementation process.

1. The purpose of the change has not been clarified or substantiated
2. The operations and patterns of work groups have been disregarded
3. Employees have not been kept informed about the change
4. Excessive work pressure is created during implementation phase of a change
5. Issues regarding job security and concomitant anxiety have not been given attention in an open, real way (Vogt and Murrell, 1990, p. 138)

2. **Interdependence.** Change in one part of a system affects every other part because every system has many interrelated parts. Elimination of the policy and procedure committee affects more than the nursing department committee structure. A practice determined by professional standards stated by the practice council is based on a model different from the typical institutional task model.

3. **Participation.** People affected by a change should participate in making the change. In addition, the sooner individuals are allowed to participate in a change process, the less resistant they will be. In a shared governance model, multiple opportunities are provided for individual participation in both unit and departmental activities.

4. **Inertia.** Once change is initiated, it will continue in the same direction, unless outside forces effectively stop the movement. Drucker's rule of twenties best expresses the principle of inertia in action:

   • Twenty percent of individuals are the first to arrive and the last to leave
   • Twenty percent of individuals are the last to arrive and the first to leave
   • The other 60 percent in the middle will go with whoever is winning (Drucker, 1974)

It is also important to remember that the group that is the last to arrive and the first to leave is often the noisiest group, although it does not usually include the majority. Because individuals operate with different rates of readiness, there is a need for multiple ways to facilitate involvement as the change moves forward.

Reality-testing comments such as the following are often erroneously labeled as resistance:

   • "I already feel overloaded; this just sounds like more time, pressure, and additional burdens."

- "What kind of help are they going to give us in making this change?"
- "I don't think they have thought it through. I can see some possible side effects that I bet they have not thought of."

Change agents must know how to analyze and manage forces operating against change and to acknowledge those who will encourage the change. The shared governance council structure fosters a gathering momentum of participation that moves change forward.

5. **Flexibility.** Adaptability must be built into the system. Shared governance, although firm in its value structure, is a flexible model in actual implementation. Rules are determined by councils.
6. **Inevitable conflict.** Change that alters roles, responsibilities, and accountability by its nature creates conflict among the individuals involved. Therefore conflict resolution skills are necessary to clarify and negotiate new roles within the shared governance model.
7. **Parallel realities.** Because reality is reflected in one's perception of the world, multiple pictures of the change process exist at any one time. A common vision of shared governance will increase speed of implementation. However, individuals voicing their differences simultaneously shape the outcome. Often these individuals are seen as "devil's advocates" but they are as crucial to the process as are cheerleaders. Both keep each other honest and in touch with the group's view of changes.
8. **Reward.** People continue to express behavior for which they receive recognition, reinforcement, and reward. It is important to determine which behaviors are rewarded and celebrated. As progress is made and tasks are accomplished, it is important to acknowledge both the individuals and teams responsible.

These principles can serve as guides in the change process, but there is no absolute rule concerning a single way to create change. A change agent sets the stage by creating conditions necessary to direct change. By providing vision, opportunities to participate, and ongoing evaluation of change, unfreezing will occur and change will begin.

In summary, people will accept an organizational change if they are

1. Involved in the process of change
2. Asked to contribute (knowledge, suggestions, feelings, opinions) to the change
3. Informed of the reasons for and advantages of the change
4. Informed with honesty about all facts of the change
5. Given concrete and specific feedback about the change
6. Respected for their feelings, whether supportive of or opposed to the change
7. Asked about and given any assistance needed to deal with the effects of the change on the job
8. Recognized appropriately for their specific contributions to the implementation of the change (Vogt and Murrell, p. 139)

These points aid in motivating staff.

Motivational Theory in Action

In America an interesting dichotomy occurs between individuals' social and work roles. The social obligation of citizens in a democracy is to participate actively in shaping and supporting social and political institutions. However, a citizen must usually spend at least eight hours a day, five days a week in a work environment where the reverse is required. The ludicrousness of this situation is best stated by Porter-O'Grady and Finnegan (1984):

> *In the work environment, people are expected to be essentially voiceless, to perform specific tasks, to defer to others in decision making and other involvement in the decision process and to subjugate their personal interests, needs, desires and personal accountability to those suggested by representatives of the larger organization. Thus, while they are asked to be responsible, participating and active citizens in a free society while not in a work setting, they are not provided the opportunity to develop and exercise the required activities in the workplace, where they will spend clearly half of their adult life . . . It is no wonder that neither managers nor workers in the United States are culturally equipped to accept diffusion of responsibility and control in the work place.*

Ways to motivate people to become involved are found in literature of organizational behavior by such authors as McClelland (1971), Hertzberg, Mausner, and Synderman (1959), and MacGregor (1960). By understanding and applying the principles of motivation and teamwork, a manager can facilitate individuals' desire to participate.

McClelland used a formula that focused on three key ingredients for aroused motivation.

$$M \times E \times I$$

M represents the basic motivational driving force of the individual. It is what activates the individual to expend energy toward an objective. According to the theory, each individual has power, achievement, and affiliation orientations; however, one of these usually is a more prominent force. Because of individual orientations, each person has a different view of opportunities to participate in shared governance.

For example, an individual who is achievement oriented would rather be in charge of a special project, whereas a power-oriented person would be interested in being a chairperson, being in charge, or being assistant nurse manager. An individual with a high orientation to affiliation would be interested in maintaining good relationships in councils, and achievers would keep the group focused on the task.

Examples of tasks to offer individuals who have a high score in certain areas are listed below:

Achievement

1. Development of a patient acuity system
2. Development of a quality assurance system
3. Development of new programs

4. Development of case management model
5. Development of education programs

Power

1. Council chairperson
2. Management advancement opportunity
3. Interdepartmental committee representative

Affiliation

1. Solving shift-to-shift communication problems
2. Encouraging celebrations
3. Being a good role model as a caring nurse

Fundamentally, McClelland (1971) agrees with McGregor (1960) and Maslow (1954). All see individuals as self-directed, and if given the opportunities to use creativity, individuals will always act in a way consistent with organizational goals. Hertzberg, Mausner, and Synderman concluded that work satisfaction is a result of opportunities to gain satisfaction from the work itself. The challenge is to ensure that both the scope of responsibility and work are themselves strongly motivating. Shared governance provides individuals with opportunities for multiple challenges, and increased participation will be seen as a reward by all three orientations.

E represents the "expectancy of achieving the goal." If individuals believe that their efforts will make a difference, they will be motivated. Participation increases when individuals realize that council decisions become policy. Such changes create the expectancy that participation works to achieve the changes. Individuals begin to believe that their vote counts.

I is "incentive value." Incentive value is the final key ingredient. Attractive incentive opportunities abound. Incentive value determines whether a person deems the opportunity worthy of the effort required. The incentive offered must meet the basic motives of the individual and be worth the time, energy, and, perhaps, funds required. As staff members determine their own schedules and play a role in determining budget expenditures, they see the value of participation.

By knowing how to stimulate individuals' enthusiasm, create an expectation that their efforts will make a difference, and provide a reward worth the participants' efforts, managers encourage people to participate.

Without effective communication, opportunities for participation may go unnoticed. Informing staff members regarding all facets of change is important in creating a climate of trust. Without trust, open participation cannot exist.

Teamwork

The magnitude of the shared governance implementation process requires a high level of participation in a concerted effort for an extended period of time. For the process to succeed, a work group needs to function as efficiently and as effectively as possible while maintaining quality patient care and active staff participation. This is not easy for even the most seasoned nurse manager. The definition of a team by Francis and Young (1979) captures the essence of a well-functioning team: "A team is an energetic group of people who are committed to achieving common objectives, who work well together and enjoy doing so, and who produce high quality results."

This definition emphasizes the need for individuals to work together for a common goal to produce quality service. For the change to shared governance to be successful, the nursing department needs to work together; teamwork is a way to both teach and lead the process.

The characteristics of a well-functioning team are listed below.* Each requires some change in the operation of the nursing department. Some characteristics focus on the task of the team, whereas others focus on the importance of the process of group functioning.

1. The team shares a sense of purpose or common goals, and each team member is willing to work toward achieving these goals.
2. The team is aware of and interested in its own process and in examining norms operating within the group.
3. The team identifies its own resources and uses them; at these times the group willingly accepts the influence and leadership of the members whose resources are relevant to the immediate task.
4. Group members continually try to listen to and clarify what is being said and to show interest in what others say and feel.
5. Differences of opinion are encouraged and freely expressed; the team does not demand narrow conformity or adherence to formats that inhibit freedom of movement and expression.
6. The team is willing to acknowledge conflict and focus on it until it is either resolved or managed in a way that does not reduce the effectiveness of the individuals involved.
7. The team exerts energy toward problem solving rather than allowing it to be drained by interpersonal issues or competitive struggles.
8. Roles are balanced and shared to facilitate both accomplishment of task and feelings of group cohesion and morale.
9. To encourage risk taking and creativity, mistakes are treated as sources of learning rather than reasons for punishment.
10. The team is responsive to the changing needs of its members and the external environment to which it is related.
11. Team members are committed to periodically evaluating the team's performance.
12. The team is attractive to its members, who identify with it and consider it a source of both professional and personal growth.
13. Developing a climate of trust is recognized as a crucial element facilitating all of the above elements (Hanson and Lubin, 1990, p. 77).

The list clearly addresses the need for a climate of open communication in which people are encouraged to be creative and to focus energy on finding

---

*Reprinted from *Organization Development Practitioner,* Spring, 1986. Used with permission.

solutions for roadblocks to the team's success. Only when all make an effort to resolve differences through honest communication can a climate of trust develop. A trusting climate encourages the surfacing of the team problems and their resolution.

The need for cooperative, interdependent behavior on the part of all group members often directs groups to investigate the team building process. Reddy and Jamison (1990) clearly state that team-building is an effort in which a "team studies its own processes of working together and acts to create a climate in which members' energies are directed toward problem solving and maximizing the use of all members' resources for this process."

Burke (1990) succinctly states the four primary purposes of team building:

1. To set goals or priorities
2. To analyze and clarify the way work is performed according to team members' roles and responsibilities
3. To examine the way the team is working—that is, its process such as norms, decision making, communications, and so forth
4. To examine relationships among the team members

A group in the team-building process begins with setting goals and priorities because problems with roles and responsibilities may result from a lack of clarity regarding team goals. The process is generally approached in the order listed. To begin by working out interpersonal relationships (step 4) may be a misuse of time and energy because the problems may be the result of a misunderstanding in the other three domains.

Role of Consultant

Does the nursing department need a consultant to facilitate the team-building process? The answer is generally *yes,* for two reasons. First, most leaders do not have the necessary process and group skills to manage their own team-building efforts. Second, without an unbiased person, team members are often reluctant to confront their own managers.

An external consultant could help the change process in several ways:

1. Consultants are free to respond to or comment on team behaviors.
2. Team members feel less threatened voicing opinions to consultants or confronting them.
3. Consultants can provide a more objective perspective on the team's operations.
4. Consultants are perceived as having greater expertise and influence than someone within the organization (Hanson and Lubin, 1990, p. 85).

Disadvantages to use of a consultant are the length of time needed for an external person to understand the work culture, its members, and how the two interact. A consultant can assist a team-building effort in the following ways*:

---

*Reprinted from *Organization Development Practitioner,* Spring, 1986. Used with permission.

1. A consultant can help team members become aware of the group process and how it functions.
2. A consultant can coach or counsel team leaders and members, both within and away from team meetings.
3. A consultant can act as a referee in conflicts among team members that should be resolved away from team meetings.
4. A consultant can discuss theory, when appropriate, to highlight or clarify team issues and problems.
5. A consultant can reinforce (support) norms of openness and authenticity among team members.
6. A consultant can assist team members to identify and develop their own resources and skills to complement and eventually supplant those of the consultant (Hanson and Lubin, 1990, pp. 85-86).

Too often, organizations allow consultants or vendors to take ownership of change. In most situations, the organizational development consultant is hired as an idea generator, discussion moderator, or planning assistant. The consultant represents an objective listener and offers solutions or cures that the organization may wish to consider. The consultant performs a midwife role; the cure is born of the organization.

Whether the team leader is an outside consultant, inside consultant, or team member who has the necessary skills, the leader needs to help the team to continually evaluate the process, not only the shared governance implementation goals, but also the team's ability to work as a unit toward that goal. The 12 characteristics of an effective team that were previously listed provide objective criteria to use in assessing the team's actual performance versus how individuals wish the team would perform. By maintaining this focus, problems become evident and suggestions can be offered for team development.

EXPECTED ROLES AND BEHAVIORS IN SHARED GOVERNANCE STRUCTURES
Establishing Goals and Priorities

In managing the changes to shared governance, seeking role clarity is a constant process. As the nursing department establishes its goals and priorities in the implementation process, the need to change decision making becomes an obvious issue. These role expectations can be clarified only when the expected outcome is known.

For example, the nurse manager's role in working with the department heads increases as the implementation process progresses. This involves a change in role for many nurse managers and for their superiors. By keeping focused on the goals, personality conflicts can sometimes be resolved more easily. If the nursing management group determines that the role of the nurse manager is to solve operational problems and that the role of directors is solving policy and system issues, both can work separately and enact their roles for the success of implementation.

The only factor that changes this problem from a simple to a complex one is the fact that different individuals have different priorities. It is therefore important that each nursing department answer the following questions:

1. What are the differences between operational and system problems?
2. What are the role expectations members have for each other?
3. How shall group members deal with the organization's response?
4. What is the plan for changing roles in the future?

The answers to these questions can guide the continuous role clarification process, which requires participation of all staff members.

Active Participation in Decisions

Establishment of priorities for predetermined goals involves active participation of all members of the nursing department. The decision-making process changes in shared governance. As many decisions as possible are made at the unit level, just as in any decentralized structure. However, in shared governance, decisions made by the staff council are the decisions that are enacted. Conflicts are mediated by the executive council, and the appropriate decision-making body is determined.

Individuals within the department have the responsibility to be effective followers and, if they desire, effective leaders. Effective followers share their opinions and relevant information with their group. They seek clarification of information so that they can understand issues and problems the nursing department is facing in implementation of a change. Effective followers also share their successes and act as resources to other members of the nursing department.

The leader's role in a shared governance structure is to facilitate a group's determination of how to achieve its goals. This involves quieting loquacious members, encouraging silent members, summarizing, and drawing the group to conclusions through consensus.

The goal of consensus building is to reach approval of a decision; it does not necessarily involve agreement. "Can I live with this decision?" is the question each individual must answer at the time of the decision. It may not be an individual's favorite choice, but it must be a decision that the individual is willing to support. This support is important when allocation of workload decisions is made.

Allocation of Workload

Decisions on accountability are determined in the council. The workload of everyone in council is determined by speed of implementation and negotiated agreements with other councils and the nursing department as a whole.

For example, the education council may decide that all staff members need training in participatory decision making. That decision clearly affects the unproductive time budget of a nurse manager. The workload of all members increases because staff members need to arrange for each others' participation. Everyone is affected by such a decision. However, it had previously been determined that the education council has the responsibility for determining the priorities of education for the staff. Therefore all criticism about the effects on the workload should be redirected to the council that took responsibility for the earlier decision.

All nursing departments complain about the additional workload of shared governance; however, all mention a benefit of this added workload: it has forced all staff members to learn to delegate. Delegation as a process assigns the authority and responsibility for completing an assignment; it involves fostering accountability in the follow-up process.

Monitoring Group Process

The task and process goal completion take different directions. The task focus is driven by the establishment of goals and priorities. Monitoring the group process needs should be an active choice.

Group process involves many dynamics, but only one will be discussed. Norms (the expected behavior of members)—functional or dysfunctional—largely determine the output of meetings.

Norms relate to groups as habits to individuals. An individual may have a habit of lateness. If there are many individuals who are repeatedly allowed to be late for meetings (shift-to-shift reports or staff or council meetings), the team has a dysfunctional norm of lateness in the department or unit. If the group is known for its innovative solutions to problems, there is a functional norm of encouraging creativity.

Monitoring the group process involves the continuous examination of dysfunctional norms that inhibit the group's work. Facilitating the group in determining ways to remove these blocks and move forward is the role of chairperson of the councils. Moving forward includes developing strategies to improve the processes of decision making and conflict resolution.

Continuous Resolution of Interpersonal and Intergroup Conflict

You need to surround yourself with able people who will argue back.
W. Beckett, Chairman, Woolworths

If the input of capable workers is not considered, the innovation necessary for any successful change will be lost. To allow people to argue with a leader facilitates a departmental or unit norm that allows open conflict resolution.

At times an outside facilitator may be necessary to maintain the group's focus on the resolution of a particularly difficult issue. For example, in the process of role clarification, the possible elimination of positions usually evolves. Individuals may not feel safe to engage in this type of discussion or one that involves questioning the "boss's decisions" without an objective person at the meeting. This is especially true if the group has a norm of nonconfrontation.

Intergroup conflict between individuals of different levels is a natural part of the second stage of team building. In this stage, conflicts over roles, rights, and values emerge. All members need to focus on the seeking of clarity of expected roles and behaviors in a nursing department through constant conflict resolution as a group and in their relationships with each other. This conflict resolution clears the path for individuals to focus on the larger issues of the change process. The next section focuses on how to obtain commitment to the ongoing process of shared governance implementation.

OBTAINING COMMITMENT

Achieving participation requires attention to soliciting ideas, encouraging discussion and debate, integrating diverse input, and managing group processes. Participation increases when subordinates have access to information and have knowledge about the situation in question. The manager needs to recognize that proposals from staff are more likely to be successfully implemented than are changes imposed by authority. In theory, people who participate in making a decision are better motivated to execute it. Staff involvement can also improve the quality of decision making because many of the participants are close to the action. Finally, participative decision making facilitates effective on-the-job training and helps subordinates develop.

Participation encourages commitment. As individuals become involved in implementation of shared governance, they begin to feel connected to other team members. When they see that their contributions are appreciated, feelings of personal worth bring a sense of fulfillment. As individuals share their expertise, often working together in teams, they begin to understand the meaning of teamwork. Involvement in councils provides opportunities for individuals and the group as a whole to commit to the process of shared governance. If the nursing department chooses the empowerment path to shared governance, well-articulated commitment will be valuable in the "ups and downs" of the change.

The nurse executive begins the process by committing to restructure the organization to a new framework. This personal commitment initiates the change to a new set of practices that requires the energies of the executive and other leaders in a nursing department. The energy becomes self-perpetuating, impelling the nursing department to continue in its new direction. This high degree of professional commitment is an essential cornerstone in achieving a shared governance framework.

The nursing administrator who makes this decision must also realize that once the door has been opened and the people begin to experience shared governance, the door can never be closed again. Therefore, the commitment is not for the short term. It is not periodic, or temporary, or just a trial. It is one that makes a statement that will have a lasting impact on the nursing organization.

Porter-O'Grady and Finnegan, 1984, p. 123

This commitment is not to be regarded lightly because it commits the organization as well as the executive. The nurse executive must begin with the person immediately superior, interpreting the shared governance concept in the most palatable way possible given the superior's manner of thinking.

Initially, commitment springs from an enthusiastic nurse executive; however, the involvement of all nursing management in sustaining commitment is crucial. Because movement from a traditional nursing organization to one of real shared governance requires 3 to 5 years for implementation, commitment will be tested many times.

One problem that may be encountered is a lack of enthusiasm at the nurse manager level, which seems to occur for two reasons. First, nurse managers are not as informed about the shared governance process as might be expected. They tend to not be included in many educational programs concerning shared governance and skill training, mostly because people believe they "already know about it." Second, the nurse managers are seen as accountable for their units, regardless of the level of functioning of the council.

For example, a physician may want a simple "yes" or "no" answer from the manager to a request for change in product; in reality, the answer requires a decision that the practice council is now responsible for making. Physicians may pressure the nurse manager for simple solutions, thereby testing the nurse manager's commitment to the process of council decisions. Closely related to commitment is the ability to visualize results of departmental change.

Envisioning

To facilitate commitment of nurse managers and staff, clear vision and conflict resolution skills are needed to deal with persons who, for various reasons, lack commitment. Envisioning is a process that can help create agreement regarding the future. The focus is on the question of "What future is desirable?" Follow the vision of a desired future with strategy for action, and the foundation is laid for decisive action to occur. Envisioning can be likened to "A large-scale brainstorming exercise in which participants have an opportunity not only to predict what will happen but to say what should happen" (HAP, 1990).

Resolving Conflict

To sustain the commitment to shared governance, the nursing department needs to continually resolve intradepartmental and interdepartmental conflicts. The unresolved conflicts naturally surface in a shared governance process. Each individual must take an active stance in the process, both in speaking and listening. Each individual should also commit to "fair fighting rules" determined by the group.

If a group commits to do whatever is necessary to succeed in implementing shared governance, the members automatically commit to resolve conflicts. Shared governance cannot occur without ongoing conflict resolution.

Communication ground rules and education about conflict resolution thus need attention early in the process. The box on p. 154 lists a department of nursing's communication ground rules. Education on conflict resolution should focus on assertiveness and negotiation skills. Self-assessment, opportunity for role play and discussion, and practical skills should be the core of the program. Dealing with difficult people and collaborating with other departments are also important.

Role of Followers

"Lead, follow or get out of my way," read a plaque on the desk of President Eisenhower. Leading and following are as important to the success of shared governance as they are in any other enterprise. Followers need to know their leader is

---

BOX 6-1

Ground Rules for Communication

---

1. There will be no cancellation of meetings
2. All members will attend the monthly administrative update meeting
3. Administrative update will be held on the first Tuesday of the month from 9:00 to 11:00 AM
4. Individuals are to submit agenda items by noon on Friday of the previous week
5. The agenda will be placed in mailboxes on the Monday before this meeting
6. Individuals will attend the meeting, send a representative, or arrange to take notes of the meeting from someone else
7. Anyone who cannot attend the meeting will inform the chairperson
8. Vice President/Director of Nursing will integrate in the seating arrangement in meetings
9. Facilitators will be appointed for each meeting to help the group stay on track, draw out silent members, and provide guidance to group members; two to three members will be assigned to provide process observation at each meeting
10. The turnaround time for distribution of the minutes of the administrative update meeting will be 1 to 2 weeks
11. The meeting will begin and end on time
12. Chairperson of meeting will state up front whether the issue is closed or open for discussion
13. No verbal attacks will be allowed
14. It is agreed that "what is said in the group stays in the group"
15. Individuals are to speak directly and honestly to others involved in a conflict; persons who do not do so will be confronted by group member(s) involved
16. Everyone is to focus on thinking before speaking
17. In meetings, individuals will listen when not speaking to the group (Used with permission from Presbyterian Medical Center of Philadelphia, Department of Nursing, 1990)

---

an honest person. Before followers can play an active role in their commitment, they need to believe their leader is an individual of integrity.

Followers also need to take an active part in determining the direction of the shared governance evolving in the department. Consensus decision making fosters the group's commitment to shared governance in two ways. First, because one member can block approval, the group is forced to actively communicate agreements and disagreements; otherwise, consensus decision making remains a cumbersome process. Second, skills that are at the core of consensus building are facilitation skills necessary for the leadership role in shared governance.

Both leading and following are active processes in the change to shared governance. The manager initially provides the leadership until others can begin to develop their leadership skills. The role of the manager in facilitating this process of consensus and empowerment is discussed next.

TRANSITIONAL ROLE OF THE MANAGER
Letting Go

Careers of most managers have been focused on taking charge, taking control, and being responsible—in other words, having the "final say" in all decisions for which they are held accountable by the organization. For example, most present quality assurance programs are more concerned with monitoring problems than with providing a forum for innovation. Until recently, control of staffing and scheduling was considered the final bastion of necessary managerial control.

It is understandable that most managers have trouble relinquishing control. To move from a role of director and controller to that of facilitator of empowerment is equivalent to a paradigm shift. The shift is best seen in communication between management and staff. Communication is no longer on a parent-to-child level but has become adult to adult. Management no longer provides a solution; staff now decides on the solution. The manager's role in this paradigm shift is one of helping the staff solve problems, giving them authority, and supporting them in accepting accountability.

Shared governance demands of a manager increased risk-taking because of the necessity for divesting management of the ultimate decision-making power. The more inflexible, dogmatic, and controlling a manager is, the more painful the process. Such managers need coaching from the nursing executive to relinquish control.

Managers also should understand the important difference between delegation and empowerment: delegation is assignment, whereas empowerment involves helping staff to accept responsibility and accountability. Delegation of duties exists simultaneously with empowerment of staff; it is an empowerment tool, but delegation is not empowerment.

Sharing Power

There are many forms of power, and principles that govern its use. In the shared governance model, the power of expertise is a dominant force. As a nursing manager gives up being the only "legitimate power" and shares decision making with practice, education, quality assurance, and governance councils, shared governance is born.

The speed with which a nurse executive and managers share power depends on the nature of the organizational culture. Some organizations publicly affirm support but continue to practice power brokering on a daily basis.

Many individuals in such organizations believe in the scarcity model of power and therefore have difficulty with the implementation of shared governance. The basic difference between scarcity models and empowerment is that the former focuses on the concept that a limited amount of power exists to be distributed among a few individuals, whereas empowerment in shared governance is based on the power sharing of all in a collaborative effort. This collaboration fosters a sense of personal power in members and power of collected energy in the change process.

For example, as education needs are determined by staff, a nurse manager no longer needs to force people to attend in-service training through legitimate power. Instead, through communication and collaboration of the education and quality assurance councils, immediate and long-term educational needs surface. A nurse manager may facilitate consensus decision making for educational priorities, but needs and solutions are developed primarily through action of the councils.

Facilitating Consensus

Consensus decision making lies somewhere between majority rule and unanimous agreement. Facilitating consensus involves helping the group reach an agreement on decisions. This requires all members to approve the decision, even though they may not agree with it. Therefore consensus decision making requires that all opinions be heard, that discussion of the issues occur, and that every member agree to support the decision.

In majority rule, individuals are pressured, either overtly or covertly, to agree with the decision. In consensus decision making, individuals are not coerced. To avoid coercion, the nurse manager must allow differences to be voiced and facilitate working through them to accomplish the goals of the group.

The transitional role of the nurse manager involves facilitating consensus in a variety of decisions. This process involves modeling the method to achieve consensus, keeping the group focused on the subject, and helping determine when and how to accomplish the chosen decision. All members should articulate concerns, each using individual skills.

The manager needs to provide information to the group so that the councils can make decisions while linking executive management to the process. The manager initially takes an active role in facilitation of group process and provides effective structure for meetings. Gradually, as their skills develop, staff members will join in facilitating others.

In the role of facilitator, the nurse manager begins to identify blocks to effective group decision making. Individuals who squash suggestions in the group need coaching. If the issue is a dysfunctional group norm rather than individuals who inhibit action, the entire group needs to hear the feedback.

For example, a nurse manager facilitates consensus in the practice council if she or he encourages several new members to talk about models of practice they experienced in institutions where they previously worked. The new members can offer a different perspective, and they can also begin to understand the practices in a new organization. Unchallenged practice standards negate the quality improvement stimulated by the quality assurance council's questions and changes.

The Manager as Teacher and Leader

The role of the nurse manager changes dramatically in a shared governance model. No longer is the role of manager to control the staff to prevent irresponsibility and sloth. That method may have been appropriate in the industrial age,

---

BOX 6-2
Knowledge Base for Managers

- Leadership behavior
- Facilitation skills
- Knowledge of how to conduct a meeting
- Coaching and mentoring behavior
- Team-building
- Conflict resolution: assertiveness and negotiation skills
- Understanding of shared governance model and process

---

when tasks were the focus. However, in the information age, the nurse manager should act not as controller but as teacher and leader. By modeling each of these roles, the nurse manager literally teaches by example. The leader facilitates the department or unit in developing a vision and in taking the steps to achieve it, helping staff to develop the shared governance structure, and involving individuals in accomplishing their vision. A leader takes responsibility to act on the issues that the councils raise. As the organization develops, the nurse manager will be needed less as a spokesperson, but for the first several years is often the voice of the unit.

Part of the leadership role is to determine learning needs of staff members. Some of their needs can be met through predetermined in-service training and continuing education and through the manager's coaching, but some needs must be programmed. The education council and the nurse manager work together to determine educational needs. Because of knowledge of and access to numerous educational resources, the nurse manager's main role is that of facilitator and link to the organization and outside resources.

Role modeling naturally occurs as a nurse manager acts as a teacher to staff. To teach, a knowledge of several important subject areas is crucial. These assets are listed in the box above.

These areas are the basis for behaviors required of a nurse manager for successful change through shared governance. However, the test of the manager's ability to empower is not her or his own functioning but the capacity of the unit or organization to respond and grow in an ever-changing world. The following contributions not only help to define the construct of empowerment but can also be used as a firm foundation for implementing it*:

1. **Values.** Argyris' (1955) classic discussion of the management dilemma— company needs versus individual development
2. **Leadership.** The discussions of Tannenbaum, Kallajian, and Weschler (1954); Bennis (1982); and Lippitt and This (1967) on the characteristics of effective group leaders

---

*Reprinted from J.F. Vogt and K.L. Murrell (1990). Empowerment in organizations: how to spark exceptional performance, San Diego, University Associates, Inc. Used with permission.

3. **Environment.** Rogers' (1961) work on the environmental climate that allows facilitative (empowering) processes to become operational
4. **Adult learning.** Knowles' (1975) description of learning as a lifelong process, and its implications for the adult learner; and the conceptualization of experimental learning (Kolb, Rubin, and McIntryre, 1971)
5. **Organizational structure.** Gibb's (1964) recognition of the relations among individual needs (e.g., trust), communication, goals, and organizational structure
6. **Systems integration.** Recognition of the connections between organizational health and individual welfare and the postwar application of systems analysis to the integration of technological and human systems (Vogt and Murrell, 1990)

All of these contributions lead to our present understanding of empowerment. A nurse manager familiar with these concepts will be able to teach and model staff empowerment behaviors.

Leadership is currently a popular written and oral subject. It has been said that the United States suffers from a leadership crisis. What is leadership, and how can the nurse manager demonstrate it?

Leading, not managing, is the goal. In the shared governance model, a nurse manager is freed to lead as councils begin to function. The time this change provides can then be used for conceptualizing, for being a leader with vision and time to consider the forces that affect the realization of the vision. Development of a vision (management of attention) is one of the leadership traits identified by Bennis and Nanus (1965). The other three leadership traits necessary for nurse managers are management of attention, management of meaning, management of trust, and management of self (Bennis and Nanus, 1985).

Having vision is the first of four leadership traits identified by Bennis and Nanus. Annual retreats for top-level nursing management and yearly evaluation and commitment for the unit-level vision are structures that support this skill.

Mentoring is the second leadership competency. Leaders make ideas tangible to others, so that others can support these ideas. A nurse manager's own clarity concerning the shared governance model and effective communication skills are keys for success.

The third competency is the management of trust. People much prefer to follow individuals they can rely on, even when they disagree with those persons' viewpoints, than follow those who shift positions frequently. A manager must be perceived as willing to uphold his or her beliefs. Regardless of the staff members' stance regarding the belief, they know the manager is consistent. Followers need this level of integrity in all who assume leadership roles in shared governance.

The fourth leadership competency is the management of self. This is the ability of a leader to know his or her own skills and to use them effectively. It is equally important for the nurse manager to demonstrate the ability to admit a mistake. Mistakes must be seen as steps to success. Such leadership empowers the work force. Empowerment is the collective effect of leadership.

WOMEN AS LEADERS

The 1990s is seen as the decade of women in leadership. This is a force supporting nurses in taking leadership roles (Naisbitt and Aburdene, 1990). To be a business leader today, it is no longer an advantage to have been socialized as a male. Women may be at a slight advantage because they need to "unlearn" old authoritarian management behaviors. This new democratic, yet demanding, leadership encourages self-management, autonomous teams, the ability to employ vision that will be the driving force in the 1990s.

Time magazine dedicated an entire issue in the fall of 1990 entitled "Women: The Road Ahead" (Time, Fall 1990). A *Time* poll of 505 men and women ages 18 to 24 by Yankelovich, Clancy, and Shulman found that four of five believed it is difficult to juggle work and family and that too much pressure is being placed on women to bear the burden. Until now, women have been silent and followed the rules. Clearly, they now want a different set of rules. It is true that women have increased their participation in medicine and management by 300% to 400% since the early '70s. However, *Fortune* magazine found in July of 1989 that in the highest echelons of corporate management, fewer than 0.5% were female. It is evident that the female majority must still find a way to survive what they may feel are uncaring institutions, exploiting employers, and deep social inequities. Harvard psychologist Carol Gilligan (1982), author of *In a Different Voice,* a landmark study of gender differences, argues that women have greater moral strengths, a stronger ethical stance, and concern for making and maintaining relationships— all qualities of a good leader.

An effective leader for the 1990s, either male or female, will set an example of excellence and be ethical, empowering, and inspiring. A leader who is a facilitator knows how to elicit answers from those who are most knowledgeable. The primary challenge of a nurse manager is to encourage professional nurses to be more self-managing and oriented toward lifelong learning.

COACHING

In terms of importance, the consensus-building skills of leaders are closely followed by the coaching role for the nurse manager. During transition, some individuals demonstrate reluctance to move forward with the model. This is especially true if the organization has experienced other changes that lacked follow-through. This coaching role involves helping develop individuals to function in the new model.

Many nursing leaders like Dorothea Dix, Clara Barton, and Elizabeth Sanger faced both internal and external resistance when they tried to implement a model that would change the practice of nursing. Their patience, persistence, and constant focus on the desired outcome helped them overcome the direst circumstances. They achieved their objectives by continuous positive focus on their goals.

Nurse managers must remember why they agreed to the implementation of shared governance—there will be days like these nursing leaders faced. At such

TABLE 1
Stages of Team Development

	Member Behaviors	Member Concerns	Leader Behaviors
Stage I Orientation to group and task	• Almost all comments directed to the leader • Direction and clarification sought • Status accorded to group members based on their roles outside the group • Members fail to listen, resulting in nonsequitur statements • Issues are discussed superficially, with much ambiguity	• Who am I in this group? • Who are the others? • Will I be accepted? • What is my role? • What tasks will I have? • Will I be capable? • Who is the leader? • Will he or she value me? • Is the leader competent?	• Provide structure by holding regular meetings and assisting task and role clarification • Encourage participation by all, domination by none • Facilitate learning about one another's areas of expertise and preferred working modes • Share all relevant information • Encourage members to ask questions of you and one another
Stage II Conflict over control among the group's members and with the leader	• Attempts made to gain influence, suggestions, proposals • Subgroups and coalitions form, with possible conflicts among them • The leader is tested and challenged (possibly covertly) • Members judge and evaluate one another and the leader, resulting in ideas being shot down • Task avoidance	• How much autonomy will I have? • Will I have influence over others? • What is my place in the pecking order? • Personal level: Who do I like? Who likes me? • Issue level: Do I have some support here?	• Engage in joint problem solving; have members give reasons why idea is useful and how to improve it • Establish a norm supporting the expression of different viewpoints • Discuss the group's decision-making process and share decision-making responsibility appropriately • Encourage members to state how they feel as well as what they think when they obviously have feelings about an issue • Provide group members with the resources needed to do their jobs, to the extent possi-

Stage	Characteristics	Questions	Leader Actions
			ble (when it is not possible, explain why)
Stage III Group formulation and solidarity	Members, with one another's support, can disagree with the leader	How close should I be to the group members?	Talk openly about your own issues and concerns
	The group laughs together; members have fun; some jokes made at the leader's expense	Can we accomplish our tasks successfully?	Have group members manage agenda items, particularly those in which you have a high stake
	A sense of "we-ness" and attention to group norms is present	How do we compare to other groups?	Give and request both positive and constructive negative feedback in the group
	The group feels superior to other groups in the organization	What is my relationship to the leader?	Assign challenging problems for consensus decisions (e.g., budget allocations)
	Members do not challenge one another as much as the leader would like		Delegate as much as the members are capable of handling; help them as necessary
Stage IV Differentiation and productivity	Roles are clear and each person's contribution is distinct	(Concerns of earlier stages have been resolved)	Jointly set goals that are challenging
	Members take the initiative and accept one another's initiative		Look for new opportunities to increase group's scope
	Open discussion and acceptance of differences among members in their backgrounds and modes of operation		Question assumptions and traditional ways of behaving
	Challenging one another leads to creative problem solving		Develop mechanisms for ongoing self-assessment by the group
	Members seek feedback from one another and from the leader to improve their performance		Appreciate each member's contribution
			Develop members to their fullest potential through task assignment and feedback

Reprinted with permission from Moosbrucker, J. (1988). "Developing a Productivity Team: Making Groups at Work Work." In W. B. Reddy and K. Jamilson (Eds.), *Team Building: Blueprints for Productivity and Satisfaction* (pp. 91-92). National Teaching Laboratories Institute.

times the nurse manager needs to encourage, enliven, console, and boost the spirits of staff if they are to move forward in the empowerment process.

For example, staff members are usually enthusiastic about the shared governance model until they first encounter resistance. This resistance can take many forms, such as poor attendance at council meetings, noncompletion of assignments, or gossip about the leaders. Nurse managers must remain objective at these times and continue to coach the members to become effective leaders and to model teaching and leading.

A nurse manager in a leadership role acts as the team coach, guiding the individual in learning new behaviors. At times the manager stands back, watches the performance, and then provides feedback to the individual. As team coach the manager also assumes responsibility for effective functioning of the work unit team.

Much of the team-building work can be done only by the manager and other persons involved in activities for which the team was formed. A team-building consultant can help with some processes and can conduct specific events for the unit, but it is the daily influence of the nurse manager on the norms and team climate that is most important.

The nurse manager's guidance and sustained effort toward realizing a team's vision makes team-building happen. The manager guides the team through the four stages of team development, monitoring and assisting the progress of the group's evolution. A group model can have three, four, or five stages; however, the model that appears most useful is listed in Table 1 (Moosbrucker, 1990).

Many nursing departments languish in Stage II because they lack conflict resolution skills and fail to understand empowerment. For example, the nurse manager who cannot abide bickering among team members stops discussions. This is avoidance of conflict rather than conflict resolution. In this stage, the nurse manager must help group members deal with their differences with one another and between the group and the leader. If discussion becomes heated, then the leader's role is to ensure that each position is heard and, as much as possible, understood.

Dealing with staff members who are not "team players" is also a crucial role of the nurse manager. If a norm develops that such individuals are allowed to be disruptive and noncooperative and not perform their share of the work, then the team will not be effective and will waste time and energy dealing with nonteam players. At least initially, a nurse manager needs to be primarily coach and teacher for these individuals. As a peer review committee forms and as the council chairs gain strength and skills, they too can help in the coaching. The nurse manager, in addition to coaching, should work closely with one to two individuals, grooming them as replacements. This process of mentoring is discussed in more detail in the next section.

MENTORING

Is mentoring becoming a lost art? In the nursing community, a lack of mentoring is evident. Perhaps this lack is part of oppressed group behavior. Inferiors do not turn to other inferiors for guidance. However, if nurses are to move forward as professionals, mentoring needs to become part of their repertoire.

What Is Mentoring?

Mentoring is a system of selection and guidance in which individuals senior in position and experience identify and educate their juniors and promote them to positions of leadership. Mentoring is supporting career advancement. Like parenting, mentoring requires sensitivity as to when to intervene and when to let go. A mentor serves as a career role model and actively advises, guides, and promotes another's career and training. Mentoring helps people adapt by increasing their confidence. It is a process by which staff members are guided, taught, and influenced in their life work in important ways.

The role of a mentor is to foster employee development through socialization and skill development. Mentors show responsibility for the career advancement of the protege. They provide opportunities to carry out activities that make the best use of a protege's ability.

Mentor Behaviors

The roles of teacher and leader in shared governance are aspects of mentoring. A list of mentor behaviors is provided below:

1. Shares career experiences as an accomplished practitioner
2. Provides ready access to organizational information
3. Channels opportunities to neophytes
4. Establishes mutual goals
5. Takes risks in people
6. Identifies talent
7. Risks emotional involvement
8. Gives constructive feedback to protegé on problem areas
9. Gives positive reinforcement (Campbell-Heider, 1986; Bidwell, 1989)

A mentor coaches, inspires, and supports the growth and development of individuals. Coaching behaviors are a major ingredient in mentoring. A list of mentor behaviors is provided below:

1. Stimulates enthusiasm
2. Maintains high expectations
3. Gives credit for performance
4. Approachable
5. Listens to new ideas
6. Encourages risk taking
7. Helps people learn from mistakes
8. Acts sensitively to feelings of others
9. Believes people can be more effective

In shared governance, the importance of offering opportunities to neophytes, listening to their ideas, and maintaining high expectations is self-evident.

Several studies on mentoring support these behaviors as being key in teaching mentoring. In the Fagin (1983) study, the traits that nurses selected as most characteristic of their mentors were the following:

- Disciplined and hard worker
- Dedicated to job
- Independent
- Honest
- Persistent and tactful

In the White (1988) study on nursing academic administrators and mentoring, the highest-rated characteristics were the following:

- Showed confidence in me
- His or her knowledge inspired me
- Encouraged me to achieve maximum potential
- Encouraged my intellectual development

Competency and intelligence were the most frequent characteristics listed of mentors. The study also showed that those who had mentors were more likely to mentor. Studies by Henning and Jardim (1977) concluded that it was essential for women to have a mentor.

The mentoring experience benefits the mentor in several ways. First is a feeling of fulfillment in seeing another nurse flourish. There is also a sense of fulfillment in contributing to the advancement of the profession. Because of the value of interdependence, the protege may act as a referral. Finally, a protege's questions act as stimulus to thought and research.

TRIALS AND TRIBULATIONS, JOYS AND ACCOMPLISHMENTS OF SHARED GOVERNANCE

As with any change, there are always unexpected problems as well as minor miracles. The implementation of shared governance reveals any unresolved problems in a nursing department and in the organization. A paternalistic culture will become evident, as will any internal strife in the nursing department and individuals who need coaching. As a nursing department reorganizes, all roles and responsibilities are questioned. People's relationships to each other change, and individuals, perhaps for the first time, begin to understand the meaning of accountability. The ripples of this change will be felt in other departments. It is important to remember that this change will create trials and tribulations for all who undertake it.

Trials take various forms. A person who is a source of annoyance or irritation may block shared governance, knowingly or unknowingly. Outdated policies and systems at times try one's endurance. The nursing department's commitment to the process will be tested many times. A few examples of typical trials faced in implementation are listed. All have been addressed previously except the last.

1. One or more nonteam players
2. Passive aggressive behavior

3. Lack of attendance or participation in meetings
4. Controlling manager
5. Lack of accountability

A nurse who accepts accountability thinks beyond his or her shift. Accountability comes from within. It cannot be taken away. For example, a clinical nurse is held accountable by law to the code of ethics and, therefore, the quality of practice. In shared governance, practice councils help individuals and departments develop methods to reward nurses for accountability. Peer review and quality assurance councils provide directions for the education a nurse needs in practicing accountability.

The joys that arise from accomplishments may seem distant at first, but they gradually replace distress, affording the participants renewed commitment. The most obvious change in staff is an increased sense of personal power. The "victim" mentality changes as nurses become assertive and negotiate with their peers and nurse manager. As they see the results of their efforts in more control over their practice environment, most exert continued effort. The expectation of peer review affords the opportunity for staff members to deal with the nonteam players.

Self-scheduling, even with its many initial trials, provides individuals with a sense of authority and control over their work life. Nurse managers are often glad to be relieved of the burden that rarely yielded any source of satisfaction other than relief upon completion. A high level of staff flexibility and sense of team participation can make this process smoother.

As the autonomy of each individual in the department increases, individuals begin to understand the nature of professionalism. High standards, shared power base, and peer feedback all facilitate individuals' accountability. Individual concerns merge with professional concerns as members of the nursing department coalesce.

As more nursing department members actively participate in implementation of shared governance, they work with people from other units. Multilevel and interconnecting work teams form to implement changes. Rapport and closeness develop as power and control struggles are resolved. This cohesion is necessary to weather the tribulations that result from such a major change.

Collegiality—the sharing of authority among colleagues—is the process and the outcome of shared governance. In this environment, shared governance flourishes. Conquering each step along the way can offer individuals a sense of accomplishment. It is crucial for all to stay focused on the goal, to remain flexible, and to celebrate accomplishments as they occur.

SUMMARY

Shared governance provides a model for continuous management of change. Lewin's model of change (1947) (unfreezing, change, and refreezing) provides a process for fostering change and maintaining equilibrium. A set of eight guidelines also helps to maintain the focus on the empowering of the nursing staff.

Empowerment requires creating and maintaining motivation in a change process; organizational and individual strategies are necessary. An overview of six points in fostering motivation in the organization is followed by a focus on McClelland's theory of motivation (1971). Managers encourage people to participate by knowing how to stimulate individuals' enthusiasm, creating an expectation that what they do will make a difference, and providing a reward worth their efforts.

Another organizational strategy is team-building. The 12 characteristics of an effective team focus on the process and the task functions that build a team. It is noted that dysfunctional group norms can block the work at hand. Consultants are often used in the team-building process because they are able to provide an objective perception of the team's operations. They also help to decrease the team members' reluctance to confront their own managers. A consultant can assist in team-building effort in six ways.

One way is clarification of roles. Role clarification is important in the team-building process to reduce intragroup and interpersonal conflict. As the shared governance process proceeds, the role of the first line manager, her/his supervisor, and the staff changes. Four questions guide the role clarification process.

For effective implementation of shared governance, the nurse manager and council chairpersons encourage active participation of all members, allocate workload, and monitor group process. Moving forward also includes developing strategies to improve the process of conflict resolution and decision making.

Research suggests that people who have helped make a decision are better motivated to execute it. Involvement in councils provides opportunities for individuals and the group to commit to the process of shared governance. To facilitate commitment of nurse managers and staff, clear vision and conflict resolution skills are needed to deal with those who lack commitment.

To sustain the commitment to shared governance, nursing departments need to continually resolve intradepartmental and interdepartmental conflicts. Communication ground rules and education on conflict resolution thus require attention early in the process. Excellent communication skills in the nurse manager help the manager deal with the inevitable conflicts and provide staff with a role model.

The transitional role of the nurse manager involves relinquishing control and moving to the role of facilitator. By facilitating consensus, the manager helps the group reach an agreement on decisions. In the role of facilitator, the nurse manager also identifies blocks to effective group decision making.

The role of the nurse manager changes dramatically in the shared governance model. The change to a leader and teacher requires education of the nurse manager to coach the staff in the roles required for the success of shared governance. A list of subjects is provided in Table I.

A leader who is a facilitator knows how to elicit answers from those who know best about their work. The primary challenge of a nurse manager is to encourage professional nurses to engage in more self-management and to be oriented toward lifelong learning. This is best accomplished through role modeling, coaching, and mentoring.

Studies indicate that those who had mentors themselves are more likely to mentor, thereby fostering a supply of nursing leaders in the organization.

Finally, there are trials and tribulations as well as joys and accomplishments in shared governance. As a nursing department reorganizes, all roles and responsibilities are questioned. People's relationships to each other change, and individuals, perhaps for the first time, begin to grasp the meaning of accountability. The "victim" mentality changes as nurses become assertive and negotiate with their peers and nurse manager. The confusion that develops from working together as a team is seen as necessary to weather the tribulations that result from such a major change.

REFERENCES

Argyris, C. (1955). Top Management Dilemma: Company Needs Versus Individual Development. *Personnel, 32*(2), 123-134.

Bennis, W. G. (1982). The Art Form of Leadership. *Training and Development Journal, 36*(4), 44-46.

Bennis, W. and Nannus, B. (1985). *Leaders: The Strategies for Taking Charge.* New York: Harper & Row.

Bidwell, A.S. (1989). Role-modeling vs. Mentoring in Nursing Education. *Image, 21*(1), 23-25.

Burke, W.W. (1990). Team Building as a Group Development. In W. Reddy, and K. Jamison (Eds.), *Team Building: Blueprints for Productivity and Satisfaction* (p. 3). San Diego: N.T.L. Institute for Applied Behavioral Sciences.

Campbell-Heider, N. (1986). Do Nurses Need Mentors? *Image, 18*(3), 110-113.

Drucker, P. (1974). *Management.* New York: Harper & Row.

Fagin, M.M. and Fagin, P.D. (1983). Mentoring Among Nurses. *Nursing and Health Care, 4*(2), 72-82.

Francis, D. and Young, D. (1979). *Improving Work Groups* (p. 8). San Diego: University Associates.

Funches, D. (1990). Co-creating Partnerships for the Future. Speech presented at meeting of Organizational Development, Philadelphia.

Gilligan, C. (1982). *In a Different Voice: Psychological Theory and Women's Development.* Cambridge: Harvard University Press.

Hanson, P.G. and Lubin, B. (1990). Team Building as Group Development. *Organization Development Practitioner,* 27-35, Spring, 1986.

"HAP" (1990). Hospital Association Undertakes Structured Brainstorming Project to Look to Pennsylvania Health Care in the Year 2000. *Pennsylvania Hospital '90,* 1(8), 4.

Henning, M. and Jardim, A. (1977). *The Managerial Woman* (2nd ed.). New York: Anchor/Doubleday.

Hertzberg, F., Mausner, B., and Snyderman, B. (1959). *Motivation to Work.* New York: John Wiley.

Kast, F. and Rosenweig, J. (1974). *Organization and Management.* (2nd ed.) (pp. 574-575). New York: McGraw-Hill.

Knowles, M. S. (1975). *Self-Directed Learning: A Guide for Learners and Teachers.* New York: Cambridge Books.

Kolb, D., Rubin; I, and McIntyre, J. (1971). *Organizaional Psychology.* Englewood Cliffs, N.J.: Prentice-Hall.

Lewin, K. (1947). Frontiers in Group Dynamics: Concepts, Method and Reality in Social Science. *Human Relations,* (1), 5-42.

Lippitt, G. L. and This, L. E. (1967). Leaders for Laboratory Training: Selected Guidelines for Group Trainers Utilizing the Laboratory Method. *Training and Development Journal,* 3, 37-39.

Maslow, A. (1954). *Motivation and Personality,* New York: Harper & Row, Publishers.

McClelland, D. (1971). That Urge to Achieve. In DA Kolb, IM Rubin, and JM McIntyre (Eds.), *Organizational Psychology.* Englewood Cliffs, N.J.: Prentice-Hall, Inc.

McGregor, D. (1960). *The Human Side of Enterprise*. New York: McGraw-Hill.

Moosbrucker, J. (1990). Developing a Productivity Team: Making Groups at Work Work. In W. Reddy and K. Jamison (Eds.), *Team Building: Blueprints for Productivity and Satisfaction* (pp. 91-92). San Diego: N.T.L. Institute for Applied Behavioral Sciences.

Naisbitt, J. and Aburdene, P. (1990). *Megatrends 2000* (pp. 216-240). Chapter 7, The 1990s: Decade of Women in Leadership. New York: William Morrow & Company.

Porter-O'Grady, T. and Finnegan, S. (1984). *Shared Governance for Nursing: A Creative Approach to Professional Accountability*. Rockville, Md.: Aspen Publications.

Reddy W. and Jamison, K. (Eds.) (1990). Team Building: Blueprints for Productivity and Satisfaction. San Diego: N.T.L. Institute for Applied Behavioral Sciences.

Rogers, C. R. (1961). *On Becoming a Person: A Therapist's View of Psychotherapy*. Boston: Houghton-Mifflin.

Tannenbaum, R., Kallajian, V., and Weschler, I. R. (1954). Training Managers for Leadership. *Personnel*, 30, 3-11.

Time. (1990). Women: The Road Ahead. Fall Special Issue. 136(19).

Vogt, J.F. and Murrell, K.L. (1990). (Adapted). Empowerment in Organizations: How to Spark Exceptional Performance. San Diego: University Associates, Inc.

White, J.F. (1988). The Complete Role of Mentoring in the Career Development and Success of Academic Nurse Administrators. Journal of Professional Nursing, 4(3), 178-185.

7 *Integrating Differentiated Practice into Shared Governance*

JoEllen Goertz Koerner

Society is changing from an industrial society to a less materialistic and more personally fulfilling, ecologically sound society. This important development in the Western world is influencing roles and relationships in deep and meaningful ways. Consumers are becoming more involved in their health, placing an increasing emphasis on wellness and the development of their full potential. The medically dominated and controlled health care system is evolving toward a primary care distributive model in which patients select care based on real or perceived needs. All these changes call for new roles and relationships among various health care providers.

Nurses have historically been educated and socialized to assist people with self-care needs, both in an institutional setting and at home. In addition to providing care at the bedside, the nurse can now assume a role that coordinates the medical and nursing plan of care to facilitate a timely, prepared discharge. The nurse can also serve as a case manager for the chronically ill, the indigent, and the elderly who lack personal or financial assistance in their lives. This role establishes a partnership with the client, providing information and assistance in reaching a fully informed decision about ongoing self-care needs. These differentiated nursing roles require varying levels of clinical and interpersonal competence. The nurse must also share in the governance of professional practice issues if a true business partnership is to be realized.

In this time of unprecedented change, all health care agencies and providers are experiencing structural, fiscal, and boundary challenges of great magnitude. Organizational life has become messy as traditional roles, relationships, functional patterns, and prevailing belief systems must be reexamined. This time of chaos also presents an opportunity for the emergence of a new paradigm that will be liberating for all of humankind.

A paradigm is a world view about the phenomena of concern to a specific discipline that guides the practitioners' inquiry and creates scientific development. Kuhn (1970) introduced the concept of a paradigm shift to describe a radical change in the fundamental framework or way of thinking through which people

169

view their world. This altered world view requires a new intuition or insight as well as the consideration of new information, so that the discipline can see old and new aspects of its world through an altered framework.

Nursing has moved from a vocation to a professional discipline whose science has become visible in the twentieth century (Parse, 1987). Perceiving nursing as a profession, different from yet complementary to medicine, is a new idea to many nurses. Viewing hospitals and human service organizations in a business context is another new notion for most practitioners. The framework for professional nursing practice must be expanded beyond clinical expertise to include relational, leadership, and management skills. Nurses will influence patient care decisions both clinically and economically as they become true business partners with other major players in the health care system. Based on social systems theory, a blueprint can be created to guide the reframing and further development of professional nursing practice through the implementation of innovation.

A SYSTEMATIC APPROACH TO REDESIGNING ORGANIZATIONS

A *system* is an orderly arrangement of components that are interrelated, interdependent, and semiautonomous. Systems theory focuses on relationships between the parts of the whole in order to understand and predict behavior. Organizations are comprised of interrelated systems; thus phenomena are viewed as parts of these nested systems that must be investigated and analyzed simultaneously to comprehend the "totality."

The traditional concept of "organization as machine" has been predominant for the past several decades. Based on the theory of behaviorism, it assumed that employee behavior could and should be controlled. Control was most efficiently accomplished by identifying and using predictable cause-and-effect relationships to reach one's goal. Such organizations preferred that people act in a predictable, routine manner, accepting direction from authority without question. Adherence to impersonal, universal rules was valued more than subjective, autonomous action.

The physical and social worlds are now viewed as much more complex. Rules that used to be stable change from one day to another. Events are seen as ambiguous rather than predictable, influenced by many sources. Many events do not take place in assembly-line fashion. As employees become more educated, organizations benefit in shared decision making, which in turn increases the number of persons who influence causes and effects. Clear, hierarchical patterns of organization are being replaced by flatter, parallel patterns. Thus as persons and forces interact they influence and modify the output so that the entire picture changes, creating a dynamic and fluid reality (Marsick, 1990).

A new metaphor of "organization as a holographic brain" is emerging in response to this rapidly changing universe. The organization is compared to a human brain as an information processor. Based on principles of cybernetics, the organization views employees as centers of intelligence that can scan the environment, learn from mistakes, and adjust goals or plans to meet changing conditions. Thus individuals are self-directed and creative in approaching situations as they occur. In addition, the brain has a *holographic capacity* in which each portion of the brain contains information about the whole. The "whole" can be seen or sensed in any isolated segment of the organism. This makes the system both self-organizing and self-correcting. Table 2 compares the concepts of organizations as machines and organizations as brains.

Nursing as a system must be viewed as part of the greater social system as well as the health care delivery system (Brooten, Human, and Naylor, 1988). Social systems theory viewed through a holographic lens can be used to study human and organizational development in conjunction with social change. When applied to nursing, it can provide a provocative way to establish a clear professional identity. The profession is then free to organize new thinking about the components of nursing practice.

MANAGEMENT OF INNOVATION

Social and economic development depends on innovation and entrepreneurship. The stimulation and management of innovation has been identified as the central concern expressed by a group of chief executives (Van de Ven, 1982). They view innovation as the major solution to the inexorable pressures of balancing the demands from expanding technology through the specialization and proliferation of tasks, the escalating costs for achieving coordination, and the need for obtaining cooperation and conflict resolution in a rapidly changing environment.

TABLE 2

Comparison of the Organization as Machine to the Organization as Brain

Organization as Machine	Organizing Concept	Organization as Brain
• Predictable, stability is norm	Environmental conditions	• Ambiguous, change is norm
• Based on goal statements	Organizational ideology	• Based on an ideal philosophy
• Fixed with rigid boundaries	Organizational structure	• Tentative with fluid boundaries
• Assembly-line production	Organizational functioning	• Self-organizing, self-correcting
• Problem-oriented, transactional	Leadership traits	• Charismatic, transformational
• Controlling, directing	Leadership style	• Empowering, consulting
• Universal rules	Leadership directives	• Standards of competence
• Task- and reward-oriented	Individual motivation	• Values and ideals oriented
• Organizational hierarchy	Individual relationships	• Professional networks
• Prescriptive, mechanistic	Individual work style	• Innovative, creative

Contemporary nursing must cope with almost daily changes in organizational life as health care delivery systems respond to new developments in science, technology, and their client base. Institutions can no longer function with operational structures and processes based on conventional wisdom. Organizations must question many assumptions on which they have built past success. This situation demands fresh, innovative ways of using human resources and structuring workers' relationships with the internal and external environment (Mitroff, 1985).

The process of *innovation* is defined as "the development and implementation of new ideas by people who over time engage in transactions with others within an institutional context" (Van de Ven, 1986). The need to stimulate, understand, and manage innovation has been widely recognized (Ouchi, 1981; Peters and Waterman, 1982; Kanter, 1983; Lawrence and Dyer, 1983).

Creating A Conceptual Framework

Nursing administrators perform as general managers, dealing with issues that are different from, and more intangible than, those of functional unit managers. Lewin and Minton (1986) call for the nursing administrator to clearly identify the key components of their responsibility, noting the relationship of individual elements to the total operations.

Without a conceptual framework and theoretical base for understanding and addressing issues and barriers, problems in nursing recycle as symptomatic solutions fail. A conceptual framework can be designed to assist with visualization of the components of nursing practice and their relationship within the health care environment (Figure 7-1). Planning sessions with management and staff could identify the desired *outputs*, products of nursing service provided to clients within a hospital. The major *inputs*, the fiscal, material, and human resources necessary to provide those services, would then be enumerated. Components that create the most enriching and efficient structure and process for professional nursing practice were identified in the Magnet Hospital Study (McClure, 1983) conducted by the American Academy of Nursing. Four major factors were noted: participative management, a comprehensive patient care delivery system, collaborative relationships, and opportunities for personal and professional growth. These components comprise the process by which the inputs are converted to the goals of the nursing practice.

Creating A Vision

Based on the conceptual framework a *vision* would be created: The Department of Nursing will restructure the delivery of hospital nursing care by integrating nurses as professional business partners through interdependent relationships supported by a shared vision, open structure, and increased autonomy. A long-range strategic plan, complete with objectives and strategies, would then be created to assist the nursing department with innovations focused on true professional practice.

The glossary of terms in Box 7-1 clarifies the vision statement.

As the definitions indicate, the overall vision is created to combine the principles of empowerment, teamwork, and business acumen so that nurses are fully inte-

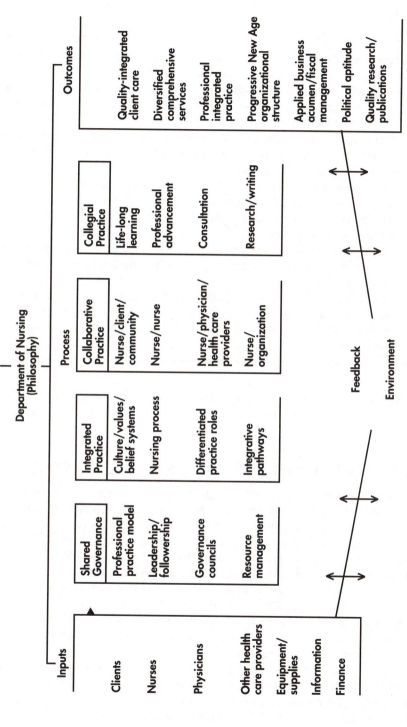

FIGURE 7-1. Conceptual framework for integrative nursing practice. (Used with permission from Sioux Valley Hospital, Sioux Falls, South Dakota.)

BOX 7-1
Glossary of Terms

Autonomy: Self-directing freedom and professional independence to influence the mobilization and allocation of resources on behalf of the patient.
Integration: The state of modifying individual goals to meet a broader objective through joining innovation and unity of effort within a given system or between related systems.
Interdependence: The state of attaining individual goals while being mutually influenced and benefited by another's contributions within a given system or between related systems.
Professional business partner: Nurses who have expanded their professional practice to include thought, behavior, and skills in business acumen. This fosters responsibility and accountability to the patient, the organization, and the society they serve.
Structure: A network of relationships among organizational positions that promotes equal opportunity and responsibility for information sharing and decision making.
Vision: A powerful mental image that clearly projects a future potential, inspiring the individuals to transform it into reality. Shared vision is the foundation for integration, unifying, and strengthening group process toward a mutual goal.

---

grated into an evolving health care industry as true professional partners to ensure their inclusion in the planning and execution of quality and cost-effective client care.

THE HUMAN CHALLENGE OF MANAGING ATTENTION

Nursing administrators occupy a unique position within the organization to identify problems and influence their resolution. They must also examine how the effects of organizational problems impact the implementation of an innovation. If the nursing administrator understands the process of innovation, she or he will understand the factors that facilitate and inhibit the progression of those innovations. Thus the administrator's management of ideas, people, transactions, and context throughout implementation of an innovation will ensure its success.

People and organizations are largely conditioned to focus on, cultivate, and protect existing practices rather than pay attention to the development of new ideas. The more successful an organization is, the more difficult it is to trigger people's attention toward new ideas, needs, and opportunities.

An innovation is a new idea that may be the recombination of old ideas, or something new and different. Although many ideas are presented in an organization, only a few receive serious consideration. If the idea is perceived as useful, it is an innovation. Ideas perceived as not useful are labeled mistakes and are automatically resisted—people prefer to invest their energies and careers in a "sure thing."

Selling The Vision

Architectural firms that design building projects create a miniature model of the finished structure. Located in a place of prominence within an organization, employees view the model and visualize the finished project, creating a common definition of the new structure's appearance as well as its relationship to the existing structure.

Creation of a conceptual model of the various elements of professional practice that are to be developed will assist staff members in conceptualizing the vision established for nursing. By identifying the various components of nursing practice and their relationship to each other, a common vision for the entire department could be created (Figure 7-2).

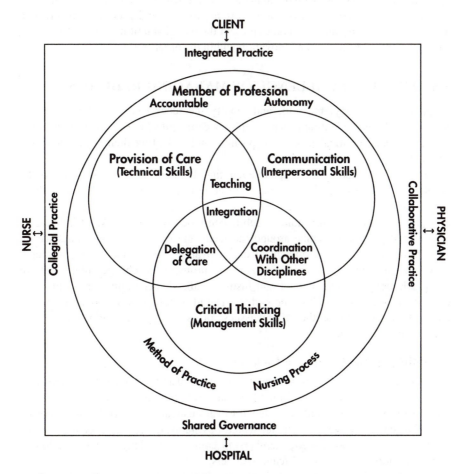

FIGURE 7-2. Professional practice model for nursing. (Used with permission from Sioux Valley Hospital, Sioux Falls, South Dakota.)

This conceptual model for professional nursing practice is based on social systems theory with a holographic focus. The center of the model depicts the role of nurse. It reflects a merging of the components of nursing practice: provision of care, management of care, and communication. The interactive roles of nursing are identified along with the public addressed: collegial practice with nurse colleagues, integrated practice with the client, collaborative practice with physicians (and other allied health personnel), and a relationship of shared governance with the hospital. Development and implementation of the components of this conceptual model would place nursing in a strategic position of business partnership and provide a framework for future research and theory development in nursing practice.

It takes a champion to move an innovative idea into action. People apply varying levels of skills, energy, and frames of reference to an idea as a result of their background, experience, and the activities that require their attention. Nursing management must be intimately involved in the generation and selling of the vision. Thus managers could be given access to a set of transparencies and a script, complete with anticipated questions and answers, to present the model at unit meetings. The vision would then be presented as an innovation within the organization.

THE PROCESS CHALLENGE OF MANAGING REDESIGN

People develop, carry, react to, and modify the ideas found in an innovation. Schon (1971) has identified that people become attached to ideas over time through a social-political process of pushing and activating their ideas into good currency.

Change is initiated by a disruptive event that threatens the social system. As the problem is recognized, ideas begin to surface to the mainstream as the result of efforts of people on the fringe (champions) who supply the energy necessary to raise the ideas into the threshold of public consciousness. Networks of individuals and interest groups galvanize around the ideas and exert their own influence on them through further development of the innovation. As the ideas are considered by people of power, legitimacy is gained to promote the change. Ideas that are acceptable become implemented and institutionalized, becoming part of the conceptual and social structure of the system. The ideas remain viable only as long as they continue to address the critical issues, or as long as the regime remains in power (Schon, 1971).

Establishing the Teams for Redesign

A model that creates and governs the practice of nursing must be designed by the individuals who are expert in the field: nurses within the institution. Thus components of the model would be assigned to various teams that work autonomously as well as collaboratively. A charter would be established for each team to outline the tasks to be accomplished, membership composition, length of time allotted, and expectations of individual team members.

Team positions could be posted, inviting staff members to apply with a statement of intent as to why they want to serve. Membership selections would be based on talent and expertise germane to the task assigned. The organization must make a commitment to value the time and expertise of individual practitioners by paying them for committee work. Team members must make a reciprocal commitment for communication with colleagues to obtain input on issues under discussion and report findings back to the team.

Nurses who participate in decision-making activities must be assisted with the development of skills in systems thinking, group process, leadership, and political acumen. Thus initial group leadership is best assumed by a nursing manager with a staff nurse serving as co-chair. The agenda and current articles pertinent to the task at hand would be sent to all team members before the initial meeting to focus awareness. Formative activities completed at early meetings could include education on the concept to be developed, creating a common understanding; establishment of group norms to clearly articulate suitable group behaviors and group decision-making processes; and the development of assumptions to clarify group beliefs regarding the component under development. As the team members become more familiar with each other and the task at hand, the ongoing leadership would be selected by the group from among the members.

Managing Attention

Empirical evidence suggests that most individuals lack the capability and inclination to deal with complexity (Tversky and Kahneman, 1974; Johnson, 1983). Allowing for individual differences, most people have a short-term memory for raw data that lasts only a few seconds. Most individuals are very efficient at processing routine tasks. Skills for these tasks are stored in subconscious memory. People do not concentrate on the repetitive tasks once they are mastered, thus freeing time and attention for unfamiliar things.

The average person begins to create stereotypes as a defense mechanism to deal with complexity when seven (plus or minus two) objects or concepts are involved in the decision (Miller, 1956). As decision complexity increases, people become more conservative and apply more subjective criteria, which are further removed from reality (Filley, House, and Kerr, 1976). Because the correctness of outcomes from innovative ideas can rarely be judged, the perceived legitimacy of the decision process becomes the dominant evaluation criteria. Thus as decision complexity increases, solutions become increasingly error prone, means become more important than ends, and rationalization replaces rational thought (March, 1981; Janis, 1982). For an innovation to receive proper attention and understanding, it must be presented in a sequenced manner that staff can assimilate.

Differentiating the Practice Roles of Nurses

The project to implement change must begin with an evaluation of nursing roles within the organization because nursing is a clinical discipline. To trigger the action threshold of the nursing staff, it is essential for management to identify and address the most significant source of dissatisfaction to nurses within the institution as well as within the total profession. Historically, nurses with different levels of education have been used interchangeably in most health care settings. Nursing practice is not systematically differentiated on the basis of basic education, prior experience, or additional contribution to the practice. Informally, the "expert" nurse has been relied on by patients, physicians, other nurses, and hospital management to a greater degree than the "novice," with little formal recognition or compensation. Professional advancement into a new role category required movement into a management role.

The current system of nursing education and licensure, which fails to differentiate the competencies and responsibilities of nurses educated in associate, diploma, and baccalaureate programs, has confused the public and the employer, while creating deep divisions within nursing (Boston, 1990). Three compelling reasons to differentiate the practice role of nurse include:

- Fragmentation of client care as a result of increasing physician subspecialization and the emergence of a decentralized, distributive health care delivery system
- Changing career expectations of graduates who seek career advancement opportunities based on education and competence
- Changing reimbursement options that demand coordinated care, thus eliminating redundancy and gaps in service

Differentiating practice roles provides the nursing profession with a vehicle to create a nursing care delivery system, based on client needs, across the health care continuum. This will position nursing as a powerful integrating force in the changing health care industry.

A pilot project invites staff members to participate in the testing and refinement of alternate care delivery systems and the inherent role changes for nursing practice. To ensure staff support and investment, units involved in a demonstration project should be self-selected through an 80% vote to participate from the membership on the unit. It is essential to attain this level of commitment from the staff to minimize the internal group pressures to maintain status quo.

Janis (1982) has suggested that innovation can only occur under conditions of moderate stress. There must also be sufficient time and an abundance of resources to help make decisions. Under conditions of tight resources or short time horizons (which produce stress), the decisions made regarding innovation will have a crisis orientation, resulting in significant implementation errors. A unit with a history of innovation, a nursing manager who has demonstrated leadership and experiences the trust of her staff, or a staff that has demonstrated involvement in professional practice activities will maximize the potential inherent in a change project of this magnitude.

Argus and Schon (1983) have identified that double-loop learning models, rather than single-loop learning, may improve the innovation process. Single-loop learning represents conventional monitoring activity, with action taken based on the findings of the monitoring system. This process may lead the organization to inertia. Double-loop learning includes the option of changing the evaluation criteria. Past performance is questioned, new assumptions are raised, and significant changes in operations can occur on an ongoing, dynamic basis.

On the basis of pilot project outcomes and the experiences of the demonstration units, a recommendation to adopt the innovation can be forwarded to the practice

(Koerner and others, 1989a). A set of guidelines and recommendations for implementation would be generated by the pilot units to be evaluated in second-generation activities regarding this concept. These recommendations and guidelines would be categorized and submitted to various committees for addition, deletion, and further refinement.

THE STRUCTURAL CHALLENGE OF MANAGING WHOLE-PART RELATIONSHIPS

A little-understood but pervasive characteristic of the innovation process is the proliferation of ideas, people, and transactions over time. With these phenomena come complexity and interdependence as well as the basic structural problem of managing good ideas into currency.

Successful implementation of innovation is not an individual activity, but rather a collective achievement. Therefore over time there is a proliferation of people (bringing diverse skills, resources, and interests) who become involved in the innovation process. The differing perceptions and frames of reference are magnified through the increase of transactions or relationships among people and organizational units that occur as the innovation unfolds. Thus the management of the innovation process can be seen as managing increasing numbers of transactions over time.

Integrating the Diverse Components of Innovation

Innovations thrive or perish depending on their acceptance or rejection by people who are affected by them. Human transactions are exchanges that tie people together within a common context. The more novel and complex the innovation, the more often trial-and-error cycles of renegotiation, recommitment, and readministration of transactions must occur. People demonstrate a conservative bias, entering into transactions with people they trust through previous successful experiences. Therefore building trust within and among groups is a key activity to foster in team-building activities.

The most effective approach to handling the complexity and interdependence is to divide the labor among specialists best qualified to perform unique tasks. The reintegration of these specialized parts will recreate the whole. The innovation could be divided among four major committees: clinical ladder committee, integrated care committee, collaborative practice committee, and collegial practice committee. Committee membership would be participative, with a staff nurse selected by each unit to be their representative. A unit manager from each division (medical-surgical, critical care, and maternal-child), a supervisor, a clinical nurse specialist, and representation from staff development would complete the committee. A clinical director and the vice president of patient services would serve in an ad hoc advisory capacity to all committees.

Clinical Ladder Committee

The concept of "differentiated practice" is currently being used in several ways. Some institutions view it as a care delivery model for primary nursing. Others use it as a staff deployment mechanism that ascribes job categories based on education and/or competence. A third approach is the use of the concept as a philosophy. The Governing Board of the National Commission on Nursing Implementation Project (NCNIP) completed 3 years of activity dedicated to creating strategies for redesign of the nursing profession. The goal for differentiated practice within the organization is stated in the NCNIP (1989) definition:

> **Differentiated practice:** In order to improve patient care, effectively utilize health care resources, and create a more satisfying work environment, roles and functions of nursing personnel should be based on education, experience, and competence, and nurses should be compensated accordingly.

Many organizations currently have some form of a clinical ladder. Based on the Benner model of novice to expert (1984), most organizations reward increasing competence in the basic role of nurse. Differentiated practice proposes two distinct career pathways, each offering a continuum of novice to expert within the role. The organizational clinical ladder committee would take the recommendations from the demonstration units, along with the job descriptions tested during the project, to refine career opportunities for the nursing practice (Primm, 1987). Their charge would be to create two distinct clinical tracks for nurses at the bedside: the associate nurse role, which provides direct care at the bedside, and the primary nurse role, which integrates the nursing and medical plan of care to facilitate a timely, well-prepared discharge. A plan for placement into the role, evaluation, and reward criteria for the practitioners plus educational plans to ensure success in the newly developed role are also needed. Although the roles are mutually valued, the competencies and salary would expand with each role (Koerner, 1990).

As discussions evolve, the staff will identify that the emerging importance of critical thinking and timely communication of information is equal to that of technical skills. The term *career pathways* may be viewed as more reflective of the totality of nursing practice than clinical ladders. At this point the committee may change its name to "career pathway committee," and broaden its charge by expanding on the best components from the previous clinical ladders concept.

As the innovation unfolds, the committee may identify that the practice role of MSN-prepared nurses must be restructured to support the evolving practice roles of nursing at the bedside (Nicholai, 1990), creating three levels of career opportunities for nurses within the organization and the community (Figure 7-3).

Dialogue may also reveal that nurses have varying needs during their professional career. Most nurses begin their career with a great deal of time and energy for their profession. Staff members will express concern that the challenge of raising children, caring for elderly parents, and managing the pressures of combining school and work may deter some of the energy previously available for their career. A pilot project on differentiated practice revealed that 40% of the nurses with BSN degrees chose to maintain their current RN position when offered expanded career opportunities (Koerner, 1989).

Thus an equitable transitional model for career advancement may best be based on *competencies* and *choice*. A nurse with the requisite competencies (as demonstrated through a factoring process) could work in the primary nurse role. In addi-

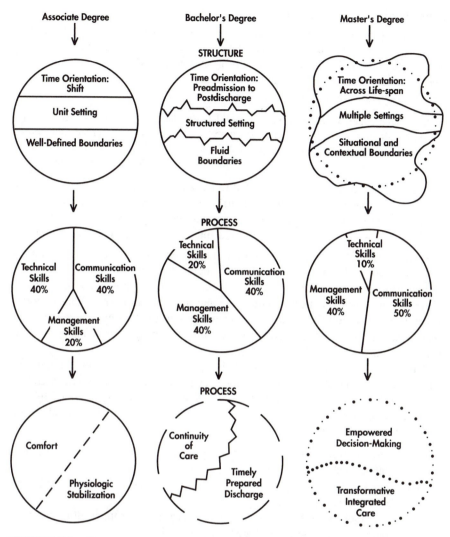

FIGURE 7-3. Framework for differentiating practice roles of nursing. (From American Academy of Nursing: Differentiating Nursing Practice: Toward the Twenty-First Century. Kansas City, Mo. American Academy of Nursing, 1991. Reprinted with permission.)

tion, that nurse may choose to return the traditional RN role and salary if life circumstances so dictate.

There is an important connection between the transactions of a group and the total organization. Transactions are the micro-elements of macro-organizational arrangements. Each month the committee members must report on progress of the group at the unit meeting. All work of the committee should be posted in an information book strategically located on the unit so that individual nurses can review and comment on the item under consideration by the committee at that time. When competencies and guidelines are adopted, the work of the committee would be ready for implementation by the nursing practice throughout the organization.

Integrated Care Committee

Demographic and economic forces are demanding changes in the structure and organization of the health care delivery system. Thus the nursing profession must establish an integrative nursing care delivery system with the following goal: nursing will integrate the care of patients to maintain quality while maximizing efficiency in resource allocation and utilization.

> **Integrated care:** A system of patient care delivery that integrates the allocation of resources (human and material) over a variety of settings and appropriate time frames through differentiation of nursing practice. Differentiation implies expansion of patient care management beyond physiologic stabilization to the entire episode of illness.

When the roles of nursing have been differentiated, the delivery of nursing care should be evaluated to clearly unite the roles into an integrated whole on behalf of the client, the professionals themselves, and the total organization.

Each unit would establish a unit-based integrated care committee to redesign the unit's care delivery system based on the revised role competencies according to established guidelines. A hospitalwide integrated care committee would also be established as a monitoring, problem-solving arena for the individual units to share innovations and concerns. Often one unit may find another moving smoothly in an area of difficulty for them. An increase in consultation by nurses (staff and management) from one unit with another will be noted, facilitating a growing sense of teamwork and professionalism.

Currently, no formal health care delivery system exists within our country. Thus "each individual or family puts together an informal set of services and facilities to meet their own needs" (Torrens, 1978). Financing is provided by personal and employer contributions or governmental funds. Services currently available include the following:

- **Environmental protection** (en masse protection; water, sewage, etc.) from the public health department.
- **Biogenetic engineering** (monoclonal antibodies, gene splicing, etc.) from geneticists and scientists.
- **Wellness promotion** activities (discretionary care) from health educators, nutritionists, exercise physiologists, and lay advisors.
- **Ambulatory care** (prevention and maintenance care) from a private physician, nurse practitioner, dentist, or psychologist.
- **Acute care** (profit or nonprofit) from a hospital setting using advanced technology, multispecialty services, and practitioners.
- **Rehabilitative care** (restorative care) from a physiatrist and multidisciplinary team.
- **Home health care** (individual support services) from case managers, visiting nurses, home care aides, and congregate living centers.
- **Extended care** (continuous care) from skilled care facilities and nursing homes.
- **Hospice care** (terminal care) from a multidisciplinary team of caregivers.

The presence of primary nursing within one agency resulted in a 150% increase in discharge referrals for some client populations (Koerner, 1989a). A need for coordination and integration of posthospital activities in a manner similar to that provided in the hospital was apparent, thus the emergence of a case management role. Table 3 explains the role functions of primary nurses and case managers.

Nursing case management is a natural extension of differentiated practice within an organizational context. Primary and associate nurses provide integrative nursing support to the client and family across the acute episode of illness within the hospital setting. Primary nurse communication occurs through the nursing process, with each nursing diagnosis resolved or referred to the primary nurse in the receiving unit. Those patients who need ongoing case management are then referred to the case manager (CNS) who provides continuing care throughout the illness episode in multiple settings. This type of care is best suited to individuals with chronic illness requiring support across the full spectrum of health care services (Figure 7-4), individuals with knowledge or financial deficits, or clients lacking support and assistance from a significant other. The following situation describes use of a case manager.

A pregnant teenager of Native American background was admitted to the hospital in premature labor. As the primary nurse worked with the client, it was discovered that the individual had no resources or support. The family had removed her from their home, and she had no fiscal or significant other support. Her situation was referred to a case manager, who made arrangements for living quarters and subsidy support upon discharge from the hospital. The mother and infant were followed after discharge, and a successful outcome was achieved for all.

TABLE 3
Comparison of the role functions of the primary nurses and the case managers

Primary Nurses	Role Function	Case Managers
Integrate medical and nursing orders into a comprehensive plan of care	**Integrator**	Integrate medical and nursing plan of care with health patterns of client
Coordinate activities of various departments on behalf of client	**Manager**	Coordinate activities of various agencies on behalf of client
Communicate wishes and fears of client and family to other health care providers	**Advocate**	Communicate unique lifestyle and cultural issues to other team members and agencies
Develop and coordinate discharge teaching activities pertinent to illness episode	**Teacher**	Consult with various professionals on complex client care needs, teach patient and family health promotion or health maintenance activities
Negotiate for changes in medical or nursing plan of care as client condition changes	**Negotiator**	Negotiate for changes in agency services or reimbursement options as client condition changes

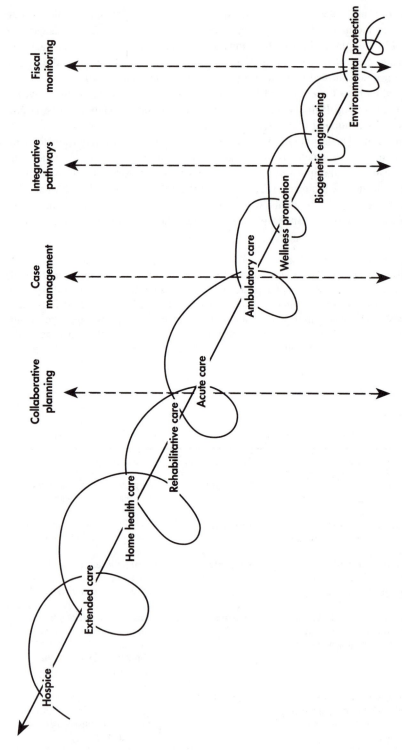

FIGURE 7-4. Continuum of health care services and integrating factors. (From *Differentiating a Nursing Practice: Toward the Twenty-First Century*. Kansas City, 1991, American Academy of Nursing. Reprinted with permission.)

The Contextual Environment

To more fully comprehend the totality of nursing, the work of nursing must be placed into the context of the entire organization and the health care industry. Gareth Morgan (1984) states that to avoid having the whole be less than the sum of its parts, it must be viewed within the concept of a hologram. This biologic brain metaphor emphasizes that organizational design for innovation is not a discrete event, but a process for integrating all the essential functions, organizational units, and resources needed to manage an innovation from beginning to end.

The holographic approach directs attention to activities that identify and combine the key resources and interdependent functions needed to develop an innovation on one organizational unit, so that it can operate as if it were autonomous (knowing that no unit is ever completely autonomous). Members of the unit are socialized to "think globally while acting locally" (Hrebiniak and Joyce, 1984). Each member comes to know his or her role and how it relates to the other specialties. Members also understand the master blueprint of the overall innovation. This facilitates interdependent action and survival of the innovation.

Critical dimensions of the institutional environment are present on the unit. The key resource for nursing practice at the unit level is the presence of a competent nursing team. The major interdisciplinary players are the physicians and other allied health personnel. Interaction among these various players permits unit members to develop and store rich patterns of information and uncertainty that are needed to detect and correct errors existing in the environment. Thus environmental scanning and clear communication become a responsibility of all unit members.

Collaborative Practice

Increasing fragmentation of patient care because of heightened acuity, shortened length of stay, increasing physician subspecialty, and consultation increases the need for shared communication, decision-making, and some standardization. The goal of collaborative practice is to integrate the nursing and medical data base and plan of care to enhance the quality of patient care.

> **Collaborative practice:** Mutual valuation of nursing and medical practice that fosters respect among the professions and potentiates the contribution of each for the benefit of the patient.

Opportunities for collaboration are strengthened through joint committee appointments of staff nurses as well as nurse managers to the hospital medical committees. Multidisciplinary grand rounds could be established in various specialties of practice. The establishment of integrative pathways (critical paths) on the major DRG categories on each unit may be done as a descriptive (not prescriptive) process to facilitate timely decision making and communication among all care providers. As trust emerges among team members, the pathway may assume a prescriptive focus to maximize cost efficiency.

The relationship that emerges between case managers and primary care physicians develops a unique characteristic of collegiality over time. As each partner learns to trust and respect the other's unique perspective of the client, true negotiation regarding interventions occurs. In one agency the ability of a case manager to influence medical orders by assisting the physician to see the uniqueness of each client resulted in reducing the cost per hospice patient for laboratory procedures from $2.46 per day to $.02 per day. The open dialogue resulted in more focused decision making for both the nurse and physician, and less cost and discomfort for the client without reducing quality of care (Slack, 1990).

Collegial Practice

The need to improve collegial relationships in nursing requires a radical change to achieve freedom from an isolating practice orientation of power and control to a professional practice model of partnership. This requires a disciplined personal commitment to the other's and to one's own continued growth. Bunkers and Ko-erner, (1990) have identified that nurses need to understand that they are part of a community of caring. They have a responsibility to pay attention to the entire community of nursing to gain improvements for all nurses.

A primary goal for collegial practice is to establish professionalism as the unifying value for nursing, and develop a nursing center to assist nurses from all settings to meet evolving clinical and scholarly (education, research, and publication) goals.

> **Collegial practice:** Mutual valuation of individual nurse practice based on scientific principles that establish credibility, and a common language that facilitates clear communication.

Nursing has had to confront both gender and class barriers in its attempts to determine its own destiny and assume a meaningful role. Class and gender issues place women in a submissive status, creating an oppressed group mentality within the profession. Because of this background, nurses have much difficulty articulating the value and worth of nursing, impacting the image of the profession and relationships within it.

In the 1980s women made a shift from people who serve others, defer to others, and define themselves through others, to people who are visible in their own right, and who stand as separate individuals while still connected to others (Eichenbaum and Orbach, 1988). Once a woman has learned to be autonomous, both her work relationships and her intimate relationships are usually healthier (Hagberg, 1984).

Facilitating collegial relationships must be a major goal of any nursing practice. Analysis of the situation reveals that trust is basically missing in many nursing relationships. Lack of clear and concise communication and misunderstanding of the various nursing roles within the organization are key elements that contribute to the existing distrust.

Two vehicles specified to facilitate clear, concise, and accurate communication are nursing diagnosis and the nursing process. Norms for communication in nursing diagnosis language and nursing process format must be established for planning, charting, and change of shift report. Collaborative, ongoing care planning and clear delegation would increase teamwork. Thus a clear norm for delegation would state that within the department of nursing, delegation occurs through nursing orders. Failure to execute a nursing order would require a variance report just as omission of a medical order, as they are mutually valued.

Mutual respect among colleagues would be further fostered through increased understanding of the various roles within the nursing department as well as individual preference for a specific role. A nursing center could be established to assist individual nurses with career planning and developmental needs. An administrative nursing director would develop the center and integrate its activities into evolving needs within the organization, as well as beyond its walls. Services offered to professionals might include:

- Career assessment activities that focus on interest inventory and job placement activities
- Formal educational opportunities in academic centers with scholarship and loan support toward an advanced degree
- Continuing education of an experiential nature through participation in fellowship and professional exchange programs, as well as traditional in-service programs
- Personal growth opportunities in leadership and team-building skills, ethical competence, and creative innovation

The nursing department may also be committed to supporting the education and practice needs of the larger profession. Affiliating and rural hospitals employ nurses with varying needs in meeting the unique health care requirements of rural communities. Activities might include:

- Educational outreach activities for professionals and the community
- Provision of nurse managers and directors in various hospitals seeking a nursing management contract, or management development programs for rural nurse managers with limited access to resources
- Fellowship programs in obstetric nursing and emergency nursing, offering affiliate nurses an intensive week of didactic and clinical experience in a low-volume, high-acuity aspect of their rural practice

Relationships with the nursing schools would also be strengthened through the development of "middleground" (Figure 7-5) (Bunkers and Koerner, 1990). Student experiences at the hospital would be enhanced through summer externships and a 6-month residency program for new graduates. Five fields for interinstitutional integration between nursing education and nursing service may be developed by:

- Staff development courses offered for college credit
- Shared faculty/joint appointment wherein educators and administrators plan and teach courses collaboratively
- Consultative services—the hospital hires faculty to design and implement research as well as consulting on specific nursing issues
- Joint decision-making with both administrative and faculty personnel serving on college curriculum and hospital management committees

Another area for further development is group practice, in which administrators and educators would carry a caseload of clients, engage in peer review and quality

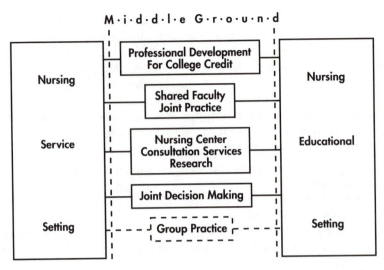

FIGURE 7-5.   A model for interinstitutional integration of professional nursing. (From Bunkers, S. and Koerner, J. [1990]. The M-I-D-D-L-E-G-R-O-U-N-D: A model for inter-institutional integration. Nursing Connections, 3[1], Spring.)

assurance, and cover another's practice when one is absent. Through collaboration among nursing peers, the integration of practice and research is strengthened in a way that can contribute much to the advancement of professional nursing.

THE STRATEGIC CHALLENGE OF INSTITUTIONAL LEADERSHIP

Innovations not only adapt to existing organizational arrangements, they also transform the structure and practices of those environments. Because innovation is not the enterprise of a single entrepreneur, the network of individuals and units that have created, adopted, and transformed the innovation into good currency must be formalized within the infrastructure of the organization. A strategic chal-lenge is the creation of an infrastructure that will maintain the innovation and the networks.

Reframing the Manager Role for an Empowered Environment

Within the organization institutional leadership is critical in creating a cultural context that fosters innovation, in addition to an established organizational strat-egy, structure, and system that maintains autonomy and accountability. There is growing recognition that innovation requires a special kind of transformational leadership:

This type of leadership offers a vision of what could be and gives a sense of purpose and meaning to those who share that vision. It builds commitment, enthusiasm, and excite-ment. It creates a hope in the future and a belief that the world is knowable, understandable, and manageable. The collective energy that transforming leadership generates, empowers those who participate in the process. There is hope, there is optimism, there is energy (Roberts, 1984).

During periods of transition the leader is charged with the creation of the organization's character and culture. This is accomplished through four main functions: defining the mission, embodying purpose into the structure and systems being designed, defending the institution's integrity, and ordering the inevitable internal conflicts that arise.

Institutional leadership is at the heart of corporate institutionalization. An organization does not become an institution until it is infused with the value of being a vehicle for group integrity. Infusion of norms and values occurs over time, in a sporadic rather than a linear fashion. This activity is the key to social integration of all members within the organization (Van de Ven, 1986).

Shared Governance

Increased autonomy and responsibility are central goals that drive nursing's quest for professionalism. Decentralization, participation in decision making, and shared governance make organizational structure and professional practice more complementary. As nursing's role in patient care increases, so must its role in hospital management. The goal for shared governance must be to position nurses as esteemed business partners who assume more responsibility in integrating the allocation of human, fiscal, and material resources for improved patient care.

Shared governance: A governance system that distributes responsibility and authority between the business organization and the professional business partner. Nursing is challenged to couple the professional good of autonomy with business acumen to become a proficient and esteemed business partner.

Shared governance may be viewed as a twofold process: the strengthening of autonomy in decision making through further decentralization, and development of business acumen to strengthen positioning within the organization.

The Movement Toward Autonomy

A central principle in the development of models and concepts is to keep the management team "one step ahead" of the staff in the process so that they can lead and facilitate staff development. Thus a long-range strategy to prepare unit managers for their new role in a shared governance structure must be executed. Staff development would be initiated *after* management education is begun.

Teamwork and Creativity

Work in any setting comprises two component parts, tasks and relationships. A harmonious relationship will facilitate the responsibilities inherent in the task. Thus nursing administration might begin the management training program with a class designed to facilitate teamwork. A class entitled "Whack on the Side of the Head" (van Oech, 1983) was developed to strengthen the creative ability and communication skills of individuals on the management team in one organization (Bunkers and Koerner, 1988). Co-taught by a nursing administrator and a professor from a local college, the course, which focused on principles of creativity and communication, was offered for college credit. Using adult learning principles and innovative teaching techniques, the class fostered new perspectives on well-known issues (i.e., the local zoo provided the setting and a manager to deliver a lecture that compared the management of a hospital unit to a zoo). During the course each member of the team created a change project for his or her unit, applying principles of design and development. Colleagues assisted in the identification of strategies for successful implementation, pledging support for co-worker success.

Management Principles

A second class on management principles was presented to the entire management team and reviewed concepts in planning, budgeting, staffing, resource allocation, quality assurance, and personnel management. Although the class was a review for many, it helped to frame those activities in the context of a health care delivery system experiencing corporate reorganization in response to changing environmental, economic, and demographic trends.

Participative Management

A third class, "Creative Nursing Administration for the 21st Century," helped the unit managers develop an understanding of the evolving need for participative management. Strategies to create a professional environment and foster staff accountability were identified (Porter-O'Grady, 1986). Needs and challenges facing managers in an empowered environment were addressed, providing them opportunity to vent their fears, frustrations, and expectations as the management process was changing.

Revitalizing Professional Commitment

The principle of temporal linkage is vital to successful implementation of an innovation. It highlights the necessity for linking past, present, and future to the innovation at hand. Celebrating the contributions of the past and integrating salient features of the current process into a future model assists people during the transition. They are then able to take investments, commitments, and values from the past into the future. Albert (1984) states that there is a need to create funerals, celebrations, and other transitional rituals that commemorate ideas, programs, and commitments that give way to new changes that must gain good currency for innovation to succeed.

The final class created for the unit managers and clinical nurse specialists, "Change, a Professional Challenge," began with a funeral. Each participant received an invitation to bring a symbol of something in nursing that they would like to release as they moved into a new model of professional practice. Managers were then taken to a local funeral home where the funeral director assisted with the burial of the old symbols of nursing and the resurrection of new, favored ways.

This three-credit-hour course was co-developed and taught by nursing educators at a local college and nursing administrators at a hospital. It focused on principles of change, personal and professional development, and situational leadership. Each individual's philosophy of nursing and future career goals were examined along with personal issues that influence career choices and decisions. The process of influencing through motivation, initiation, facilitation, and integration was examined (Hersey and Duldt, 1989). After this group completed the class it was offered to supervisors within the organization. Staff nurses were then offered the class, which meets the "Introduction to Baccalaureate Nursing" course requirements for BSN degree completion.

Strengthening Staff Participation

While the management team is being reoriented, the staff must be introduced to activities that foster their participation in decision making. Committee work designed in a team-building format would establish staff accountability. As openings are posted for the first design team, there may be an apparent lack of interest in participation by the staff, with few people applying for the positions. A certain skepticism and mistrust exist among staff nurses who believe that nothing makes a difference, that their input has not been heeded in nursing's past. If this phenomenon occurs, individuals with a track record for innovation and participation may be invited to join the committee. As the first round of committee work is completed with results valued and implemented, an increase in staff participation will be noted. Thus a "new reality" would emerge for staff-manager collaboration in decision making.

Introducing Business Principles

"Ecology of Excellence" is a business program developed by an innovative nursing leader, Donna Davidson, and Dr. Frank Steiner (Steiner, 1986). It combines principles of empowerment, teamwork, and business to create a business partner for the entire health care setting. The program teaches all hospital staff a process that balances the quality of worklife with business performance, creating a corporate culture of excellence.

A business curriculum would teach the concepts of true communication, team leadership, idea marketing, wise negotiation, and intrabusiness skills. Ongoing activities would find staff creating work teams based on the Myers-Briggs inventory to address issues of concern and ideas for new program development. Interface agreements would be developed for problem areas within the organization by the parties in conflict. First-party communication would replace the nonproductive third-party communication so prevalent in practice today. Staff members could present any request desired after a cost-benefit analysis had been completed. Thus increased budgeting and systems information would be made available to staff members so they could evaluate the impact of their request on the organization, the client, and others within the institution.

A final feature of a business program is the development of baselines to evaluate and monitor the cost and quality outcomes of caregiver performance and care provided. Management of issues that impact quality and cost would be transferred to the units. Staff would interview new business partners for hire, make purchasing decisions with their capital budget, and track lost charges and other activities that have a fiscal impact on both the client and the organization.

THE INTEGRATIVE CHALLENGE OF REUNITING THE WHOLE

After management and staff have matured to the point that shared governance would be successful, formalization of an infrastructure to honor and support the various components developed by staff through their innovative efforts would occur. The goal would be to create an infrastructure that integrates the various components of nursing practice while supporting ongoing innovation.

Alpert (1984) states that innovation is an institutional success to the degree that it exhibits authenticity, functionality, and flexibility over time. Authenticity requires that the innovation embody the organization's ideas. The organizational chart for the nursing department must reflect the new philosophy (Figure 7-6). An innovative, organizational model places the client at the center of the chart. The circular design reflects removal of hierarchy, depicting instead mutual valuing of all care delivery roles. Placement of the administration at the bottom of the chart identifies a role change of management from controlling, directing, and supervising to one of facilitating, coordinating, integrating, and supporting.

Functionality requires that the innovations work. Baseline data must be generated at the onset of the innovation in several major categories: patient, physician, and nurse satisfaction; cost and quality indicators; staff turnover; and informal assessment of quality of worklife experienced by the staff. Indicators in each area must be maintained or enhanced, especially as staff became more expert in a specific innovation.

Flexibility requires that the innovations incorporate input and suggestions from the institution's membership. Thus the governance model may centralize financial allotment, staffing philosophy, and policy formulation for the nursing department. Budget allocation, staffing patterns, quality assurance activities, standard development, integrated care delivery activities, peer evaluation, and continuing education activities would be decentralized to the unit level.

Three cybernetic principles based on the holographic metaphor have been identified by Morgan (1984) as essential in an infrastructure to address problems of managing attention, ideas, and whole-parts relationships over time. First, organizational members must develop the capacity to control and regulate their behavior through ongoing feedback. The organization must have values and standards that define the critical limits within which to function. Second, double-loop learning principles should be used so that the organization can detect and correct errors in the operating norms themselves. This focus permits the organization to adjust to changing environmental and professional technologies and ideologies. Finally, maintaining a certain degree of uncertainty, diversity, and turbulence maintains a bias for creativity. This could best be accomplished by developing a tolerance for ambiguity and risk-taking. Innovation would thus be enhanced and ongoing. These principles must be woven into the shared governance model.

All members of the nursing department would become members of the con-

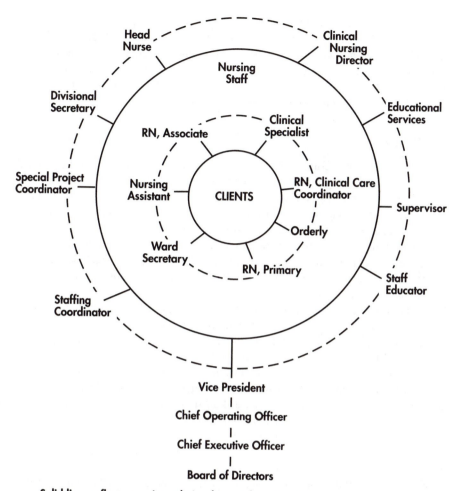

FIGURE 7-6. Department of nursing divisional chart. (Used with permission from Sioux Valley Hospital, Sioux Falls, South Dakota.)

gress (nursing practice) on the basis of credentials, in a manner similar to that of medical staff. After an initial interview with a staff nurse, the applicant would go through an admissions process based on criteria for professional expertise developed by staff. Professional portfolios would be maintained by each nurse in practice to demonstrate proficiency in nursing process for peer evaluation and further professional development.

Four councils would coordinate activities for the nursing department. The council on practice would establish nursing standards; the council on management would support those standards through allocation of fiscal and human resources; the council on education would educate to those standards; and the council on quality assurance would measure standards of professional performance and quality outcomes for the client (Porter-O'Grady and Finnegan, 1984). Unit-based councils would be micro-elements of the departmental councils. The nursing executive council, composed of the departmental council chairpersons, clinical directors, and the vice president of patient services would monitor and facilitate the activities of the various councils and the congress. Bylaws would govern the activities of this model based on professional accountability.

SUMMARY

A sense of crisis has erupted in the nursing profession as a result of heightened aspirations for nursing's role along with recognition of inadequacies in performance and opportunity. Conflict exists within nursing because of a lack of unifying values and vision. Nurses must accept and value themselves as true autonomous professionals. They must move from the current procedural orientation that reinforces division, to a professional orientation that is concerned with the essence of nursing. Enhancement of professional opportunity and accountability must be the primary motive underlying the creation and implementation of an innovation for nursing practice.

Development and implementation of an innovation based on systems theory, using the holographic brain metaphor, will assist transformation of the profession. Cybernetic principles, woven into an infrastructure, would ensure ongoing maintenance and further development of the model established.

Nursing must accept and value the institution as an esteemed arena for practice if the institution is to accept and support the profession as a valued partner in business. Gilb (1985) has observed that freedom in a complex, interdependent economy is derived through organizations. Without an organization to define and sustain the area of freedom, the individual professional is seldom free. Thus the practice role of nurse must be differentiated and placed within an organizational context, or informally connected to it.

Nurses must become autonomous professional business partners with other major players in the health care system to strengthen hospital nursing and improve patient care. Recognizing the importance of nursing to quality patient care, organizations must support the nursing department in creating a practice model that positions nurses as esteemed professional business partners within its walls and beyond. Professional nursing practice must also be expanded to include political acumen and business skills that influence patient care decisions, both clinically and economically.

Four major partnerships for nursing are essential for ongoing success: **integrated practice,** partnerships with the clients served within the organization and external to it; **shared governance,** a partnership with the hospital; **collegial practice,** partnerships among the nurses themselves both within the institution and external to it; and **collaborative practice,** a partnership with physicians and allied health colleagues.

Professional nursing business partners must be placed in a strategic position within the hospital and the larger health care community. An integrative care delivery model would create a foundation for future research and theory development in nursing practice. By combining the strengths of professional practice and a business acumen that influences quality and cost-conscious decisions, nursing will become a highly influential and valued integrative link between the client and the health care industry in this time of unprecedented change.

Nursing administrators must accept the challenging role of transformative leadership in redesigning the position of nursing within their organization as health care delivery is transformed. Their vision and courage can liberate nursing from limiting thoughts and actions. As nurses' imaginations are freed, fear, closed thinking, and poverty of spirit will be abandoned. This is the key to successful transformation of nursing for the twenty-first century.

REFERENCES

Albert, S. (1984). A Design Model for Successful Transitions. In J. Kimberly and R. Quinn (Eds.), *Managing Organizational Transitions* (pp. 169-199). 1984. Homewood, Ill.: Irwin Press.

Argus, R. and Schon, D. (1983). *Reasoning, Learning and Action*. San Francisco: Jossey-Bass.

Ashleym J. This I Believe About Power in Nursing. *Nursing Outlook, (21),* 11, 737-641.

Bates, B. (1970). Doctor and Nurse: Changing Roles and Relationships. *New England Medical Journal, 283,* 3, 129-134.

Benner, P. (1984). *Novice to Expert*. Menlo Park, Calif.: Addison Wesley.

Boston, C. (1990). Introduction. *Current Issues and Perspectives on Differentiated Practice*. AONE, Chicago: AHA Catalog No. 154830, 1-5.

Brooten, D., Human, L., and Naylor, M. (1988). *Leadership for Change*. Philadelphia: J.B. Lippincott Co.

Bunkers, S. and Koerner, J. (1988). Making the Glue Stick: A Group Experience. *Journal of Nursing Administration. 19,*(2), 41.

Bunkers, S. and Koerner, J. (1990). The M-I-D-D-L-E-G-R-O-U-N-D: A Model for Inter-institutional Integration. *Nursing Connections, 3,*(1), Spring.

Deane, C. and Campbell, J. (1985). Developing Professional Effectiveness in Nursing. Reston, Va.: Reston Publishing Co.

Eichenbaum, L. and Orbach, S. (1988). *Between Women*. New York: Viking Penguin Inc.

Fiesta, J. (1983). *The Law and Liability: A Guide for Nurses*. New York: John Wiley & Sons.

Filley, House, and Kerr. (1976). *Managerial Process and Organizational Behavior*. Glenview, Ill.: Scott Foresman.

Gilb, A. (1985). *Hidden Hierarchies*. New York: Harper & Row.

Griffin, A.P. (1980). Philosophy and Nursing. *Journal of Advanced Nursing, 5,*(3), 261-272.

Hagberg, J. (1984). *Real Power*. Minneapolis, Minn.: Winston Press.

Hersey, P. and Duldt, B. (1989). *Situational Leadership in Nursing*. East Norwalk, Conn.: Appleton & Lange.

Hrebiniak, L. and Joyce, W. (1984). *Implementing Strategy*. New York: Macmillan, p. 8

Janis, I. (1982). *Groupthink* (2nd ed.). Boston: Houghton Mifflin.

Johnson, P.E. (1983). The Expert Mind: A New Challenge for the Information Scientist. In M.A. Bemmelsmans (Ed.), *Beyond Productivity: Information Systems Development for Organizational Effectiveness*. Netherlands: North Holland Publishing.

Kanter, R. (1983). *The Changemasters*. New York: Simon & Schuster.

Koerner, J. (1989). Implications of Differentiated Practice Models for Nurse Executives. *Aspen Advisor for Nurse Executives, 4,*(12), 1, 6-8.

Koerner, J. and others. (1989). Implementing Differentiated Practice, the Sioux Valley Hospital Experience. *Journal of Nursing Administration, 19,*(2), 13-20.

Koerner, J. (1990). Differentiated Practice: Relevance in Today's Environment. *Current Issues and Perspectives on Differentiated Practice* (pp. 35-51). Chicago: American Hospital Association Catalog No. 154830.

Kuhn, T.J. (1970). *The Structure of Scientific Revolutions*. Chicago: Chicago University Press.

Lawrence, P. and Dyer, P. (1983). *Renewing American Industry*. New York: Free Press.

Leddy, S. and Pepper, J. (1989). *Conceptual Bases of Professional Nursing*. Philadelphia: J.B. Lippincott.

Lewin, A.Y. and Minton, J.W. (1986). Organizational Effectiveness: Another Look, and an Agenda for Research. *Management Science, 32,*(5), 5.

March, J.G. (1981). Decisions in Organizations and Theories of Choice. In A. Van de Ven and W.F. Joyce (Eds.), *Perspectives on Organizational Design and Behavior.* New York: Wiley & Sons.

Marsick, V.J. (1990). Altering the Paradigm for Theory Building and Research in Human Resource Development. *Human Resource Development Quarterly, 1,*(1), 5-34.

McClure, M. and others. (1983). *Magnet Hospitals: Attraction and Retention of Professional Nurses.* Kansas City, Mo.: American Nurses Association.

Miller, G.A. (1956). The Magical Number Seven, Plus or Minus Two: Some Limits on Our Capacity for Processing Information. *Psychology Review, 63,* 81-97.

Mitroff, I. (1985). Why Our Old Pictures of the World Do Not Work Anymore. In E.E. Lawler III, A.M. Mohrman, Jr., G.E. Ledford, Jr. T.G. Commings and Associates (Eds.), *Doing Research That Is Useful for Theory and Practice* (pp. 18-44). San Francisco: Jossey-Bass Company.

Morgan, G. (1984a). Action Learning: A Holographic Metaphor for Guiding Social Change. *Human Relations, 36,*(37), 1-28.

Morgan, G. (1984b). *Beyond Methods,* Beverly Hills, Calif.: Sage.

Nicholai, C. (1990). Weighting Role Competencies Based on Job Role. *Nursing Career Pathway Project.* Sioux Falls, S.D.: Sioux Valley Hospital.

Ouchi, W. (1981). *Theory Z.* Reading, Mass.: Addison-Wesley.

Parse, R.R. (1987). *Nursing Science: Major Paradigms, Theories and Critiques.* Philadelphia: W.B. Saunders Co.

Pelz, D. and Andrews, F. (1966). *Scientists in Organizations.* New York: Wiley & Sons.

Peters, T. and Waterman, R. *In Search of Excellence: Lessons From America's Best-run Companies.* New York: Harper & Row.

Porter-O'Grady, T. and Finnegan, S. (1984). *Shared Governance for Nursing.* Rockville, Md.: Aspen Publishers, Inc.

Porter-O'Grady, T. (1986). Creative Nursing Administration: Participative Management Into the 21st Century. Rockville, Md.: Aspen Publishers, Inc.

Primm, P. (1987). Differentiated Practice for ADN and BSN Prepared Nurses. *Journal of Professional Nursing, 15,*(4), 218-225.

Roberts, E. (1984). *A Woman's Place: An Oral History of Working.* San Francisco: Jossey-Bass.

Schon, D. (1971). *Beyond the Stable State.* New York: Norton Publishing.

Slack, C. (1990). Utilization Review of Hospice Program: Fiscal Year 1989-1990. *Annual Report to Midwest Health Inc.* Sioux Falls, S.D.: Sioux Valley Hospital.

Statewide Project Steering Committee. (1990). The South Dakota Experience. *Current Issues and Perspectives on Differentiated Practice* (pp. 53-67). Chicago: American Hospital Association Catalog No. 154830.

Steiner, F. (1986). *Ecology of Excellence.* Corrales, N.M.: Educational Professional Services Inc.

Stenvig, T. and Koerner, J. (1987). State Collaboration for Nursing in South Dakota. *Nurses in Agreement: Controlling Our Future* (pp. 85-93). Indianapolis: MAIN.

Styles, G. (1982). *Towards a New Endowment.* 1982. St. Louis, Mo.: C.V. Mosby Company.

Torrens, P.R. (1978). *The American Health Care System: Issues and Problems* (p. 33). St. Louis, Mo.: C.V. Mosby Company.

Tversky, Q. and Kahneman, D. (1974). Judgment Under Uncertainty: Heuristics and Biases. *Science, 185,* 1124-1131.

van Oech, R.A. (1983). *A Whack on the Side of the Head.* New York: Warner Books.

Van de Ven, A. (1982). Strategic Management Concerns Among CEO's: A Preliminary Research Agenda. Presented at Strategic Management Colloquium, University of Minnesota, Minneapolis, October.

Van de Ven, A. (1986). Central Problems in the Management of an Innovation. *Management Science, 32,*(5), 590-607.

Van de Ven, A. (1989). *Nursing Practice Patterns.* Milwaukee: National Commission on Nursing Implementation Project.

8

Structure, Accreditation, and Bylaws: Creating a Framework for Governance

Susan H. Cummings
Jim O'Malley

MOVING FROM MANAGEMENT TO GOVERNANCE

Decentralizing structures and systems and developing high-performing work groups is the cornerstone to successful implementation of a shared governance model. Transition from hierarchical centralized structures reduces the layers within the organization to successfully move decision making to the point of service. In the transition from management to governance, managers share power in a highly developed partnership based on defined accountability with the nursing staff. This selective vertical and horizontal decentralization disperses power within the organization to managers and staff who work on teams within the redesigned organization. Inherent in this new structure is the potential for fragmentation and the need for coordination through centralization of defined functions to ensure desired outcome attainment for the entire system.

For the system to be successful, coordination must be individualized by function and clinical issues and be assigned to the appropriate level of expertise within the nursing organization. Managers in this new governance structure "manage" by coordinating, integrating, and facilitating within the context of a peer liaison–consultative role. Power within this structure rests wherever the relative expertise lies and is not vested in one person or group. Operating "ad hocracies" develop the ability to solve problems directly on behalf of their constituencies. Within these models specialized skills of operating and administrative work are blended so that it is often difficult to distinguish planning and design from implementation (Mintzberg, 1989). In these new structures there is equity among group members. Managers derive their influence from their expertise and interpersonal relationships rather than their position. Organizations will no longer have two-tiered management and staff systems. These hierarchical systems will be abandoned and new structures and systems related to coordination will emerge.

Nursing Practice Accountability

A challenge for these systems that place authority and accountability with groups of practicing staff nurses is to ensure achievement of true behavioral accountability for clinical practice, and quality outcomes. A traditional and beaurocratic viewpoint that "no one ever holds groups accountable for their work" (Jaques, 1990, p. 128) must be considered as shared governance is implemented. Belief in this assumption focuses on the concept that group authority without accountability is dysfunctional and that accountability cannot rest with groups. Nursing has begun to challenge these assumptions by shattering the traditional structures, permitting staff to take risks, and placing accountability for both the process and outcomes of nursing practice with the collective group of practicing clinical nurses. Accountability will become increasingly important as consumer expectations increase for patient-centered services that result in predetermined quality outcomes at a predetermined cost. In the governance systems of the future, only those who are responsible for providing nursing practice will have the authority and accountability to manage it.

High-Performing Work Groups

Development of high-performing work groups provides some insights into the transition from traditional management structures to shared governance systems. The origin of high-performing work groups is derived from a group of individuals who initially have individual goals and are beginning the process of identifying their purpose, responsibilities, and norms for group behaviors. The group expects the leader to provide direction and assume accountability and authority for group functions. These groups frequently expect the manager to assume this leadership role, a behavior counterproductive to the successful transition to governance. Often this period can be "stormy" as functions are realigned with clinical nursing staff and the manager's role undergoes marked redefinition and clarification. The final stage of this process is development of a group that is able to focus energy, respond quickly, and assume behaviorally based accountability. Internalization of group purpose by individuals and the collective group is critical to success. Rewards are shared by the group and are often intangibles such as group decisions that have been effectively implemented to improve nursing practice. Group growth does not proceed in a straight line and can be impacted by changes in membership, group leadership, and new challenges and opportunities.

Characteristics of these high-performing work groups (Bukholtz and Roth, 1986) include:

1. A defined common purpose
2. Sharing responsibility among all members
3. Open, trusting communication and relationships
4. Challenges seen as growth opportunities
5. Individual and group empowerment
6. An outcome focus
7. Synergy through use of strengths
8. Ability to make expeditious decisions

Managers' and staff growth must be parallel for success of shared governance structures. A primary focus of management is to provide opportunities for employee growth as they relinquish legitimate power and authority to clinical nurses. Stages of growth can be compared to biologic growth and development, with the nursing staff moving from dependence to interdependence and managers from controlling to influencing to ultimately a true partnership relationship.

The ideal role for the manager in this partnership relationship is one of consultation, integration, and coordination. Upward and lateral communication are the norms in this interdependent relationship. Transactions are based on personal power and the manager's knowledge, rather than on legitimate power based on the manager's role. Performance results are stimulated by the interdependence and commitment to communication and high-level involvement by all participants. Critical to success of this transition for the manager is not only to "talk the talk" but also to "walk the walk." Successful managers focus on empowering, serving the nursing staff as internal customers, and contributing to individual and group growth. The true mark of success is that staff members will surpass the leader if development has truly been successful.

Environments must be created in which teams of nursing staff collaborate with the manager to manage the unit. All members of the group develop a sense of responsibility, become committed to identifying and solving problems that impact their practice and patient outcomes, and feel responsible for coordination. Strengths are complemented, weaknesses minimized, and all are empowered to translate intention into reality within the new structure. One of the hallmarks of success in this transition is that the work group functions equally well with or without the manager. All must feel ownership, accountability, and autonomy for the outcomes, both individually and collectively.

The manager facilitates shared responsibilities; thus the nursing staff members help each other grow as much as the manager does. Shared responsibility can be nurtured by communication—horizontally between the nursing staff, and vertically between the staff and manager and manager and staff. Information sharing and the effective use of information by the team in problem solving are dependent on the team's stage of development. For example, in our setting the nurse executive shared fiscal data, productivity, and skill mix data with the Council on Clinical Practice during our first year of shared governance as the budgetary process was in progress. Staff was somewhat overwhelmed by the data, even after explanation and interpretation of it. Two years later the nursing staff has identified roles and redefined the nursing care delivery system, making recommendations to managers and the nurse executive within the boundaries of available human and fiscal resources.

Regardless of the stage of group development, staff nurses often know more than the manager about the patient and how to best provide care and ensure quality, cost-efficient outcomes. Staff must be empowered to solve problems interdependently.

A clearly defined purpose and vision guide the direction of the work group. Miller's (1984) strategic culture-building model, which addresses the current and future external environments, current and future organizational culture, and current and future definitions of who we are and how we are organized, can provide a model for defining the purpose. These issues must be addressed by all within the system before the formalized governance structure bylaws can be developed. This purpose will eventually provide a context for decision making, and a standard for evaluation and a focus for shared responsibility.

The McKinsey 7-S framework reminds managers that the seemingly irrational, intuitive aspects of the organization are actually important to the health and success of the organization. This framework (Peters and Waterman, 1982) examines shared values, structure, strategy, systems, style, staff, and skills. Centering around shared values forces executives and managers to focus on concepts related to the organization and staff that must be realigned in the transition from management to governance.

Health care managers of the 1990s should focus on this framework from the perspective of developing the staff by providing education about the skills necessary to successfully participate in a professional governance structure. Managerial skills and styles must also be redefined to facilitate this process. Shared values about people and the roles they play in the success of the organization will be equally important. Effective change that results in implementing organizational strategies for market-driven quality care and services will be supported by decentralized structures that use individual values to support individual, group, and organizational growth. Human technology changes are vital for health care organizations to obtain strategic advantage in the marketplace. These changes need the ongoing support of systems that provide sophisticated information to enhance data management and facilitate group problem solving.

A successful human culture in which employees love their work can be facilitated by the transformation from management to governance. As the system moves toward a governance model in which the role of the manager is that of consultant, a series of processes is vital to the success of developing a professional leadership model. These include:

1. Planned change focusing on agreement of a shared vision or purpose by key stakeholders
2. Education and skills development for all involved in the systems change
3. Coaching through team meetings and problem-solving sessions
4. Reinforcement of new behaviors

Another transition from management to governance is a concept called *team learning,* defined by Senge (1990) as the process of developing the team so that the shared vision is implemented by building on the ability of the team to attain the vision. Because most decisions in today's health care organizations are translated into actions by teams, one of the tasks for successful transition from management to governance will be the development of team learning, which will markedly impact organizational outcomes. Team learning and interaction allow better solutions to complex issues because of collective creativity and provide for coordinated activity that synergistically capitalizes on individual strengths. This process involves trust, team communication with a focus on active listening, and discussion focusing on divergent and complex points of view.

Relinquishment of authority and control to the staff by managers is facilitated during the transition to team learning. Team learning negates systems that control behavior, and focuses on shared visions, understandings, and decentralization as the forum for decision making. During this process managers are researchers and designers (Senge, 1990). Successful managers in the learning organization will understand the organizational system and driving forces that impact change and will create the learning necessary for them to be understood.

Motivation, commitment, and rewards are concepts inherent in the transition to an accountability-based shared governance model. Team energy provides the motivation to continue the development of the governance process. Early in the process small successes emphasize that staff members have assumed accountability for their professional practice, peer relations, and governance. For example, in our setting, staff members had an early success in initiating and implementing a nursing care delivery system change that solidified their role in decision making, and the role of the nursing management in the partnership. Commitment increases as the system matures and more staff members have opportunity to operationalize the bylaws and actively participate in the system. Power increases within the governance system as shared values are operationalized and goals are attained.

Rewards are intangible and are often manifest as staff decisions directly and positively impact patient care. As the governance structure successfully handles complex, difficult issues, individual and group professional growth is noted throughout the organization.

SHARED GOVERNANCE AND JCAHO NURSING STANDARDS

The Joint Commission on Accreditation of Health Care Organizations (JCAHO) agenda for change focuses on quality and clinical and organizational outcome measurement. The philosophic base for the agenda for change is founded on the concepts of continuous quality improvement with the needed transition from the process to outcome. Accountability-based shared governance models are a natural vehicle for compliance with these new standards.

The revised JCAHO nursing standards provide an exciting opportunity for nursing by clearly outlining what patients should receive as a result of nursing care. Although the standards provide a broad framework for nursing practice within a health care setting, they do not dogmatically describe the structure and process of the nursing service but focus more on outcomes of nursing care. Nursing care standards (Joint Commission on Accreditation of Health Care Organizations, 1991) state:

1. Patients receive nursing care based on a documented assessment of their needs. (p. 131)
2. All members of the nursing staff are competent to fulfill their assigned responsibilities. (p. 133)
3. The nurse executive and other appropriate registered nurses develop hospital-wide patient care programs, policies and procedures that describe how the nursing care needs of patient or patient populations are assessed, evaluated and met. (p. 134)

4. The hospital's plan for nursing care is designated to support improvement and innovation in nursing practice and is based on both the needs of patients to be served and the hospital's mission. (p. 136)
5. The nurse executive and other nursing leaders participate with leaders from the governing body, management, medical staff, and clinical areas in the hospital's decision-making structures and processes. (p. 137)
6. As part of the hospital's quality assurance program, the quality and appropriateness of the patient care provided by all members of the nursing staff are monitored and evaluated . . . (p. 138)

The standards incorporate the concepts of professional accountabilities related to practice, quality, competence, resource usage, and research. The parallel accountabilities and authority reflected in nursing staff bylaws complement and mirror the new JCAHO standards.

In our setting, measuring attainment of the standards provided an additional opportunity to strengthen the professional governance model as we prepared for our triennial accreditation survey by developing action plans based on opportunities for improvement identified during self-assessment using the JCAHO standards. Action plans were implemented in collaboration with the nurse executive and nurse managers who ensured resource availability. Nursing management provided coordination, facilitation, and integration during the preparation process.

The decentralized unit-based accreditation visit provided the nursing staff with the opportunity to review their nursing practice, policies, orientation/education/ competency documentation and quality assessment, and improvement activities directly with the nurse surveyor. Staff ownership of accountabilities and articulation of practice decisions facilitated positive interactions during the on-site visit. Examples of systems developed as outcomes of shared governance in our setting that incorporated our nursing theoretical model and facilitated compliance with JCAHO standards included:

- Competency-based orientations and skill assessment
- Unit-based education for patients and staff
- Professional review
- Professional practice model
- Outcome-focused care planning/documentation
- Identification of professional references for standards
- Unit-based quality assessment and improvement activities
- Staff-directed selection of nursing staff

In the final analysis, the philosophy and style of nursing management determine how the accreditation standards are put into operation in a health care setting. Sharing power within clearly defined boundaries will be imperative as nursing moves to staff empowerment models and employee involvement systems.

The organizational culture within a health care institution and the level of maturity in development of the shared governance model will assist the nurse executive in determining the most appropriate processes to ensure that the responsibility, authority, and accountability for nursing practice reside with the nursing staff. Nursing leadership can most effectively use the professional governance structure within a consultative model for ongoing interactions with the professional nursing staff. Early in the development of a shared governance model, the nursing executive often provides focused direction for staff but as the staff matures in governance activities, the nurse executive's role moves to one of providing feedback, listening, and asking questions. Staff participation in forums within the health care organization must be facilitated by the nurse executive.

BYLAWS FOR THE NURSING ORGANIZATION

Bylaws define how a professional nursing system operates and also legitimize the nursing structure within the organization. Bylaws are critical to a shared governance model's success. They lend credibility and provide parameters for practice and structural operation just as medical staff bylaws provide a framework for the organization of medical practice within an organization. It is the premise of transitional professional governance models that decisions should be made by those who use the resources, whether they be within the nurse manager–nurse executive relationship, or the nursing staff–nurse manager relationship or the nursing staff–patient relationship. Bylaws, a set of shared values and guidelines about the discipline of nursing that include details about its execution within a setting, can provide a framework in which practice accountability and autonomy at the professional staff nurse level take place.

Bylaws are the rules and regulations adopted by the nursing organization for its governance. They reflect expectations in the interdependent relationship of governance related to performance for professional practice and the manager's role in creating an environment that supports professional practice. Bylaws are a written manifestation of the structure that flows from the organization and replace rigid, administratively generated policies and procedures. Bylaws must clearly describe the structure, functions, and operations of nursing within the health care organization. Provision should be made so that bylaws cannot be amended unilaterally by either the organization or the clinical nursing staff. Refer to Appendix 8-1 for an example of bylaws.

A framework for accountability-based decision making centered on the innate human desire to succeed is created within which the nursing staff can act with a reasonable degree of autonomy for professional obligations to the organization related to patient care. Articles of the bylaws identified by Porter-O'Grady and Finnegan (1984) include the following:

1. Preamble
2. Role
3. Services
4. Membership
5. Governance
6. Discipline and removal
7. Organizational coordination
8. Bylaws revision
9. Rules and regulations
10. Adoption (pp. 168-169)

Bylaw Development

The development of bylaws is based on identification and integration of professional accountabilities related to practice, quality, competence, resource utilization, and research. These accountabilities must be clearly defined with the professional nursing organization as a prerequisite to the process of bylaws development. Issues that serve as a foundation to bylaw development within the context of a professional organization are multifaceted and include:

Practice
- What is it nurses do?
- What is nursing practice?
- What are the outcomes of nursing?
- What effect does nursing practice have on clinical and organizational outcomes?

Quality
- How do we define quality?
- What is the quality of service that nurses provide?
- How is the quality of the provider of service ensured?
- How is quality of service measured?
- How are quality assurance and quality improvement ensured within nursing and the health care organization?

Competence
- How is a prior competence assessed?
- What are the organization's standards of competence?
- How do professional nurses within the organization fulfill their obligation to teach each other?
- What are the organization's beliefs about ensuring continuing competence?
- What are nursing's beliefs about lifelong learning for professionals and how are they supported within the organization?

Resource issues
- How will resource accountabilities be integrated with clinical accountabilities for practice, quality, competence, and research?
- What is management's accountability for human, material, fiscal, support, and systems resources?
- How is management accountability related to resources in operation within the organization?

Research
- How does nursing develop new knowledge?
- How does nursing verify existing knowledge?
- What are the role and responsibility of the practicing professional nurse in these processes?
- How do these processes impact nursing practice and clinical outcomes?

A clear organizational commitment to professional governance and the definition of accountabilities are essential steps in the development of formal bylaws.

Although bylaws may be developed before the implementation of a professional governance structure, their development and implementation are often delayed until the model has been implemented to allow ample experience with the governance structure.

Often, in the evolution of professional governance within an institution, both the professional nursing staff and nurse executive have begun to address the political issues of obtaining support and approval for the bylaws. Clearly defined bylaws outline the professional governance activities of nursing and their format needs to be fully integrated with professional nursing responsibilities, authorities, and accountabilities. Administrative support and approval are fostered by ongoing communication with key stakeholders about the development of the professional governance model and their relationship to successful outcome attainment consistent with the mission of the institution.

Bylaws should be as simple as possible. Although each organization's bylaws will be unique, an overview of their generic elements may be useful to those who are beginning the development process. Bylaws must be written and owned by the professional staff. In most settings this is an evolutionary process with growth of the professional organization reflected in bylaws development.

Development of Bylaws Articles

Preamble.   The preamble includes information related to the purpose, philosophy, and objectives of the organization. This section provides a clear understanding of the role and function of the organization and what it means to the individual nurse. Issues to be addressed during development of the preamble of the bylaws include:

- Why are bylaws being written?
- What is the purpose of nursing within the institution?
- What is the philosophy of nursing within the organization?
- How is nursing defined within the organization?
- What are the objectives for the organization?
- Are the objectives stated so they reflect the accountabilities of nursing within the hospital?
- What framework best states the nursing organization's objectives from a short- and long-term perspective?

Role.   As defined in the nursing organization's bylaws, *role* determines the authority and thereby the accountability for professional nursing. Role functions and activities of the professional nurse are stated as they relate to accomplishing the purpose, critical objectives, and philosophy of the organization. Role identification, expectations, authority, and accountabilities must address:

- What authority and accountability for practice is stated in the nurse practice act?
- What other internal or external standards guide the nurse's authority and accountability for clinical nursing services?
- What are the responsibilities, authorities, and accountabilities of the professional nurse in the organization for clinical nursing services?

- How are nursing services structured to meet individual patient and significant others' needs?
- How are nursing services structured to facilitate the nurses' management of resources to provide quality, cost-efficient, coordinated care and leadership development for the nurse?
- How does the nurse develop interfaces to facilitate patient and organizational outcomes?
- What is the nurse's role related to participation in organizational forums within the health care organization?

Definition of services. Professional nursing services as defined in the bylaws assist those who read them in clarifying the role of nursing within the organization. A synopsis of the nursing organization's scope of care as articulated in the quality assurance plan may be easily translated into this segment of the bylaws. Considerations include:

- What are the primary services provided?
- Who provides them?
- When are they provided?
- Where are they provided?
- What population of patients receives them?
- What is the conceptual framework for nursing practice?
- What is the nursing care delivery system?
- What are the professional nurses' accountabilities for patient care within the scope of nursing services provided?

Membership. Nursing staff membership as a privilege rather than as a condition of employment is a relatively new concept for most nursing organizations. Specifics related to credentials, privileges, tenure, removal, and obligations of accountability will be reviewed later in this chapter. Membership issues include:

- Who will be granted privileges?
- What are the criteria and qualifications for membership?
- What will be the process for granting privileges?
- What will be the duration of privileges?
- What are the conditions for reappointment?
- What are the types of membership to be granted (i.e., provisional, consulting, full)?
- What are the specific role activities, authorities, responsibilities, and accountabilities for each type of membership?
- Who will be responsible for the process of granting membership?
- How does the membership process interface with human resources within the larger organization?

Governance. The governance article in the bylaws clearly defines the role, activities, process, responsibilities, and membership of the bodies that comprise the governance structure. If a councilor model of shared governance is selected, councils can be aligned based on accountabilities of the professional nurse. These councils are responsible for the operation and integration of the professional nursing organization as it organizes, manages, and evaluates delivery of nursing care services within the organization. Basic issues to be addressed are:

- What governance structure best supports the purpose and attainment of the critical objectives of the nursing organization?
- What is the role of each governing group within the governance model?
- What are the authorities and accountabilities of each council or governing group in the governance system?
- How will the business of the governing group be conducted?
- How are members and officers of the governance selected and how long will they serve?
- How is membership rotated so that new members are integrated into the group's work?
- What are the expectations for attendance?
- How are decisions made between scheduled meetings?
- How are task forces and subcommittees appointed and what is their accountability within the governance structure?
- How will the performance of the governing group be measured and what is the relationship of the councils to each other related to integrative and coordinating functions?

Discipline and removal.   Discipline and removal from the professional nursing staff are discussed in conjunction with the credentials process. It is imperative that these processes are clearly defined in the bylaws and are implemented within the health care organization's framework, reflect the organization's human resource policies and integrate with them, and meet state and institutional requirements.

Consultation from the hospital's legal counsel and human resource department is imperative in development of this article of the bylaws.

This article of the bylaws has been expanded in some organizations to include information about career advancement and professional review processes. These processes may include advancement from one level of professional nursing practice to another. They may also include information about the professional review process at the time of annual performance evaluation.

Organizational Coordination

This article of the bylaws addresses organizational coordination and governance of the professional nursing organization from the perspective of the role of nursing administration, the coordinating council or body, and the professional nursing staff as a whole. Critical to the development of this section of the bylaws is a clear definition of the role of the nurse executive related to responsibilities and accountabilities to the hospital administrator of the organization for the coordination, integration, and administration of nursing. The nurse executive also has responsibility for ensuring that bylaws are promulgated to staff, and that they are followed according to the existing rules, regulations, policies, and procedures of the particular institution.

The role of the nurse manager on behalf of the nursing staff to coordinate the nursing service is one that supports the staff's accountability for nursing practice. The primary role of nursing management is to support the work of nursing within the clinical system by integrating, coordinating, and facilitating human, material, fiscal, and systems resources. In this new forum the nurse executive's role in organizational coordination is to provide corporate perspective by clearly expressing visions and supporting staff involvement in forums that facilitate professional governance at all levels of the organization. This ultimately ensures that the corporate or organizational needs for nursing care services are met.

Regardless of the type of governance structure the role, power and authority, membership, and meeting times of the coordinating governing group are clearly delineated in the bylaws. Clear definition of the role of the council chairpersons and the coordinating council for the decision-making process is critical to a governance model's successful function.

The article on organizational coordination also elaborates on the role of the professional nursing staff in decisions affecting it and discusses the purpose, frequency, and procedures for meetings of the professional nursing staff.

Bylaws Revision

Bylaws adoption and subsequent revision or amendment are accomplished by processes that allow for review of the proposed changes by the professional nursing staff and nurse executive before formal approval. Often bylaws in a councilor model of governance state that any member of the professional nursing organization may submit a recommendation to a council chairperson, who will then present the bylaws changes to the coordinating council for review and inclusion on the agenda of a regularly scheduled meeting of the professional nursing staff. Changes are usually approved by a two-thirds majority of staff. In most organizations bylaws are reviewed and revisions or amendments are approved at the annual meeting. Changes often reflect growth within the professional nursing organization or reflect organizational changes impacting the nursing organization.

Rules and Regulations

This section of the bylaws grants permission to the councils or governing groups to develop rules and regulations. Rules and regulations are developed by individual councils or governing groups. These rules and regulations define activities and enable the council or governing group to implement its work consistent with the bylaws. Rules and regulations are often approved by the coordinating council or governance body before implementation and are not attached to the bylaws of the nursing organization.

Adoption

This bylaws section states the process for approval of the bylaws by the professional staff and a section for appropriate signatures, including the president of the nursing staff, and appropriate executive and/or administrative signatures within the institution. Bylaws usually are approved by a two-thirds majority of the nursing staff at the regularly scheduled annual meeting. Ample time for all members to review bylaws before the meeting is imperative to the success of their adoption.

Bylaws create the setting for "win-win" agreements (Covey, 1989), one of the characteristics of organizational effectiveness in professional governance models. Clearly defining the framework and obtaining consensus before implementation creates an environment for success and clearly delineates standards against which individual, group, and system outcomes can be measured. Five elements cited by Covey as crucial to win-win agreements are:

- *"Desired results* (not methods) identify what is to be done and when.
- *Guidelines* specify the parameters (principles, policies, etc.) within which results are to be accomplished.
- *Resources* identify the human, financial, technical, or organizational support available to help accomplish the results.
- *Accountability* sets up the standards of performance and time of evaluation.
- *Consequences* specify—good and bad, natural and logical—what does and will happen as a result of evaluation." (p. 223)

It is evident in this framework that methods are not delineated. Bylaws, like win-win agreements, focus on results, boundaries, availability of resources, the meaning of accountability, and the consequences of performance. Bylaws operate on the basic assumption that the professional nurse is capable of self-direction and performance control and can be self-governed to do whatever is necessary within established guidelines to attain the desired outcomes. The consensus or mutual endorsement of the bylaws by nursing staff and the organization, coupled with involvement in their development, cements and broadens nursing's contract with society.

Bylaws provide basic guidelines and must be adaptable and flexible to the developmental stage of the professional governance structure within the organization. Initially more guidelines, visible resource availability, and systems performance evaluation may be necessary for successful development of true professional governance systems. As the governance model matures, fewer guidelines, less frequent accountability measurements, and longer-term intrinsic rewards will be supported by the bylaws. Ultimately the bylaws become internalized and are inherent in the governing process.

When bylaws are implemented, all systems within the organization must support the win-win situation that must occur for professional governance system success. Systems traditionally within the realm of the manager—job design, organizational structures, role definition, communication, budgeting, compensation, planning, operational activities, information, hiring, education, development, and evaluation—must be integrated for governance to be a success. Accountability is fostered by the bylaws and the basic nature of humans in their motivation to do whatever is necessary to accomplish desired results within the parameters of the system. This is further supported when individuals have input into the development of the system, have agreed to support it, and have received ongoing performance feedback to celebrate success or make necessary performance corrections.

During the development of bylaws nurses within an organization participate in the development and operation of the professional governance structure. As each section unfolds, the structure, responsibilities, and accountabilities within the setting are further clarified. An example of bylaws is included in the Appendix as a possible guide for organizational thinking as bylaws are developed and sanctioned.

Definition of nursing staff membership, credentials, tenure, removal, and obligations of accountability are new concepts in most nursing organizations and will be discussed as they relate to bylaw development and implementation. Because the nursing staff has responsibility for peer-based activities of performance evaluation, competency, and accountability within the professional governance framework, it is imperative that members share in the credentialing process as well. Credentialing is a function of professionals for the appointment of staff that is clearly denoted in staff bylaws and supported by regulatory and accrediting bodies. Within the framework of the bylaws nursing staff membership should be clearly defined. Staff membership is granted by the nursing organization in accordance with the bylaws, rules and regulations, and policies of the nursing staff and the hospital. Each applicant for membership is oriented to the bylaws and agrees that his or her practice shall be bound by them. Criteria in the bylaws clearly delineate licensure, as well as education and professional experience requirements. Bylaws may also elaborate on the hospital's ability to provide resources for applicants as they participate in fulfilling their obligation to the institution in providing quality-based and cost-efficient care. In addition, each applicant for nursing staff membership consents to review of records and documents pertaining to licensure, experience, education, and other evidence of competencies. The process usually includes a personal interview to determine eligibility for nursing staff membership.

Peer recommendations can be part of the staff involvement process in recommendations for nursing staff membership. In some settings establishment of credentials begins at the initial formal contact of the nurse applicant with the organization as staff assumes accountability and responsibility for the interview and selection process of staff. Managers in this process act as consultants and facilitators to staff to ensure compliance with institutional and legal mandates related to hiring. In other settings applicants' credentials reviews are handled entirely by a credentials committee, a group reporting to the quality assurance body within the governance structure.

Accountability is fostered within the system by the credentialing process. Nurses within the system are accountable for selection of staff members who they think will abide by the bylaws. Applicants who are bound by the bylaws as a condition of nursing staff membership will also be charged with accountability within the governance structure. Professional nurses who have been appointed in any membership category are oriented to the bylaws and accept the professional obligations stated in them as an expectation of clinical privileges.

The tenet of accountability in the process of professional governance is based on the innate desire to succeed and be responsible for achievement of mutually endorsed goals and responsibilities by those participating in the system. The following checks must be built into the bylaws structure related to credentials and privileges:

1. Expeditious review of applications
2. Delineation of additional organization approvals

3. Periodic review and reappointment process
4. An appeals process

If nursing seeks approval of the governing board for its bylaws, then the issue of approval from the governing board for applications for staff appointments must be addressed.

As nursing moves into the twenty-first century and continues its development as a profession, nursing organizations within health care institutions may explore the possibility of board approval of bylaws to obtain legal support for governance. Dialogue between executives and the board will determine the feasibility of the process and delineate issues to be discussed and approval processes. This approval by the board will cement the responsibility of nursing as a profession with its rights, obligations, and responsibilities within the health care organization.

Active credentials review must be an ongoing process. The requirements for reappointment and advancement within categories of nursing membership within the organization must be clearly delineated in the bylaws. Attainment of performance-based criteria by professional nurses provides the foundation for advancement within the system. Career advancement programs, peer review systems for performance evaluation, and appeals and grievance processes will need to be integrated within the organization with the credentialing process as the professional governance model unfolds. Part of the process of definition of accountability is the development of systems and processes for disciplinary action if obligations and responsibilities are not fulfilled by the professional nurse. These processes often reflect the organization's human resource policies related to these situations and are implemented within the health care organization's framework. If additional processes are developed within nursing, they must also be integrated with human resources.

All nurses (Porter-O'Grady, 1985) whose primary role is clinical nursing practice need to be integrated within the credentialing process. A system must be developed to ensure that this occurs and that all nurses currently employed in the setting as well as those who will be employed in the future in expanded roles participate in the process.

Granting of privileges is an important cornerstone in establishing accountability within the professional governance framework. It is imperative that the bylaws be clearly followed, decisions made expeditiously, and that documentation of reasons for action be related to patient care issues within the efficient operation of the nursing organization. These parameters should be integrated in professional staff governance activities whether they be related to initial application for membership, reappointment, performance review, or the grievance and appeal process. Only if the bylaws clearly address the basic concerns of the hospital and its nursing staff and clearly delineate that the procedure of earning credentials and granting of privileges is applied equitably will the process be insulated from attack. Immunity from liability should be included in the bylaws for those on the review committee. This issue can be discussed with hospital counsel to ensure compliance with state law.

Nursing staff bylaws clearly delineate the role of the professional nurse with clinical privileges in the care of patients throughout the system. Bylaws state parameters, rules and regulations, and either general or specific policies that support the nursing organization and the institution. The bylaws are designed to provide a framework for structuring the ongoing work of the nursing organization as it defines, delineates, implements, and evaluates activities related to the provision of patient care including individual professional development, peer relationships, and the governance structure. Periodic scheduled review of the bylaws ensures the opportunity to reconfirm important aspects about the function and structure of the nursing organization as well as ensuring that the bylaws reflect current practice with respect to the organization and its functions.

Bylaws development, as with any other major change in the organization involving a redefinition of the organizational culture, is facilitated by stakeholder analysis in the developmental process. Key stakeholders in this process of development of bylaws for the professional governance system in nursing include professional nursing staff, nurse managers, nurse executives, organizational administration, physicians, and possibly consumers. Professional nursing staff and nursing management must advocate the governance concept and development of bylaws necessary to support it or the transformation to professional governance will perish. During the planning phase, systems outcomes and criteria for measurement must be defined. Early in the process, after the initial buy-in at the nurse staff level, a political analysis of the organization will provide information about when and how to involve the medical staff, hospital administration, human resources personnel, and legal consultation in the development, approval, and implementation process of the bylaws. Validation of bylaws by key stakeholders within the organization provides additional credence for nursing professional governance and the belief that nursing can be responsible for its professional practice. The framework has been delineated and expectations for success of the model established by the bylaw process.

Resources will be invaluable to the nursing staff, nurse managers, and executive team as bylaws are developed to ensure that the mission, goals, and governance structure are feasible within the constraints of resource allocation. They must also meet criteria established by regulatory and accrediting bodies including but not limited to the state board of registered nursing, the labor board, and federal and state statutes, as well as the organization's insurer and the hospital's legal counsel. Hospital legal counsel should review bylaws before implementation to ensure they are in compliance with current state laws. Although the primary responsibility for development of bylaws rests with the professional staff, judicious use of resources ensures their development and implementation to facilitate positive outcomes for all stakeholders. The consultative and review process is inherent in the development of bylaws that support a system that fosters professional autonomy and accountability.

Development of bylaws and a professional governance model is a long and tedious process. Staff involvement, communication, education, staff and organizational approval, and building stakeholder support for the concept are critical to its success. The professional governance system must be based on organizational values consistent with common goals and supported by a strategic plan. Bylaws support the vision, values, and structure of professional governance to become a reality.

GOVERNANCE ISSUES

Professional governance models for nursing are transitional leadership models that will lead the profession into the twenty-first century. Several issues arise regarding the implementation of nursing governance functions within and perhaps outside the traditional boundaries of organizational structures.

Nurse Participation in Hospital Governance

One of the fundamental issues addressed is the need for nursing representation on the hospital governing board. Governing boards have been involved with medical staff issues and participation historically but not *with* nursing, whose role within the organization is critical to attainment of quality, cost-efficient clinical and organizational outcomes. A paradigm shift is beginning as "successful institutions see leadership as a critical mass that brings in components from governance, management, medical staff and patient services especially nursing" (Chapman-Cliburn, 1989, p. 48). Board members are beginning to seek advice from people other than the chief executive officer and are beginning to interact with senior and middle managers within the institution.

Several models have been implemented to foster productive, successful relationships between nursing services and the board of trustees or governing board of a health care institution. Sands (1990) states that board members who are nurses are the exception to the rule and that open relationships between nurse trustees and nurse executives can benefit the institution by better facilitation of information to the board. These open relationships, which enhance the nurse trustee's and nurse executive's perspective, can strengthen nursing's position within the institution while positively impacting hospital governance.

Smith (1986) cites that nurses "need direct access, indeed membership on hospital boards to represent themselves in a publicly responsible manner and to see that nursing resources are committed within justly accountable bounds. They need to be a visible presence just as physicians do." (p. 48). It is unclear whether future access to and participation on governing boards will be through nursing staff members who are independent and contract directly with a hospital for the provision of clinical nursing services and are organized in a self-governance model through nurse executives or through nursing representatives from the professional governance structure. Regardless of the model for participation in governance activities of the institution at the board level, nurses must learn new social and political behaviors. Translation of the clinical perspective must be succinctly presented, often in the language of economics and politics. Learning to function within this new political and power structure will challenge nurse executives and the professional nurses who deliver clinical services as nursing moves into more developed and sophisticated governance models.

Joel Edelman, president of Rose Medical Center in Denver, has stated "So too, then must nurses collectively generate a new spirit of self-sufficiency, self-determination and accountability" (Johnson, 1988, p. 8). Johnson, who has been a member of the board of trustees at Rose Medical Center for 10 years, identifies her role predominantly as that of a community lay person who shares an invaluable perspective of the practicing nurse and nurse executive. Since 1988 the president of Rose Medical Center's Nursing Congress has also been a board member.

Nursing within the institution has recognized participation on this forum as an opportunity to address professional issues and influence positively the quality of care within the rapidly changing health care environment. Another positive outcome of staff nursing representation on the board has been increased confidence in nursing abilities and increased power for nursing within the institution. Conversely, nurses in these governance structures have become increasingly accountable for their practice and governance activities, a quantum leap for nurses in most institutions. One of the major benefits of representation on the board by the president of the Nursing Congress at Rose Medical Center has been presentation of the unique view of a practicing professional nurse to the governing body as well as enhanced two-way communication between the board and practicing nurses who now have a better understanding of the rationale behind some of the decisions made in the current turbulent health care environment. As a professional group with employee status within a given organization, nurses need to address the issue of appropriateness of sitting on the board of directors of their employing organization. Perhaps nursing's collective needs could be more objectively and systematically represented and advocated by a nurse who is a true community member and not bound or limited by employment status.

New Roles and Focus

Governance seems to be undergoing a metamorphosis from the governing bodies of the past that provided advice and counsel, discipline value, and acted in crisis situations. Carver (1990) presents a model of governance that helps boards focus on leadership responsibilities for policy making, articulating the organization's mission, and sustaining the vision. Inherent in this process are strategies of boards to create goal-dominated policies and work with management to ensure their achievement.

Fundamental to a discussion of new roles for governance boards and nursing's potential role in that arena is the need to address a parallel between medical practice in organized settings and nursing practice. During this century medicine has sought to strengthen and preserve the independent practitioner with an active voice in the definition of policy and procedures. Today more than 25% of physicians are employed by institutions (Osmond, 1980), and doctors are coping with issues of subordinancy over which the profession once had control. The role of medical director has emerged from this change in the organization of medical practice. The medical director is a liaison between the staff and administration and must establish power in both clinical and administrative arenas to be effective. Physicians (Astrachan and Astrachan, 1989) often assume these roles of authority and accountability with increasingly less time and opportunity to attain managerial competency. These organizational changes affect power, authority, accountability, and responsibility within the organization. As roles continue to change, physicians must be integrated into the organization so that both organizational and professional goals can be attained. Apparent in these new structures for employed physicians is the movement of autonomy over practice from individuals to the group. It also has become apparent that management and governance education must be provided if physicians are to be expected to participate responsibly within governance models.

Organizational structures impact both nurses' and physicians' autonomy, authority, accountability, and effectiveness. Governance models must be implemented that meet both patient and professional needs and outcomes for nurses and physicians within the health care organization of the future. Some issues that should be addressed include:

- What structures positively influence professional behaviors?
- How do these structures impact quality of care?
- How do organizations ensure group as well as individual accountability?
- Which models decrease professional stress?

The solution to these issues is highly complex and will become easier as more experience is gained with governance models in nursing and health care.

Shortell (1989) identifies new roles for participants in hospital governance of risk-taker, strategic director, expert mentor, and evaluator. He articulates that hospital boards of the future will be effective if they are able to:

1. Manage a diverse group of stakeholders
2. Involve physicians in the management and governance process
3. Meet the governance needs of multi-institutional systems and hospital restructures
4. Meet the challenges of diversification and vertical integration
5. Understand strategy formation and implementation as interdependent and interrelated processes (p. 7).

Hospital governance will be impacted in the future by health care shifts from a product-driven, professionally dominated, focus, operational base to a market-driven, customer-dominated focus, strategic management base. To be successful in this transitional environment, interrelatedness and interactions must occur among the professional staff of health care organizations, management, and the board. Nurses may soon assume hospital governance roles just as physicians currently do. Roles stated by Shortell (1989) are applicable to professional governance models within the nursing organization.

Individual participants in governance must be able to not only process information but also make strategic decisions expeditiously. Participants will have clearly defined roles and will participate in outcome-focused, criterion-based evaluation of their individual roles as well as the governance system.

Participation in governance, whether within the nursing organization or broader health care organization, will require nurses to have a broad base of industry and organizational knowledge in addition to their clinical knowledge. They will also need to structure their governance models to facilitate rapid decision-making through empowerment of committees and subcommittees, and to move toward an outcome orientation with less preoccupation and valuing of process issues. Inherent to success of governance activities in these new models will be:

- Clearly defined parameters of autonomy and accountability for decision making
- Involvement of nursing professionals, who may either be employees of the hospital or independent practitioners contracting for the provision of clinical services

- The definition of nursing governance models within multiple hospital systems
- The redefinition of nursing governance in vertically integrative and diversified systems
- The ability of nurses to participate in planned strategy formation and serendipitous processes related to opportunities

Trust and information sharing will be vital for all participants at all levels within the professional governance model for nursing. A major thrust now and in the future will be balancing the accountabilities for meeting societal expectations for quality, cost-efficient care with implementation of the organization's mission, values, and philosophy.

Governance tasks are inherently different from other management functions. Mueller (1981) ascertained that governance is an unfolding "driven by soft realms of thought and deportment. They are value laden, subjective, intuitive and characteristic of the art forms dealing with social interaction" (p. XII). Carver (1990) describes a governance model as a framework that organizes thoughts, activities, structures, and relationships of governance bodies. He hypothesizes that an effective model of governance should accomplish all of the following:

1. Cradle a vision
2. Address fundamental values
3. Demand an external focus
4. Establish an outcome-focused mission as the central organizing force
5. Separate large from small issues
6. Think in the future
7. Create rather than react
8. Facilitate diversity and oneness
9. Define stakeholder relationships
10. Define self-discipline
11. Delineate the governing body's role on specific issues
12. Determine appropriate information needs
13. Balance tight and loose control
14. Use time productively

Louden (1975) adds that "if we do not concern ourselves with how we can rule organizations, the organization will rule us" (p. 117). Nursing has the opportunity to implement professional governance models that exemplify the characteristics of futuristic models. Consideration of these facets of governance identified by Carver (1990) is clearly imbedded in bylaws of nursing organizations. Nursing is just beginning to address the issues of bylaw and shared decision-making implementation outside the nursing organizational structure within the broader organizational context.

As nursing moves into a broader arena of governance activities, it will be imperative that roles within the leadership team be clearly delineated. Multiple levels of leadership teams exist within the professional governance structure. The nurse executive and president of the nursing staff constitute a leadership team as do the nursing president and council chairpersons on the coordinating council. As with any successful team, the roles, responsibilities, and accountabilities are clearly defined at the outset.

Evaluation is a relatively new concept in the broader governance process. Nurses within governance structures must develop creative methodologies to quantitatively and qualitatively assess individual and group performance that continually focuses on the following questions: How are we doing? What do we want to accomplish? How are we achieving it?

Traditionally, such evaluations focused on process and evaluative criteria have not been clearly defined. Models must be developed to address the question of whether the outcomes are worth the cost.

Mutual respect, support, and the ability of all participants to implement their responsibilities within a framework of defined control, responsibility, authority, and accountability result in the synergy characteristic of the high-performing work team. Creating a holistic integrated framework of values that encompass the organization is also a governance responsibility and often results in interpersonal challenges as individual members interact to convert divergence into a single viewpoint. This phenomenon is clearly observable as professional nursing staff members move toward governance—at the councilor or coordinating level, or within the larger health care organization.

Carver (1990) cites six strategies that apply to nurses who are participants in professional governance models. He advises participants to be obsessed with human benefits, think in the future, communicate concisely, be innovative in the selection and education of participants, rise above traditional thought, and continue to improve quality.

In summary, governance is really about empowerment. It is about risk, error, responsibility, authority, accountability, and trust. It concerns focusing on the bigger issues, defining and implementing visions within defined boundaries, thereby controlling the amount of risk. It is about flattening hierarchy and creating new roles and new partnerships at all levels within the organization. Governance is about structural systems and shared values that support professional nursing practice within a shared decision-making framework as nursing moves toward self-governance models in the twenty-first century. One final word about bylaws in professional governance models—they may be a hindrance, especially if they describe a framework that the professional nursing organization has already outgrown.

SUMMARY

Professional nursing shared governance models are transitional designs that will successfully position nursing as the primary professional organization within the health care setting. This position is particularly crucial as nursing moves through the 1990s and completes the redesign process of the health care organization. Central to successful development and implementation of shared governance models is the acquisition of new roles and values that redefine staff, manager, and executive roles within the nursing organization of the future. Staff empowerment models of the future must be designed to ensure partnerships between management and all levels of staff within the organization. These designs should drive decentralization of decision making related to the work of nursing to the point of service: the professional nurse level. Definition and formal sanctioning of professional governance models are supported by bylaws that clearly articulate the framework for the professional nursing organization and delineate responsibility, authority, and accountability for the practice of nursing. Professional governance models provide the support for internal and external standards and the accreditation process. A multitude of interesting and complex issues regarding the implementation of nursing governance models within and perhaps outside the traditional structures of health care organizations will need to be addressed as nursing governance models mature and as the very essence of the industry undergoes radical transformation.

REFERENCES

Accreditation Manual for Hospitals Vol. 1. (1991) Oakbrook Terrace, Ill.: Joint Commission on Accreditation of Healthcare Organizations.

Astrachen, J. and Astrachen, B. (1989). Medical Practice in Organized Settings: Redefining Medical Autonomy. *Archives of Internal Medicine,* 149, 1509-1513.

Belasco, J. (1989). Masters of Empowerment. *Executive Excellence,* 6(3), 11-12.

Bennis, W. and Nanus, B. (1985). *The Strategies for Taking Charge.* New York: Harper & Row.

Bridges, W. (1980). *Making Sense of Life's Transitions.* New York: Addison-Wesley.

Bukholtz, S. and Roth, T. (1986). *Creating the High Performing Work Team.* New York: John Wiley & Sons.

Carver, J. (1990). *Boards That Make a Difference.* San Francisco: Jossey Bass Publishers.

Chapman-Cliburn, G. (1988). Are Boards Gaining More Control Over Executive Decisions. *Hospitals,* 62(23), 44-48.

Covey, S. (1989). *Seven Habits of Highly Effective People.* New York: Simon & Schuster.

Crosby, B. (1986). Employee Involvement: Why it Fails, What it Takes to Succeed. *Personnel Administrator,* 31(2), 105-106.

Jacques (1990). In Praise of Hierarchy. *Harvard Business Review,* 68(1), 127-133.

Johnson, L. (1988). A Place At The Table: When Nurses Are Members of a Medical Center Governing Board. *Aspen's Advisor for Nurse Executives,* 4(1), 6-8.

Louden, J.K. (1975). *The Effective Director in Action* (p. 117). New York: AMACOM.

Mace, M. (1990). Excerpts From the President and the Board of Directors. *Harvard Business Review,* 68(6), 37.

Miller, L. (1984) *American Spirit: Visions of a New Corporate Culture.* New York: W. Morrow.

Miller, L. (1988). *Barbarians to Bureaucrats: Corporate Life Cycles Strategies: Lessons From the Rise and Fall of Civilizations.* New York: Clarkson N. Potter.

Mintzberg, H. (1989). *Mintzberg on Management.* New York: Free Press.

Mueller, R.K. (1981). *The Incomplete Board: The Unfolding of Corporate Governance.* Lexington, Mass.: Heath.

Osmond, H. (1980). God and the Doctor. *New England Journal of Medicine,* 302, 555-558.

Peters, T. and Waterman, R., Jr., (1982). *In Search of Excellence.* New York: Warner Books.

Porter-O'Grady, T. (1990). *Reorganization of Nursing Practice: Creating the Corporate Venture.* Rockville, Md.: Aspen Publications.

Porter-O'Grady, T. (1985) Credentialing, Privileging and Nursing Bylaws: Assuring Accountability. *Journal of Nursing Administration,* 15(12), 23-27.

Porter-O'Grady, T. and Finnegan, S. (1984). *Shared Governance for Nursing: A Creative Approach to Professional Accountability.* Rockville, Md.: Aspen Systems.

Sands, R. (1990). Hospital Governance: Nurse Trustee Vis-a-vis Nurse Executive. *Nursing Management,* 21(12), 14-15.

Schein, E. (1965). *Organizational Psychology.* Englewood Cliffs, N.J.: Prentice-Hall.

Senge, P. (1990). *The Fifth Discipline: The Art and Practice of the Learning Organization.* New York: Currency Doubleday.

Shortell, S.M. (1989). New Directions in Hospital Governance. *Hospital and Health Services Administration,* 34(1), 7-23.

Smith, E.D. (1986) Nurse Trustee: Getting Power Over Policy. *Nursing Management,* 17(9), 48-50.

Tichy, N. and Ulrich, D. The Leadership Challenge—A Call for the Transformational Leader. *Sloan Management Review,* 25, 59-68.

Bylaws
Professional Nursing Staff
Suburban Hospital

ARTICLE I: PREAMBLE
Section 1—Purpose of the Bylaws

These bylaws describe the governance structure of the Department of Nursing and provide a framework for its operation. They describe the organization and the accountability of the professional nursing staff within a shared governance model.

Section 2—Definition of Nursing

Nursing is the diagnosis and treatment of human responses to actual or potential health problems.

Section 3—Philosophy of Nursing

We believe that the patient is the central figure in the hospital. The primary efforts of Nursing are directed toward meeting the patient's individual needs in relation to promotion of health, prevention of disease, and care of the dying. These needs are met without regard to race, creed, sex, disease process, or age through the coordinated and collaborative efforts of Nursing, Medicine, and other allied health professions.

We believe that all patients are entitled to the full scope of nursing. Therefore, we believe in two mutually valued levels of professional nursing practice. Nursing practice is differentiated between the Case Manager and Case Associate roles. Through these differentiated levels of nursing practice, all patients receive both the collaborative and independent aspects of nursing care.

We believe that patients and their families/significant others are to be treated with kindness, respect, and understanding. Both patients and their families/significant others are constantly involved in the patient's care and are kept informed about the patient's progress. The patient is encouraged to communicate concerns, questions, and feelings to the staff. We value the right of each patient and his/her family/significant others to understand the prescribed regimen to be followed upon return to the community. These instructions, therefore, are provided to each patient prior to discharge.

The nursing care delivery system used at Suburban Hospital is Differentiated Case Management. The Nursing Department believes in strengthening this deliv-

Reprinted with permission from Suburban Hospital, Bethesda, Maryland.

ery system through an integrated Quality Assurance Program. We believe in and support improvements in nursing practice which are based on the results of nursing research.

We believe that the practice of Nursing requires a commitment to continued professional growth through orientation, inservice, and continuing education. We support contributions to nursing education through affiliations with Schools of Nursing. We believe in a strong link between the service setting and academia in which both institutions share expertise and resources.

We believe that professional nurses accept accountability for the quality of care provided as well as the ethical and legal responsibilities involved in their practice.

We believe that it is the responsibility of Nursing Administration to identify and provide human and material resources as well as an administrative climate conducive to delivering quality care to patients.

We believe that nurse managers apply concepts of human relations and business in planning and operationalizing health care. Each manager is a developer of others. It is an expectation, therefore, that our managers be consistent in their efforts to assist their staff to learn responsible decision making. We believe that whenever appropriate, decisions should be made at the lowest possible level of the organization.

We believe that it is the responsibility of the nursing staff to utilize all the human and material resources provided in order to deliver effective and efficient care.

We believe in a working environment which is supportive to the professional, emotional, and social growth of all its employees. We recognize the need to keep abreast of local, state, and national trends in health care. We believe that Nursing must be informed, flexible, and responsive to these changes. Leadership within Nursing motivates change, promotes decision making, and fosters conflict resolution.

We believe in the value of shared governance in decision-making. Within the formal structure, councils have been established to empower the staff with the authority, autonomy, and control that is consistent with a professionally based practice model. These councils are as follows: Nursing Practice, Nursing Quality Assurance, Nursing Professional Development, and Nursing Management. A Coordinating Council guides these four councils. Involvement, authority, and accountability are broadly based in the councils and in the department.

We believe that open communication fosters ongoing cooperative relationships within the Department of Nursing and within the institution.

We believe that the values of compassion and caring should be extended to all persons associated with the hospital.

Section 4—Purpose of the Department of Nursing

1. To provide to the patient, at a reasonable cost, quality nursing care that can be evaluated and is consistent with the hospital's strategic plan.
2. To create a working milieu that encourages professional growth and personal satisfaction for its practitioners.

Section 5—Objectives of the Department of Nursing

OBJECTIVE 1: NURSING PRACTICE PERFORMANCE

To provide individualized, quality care to each patient.
Standards
A. At the time of admission, the current status of the patient's biopsychosocial needs are assessed by a registered nurse and documented on the Current Status Data Base form. The initial assessment must be completed within 1 hour of admission except where unit-based standards indicate otherwise.
B. Current status data are analyzed by a registered nurse and the appropriate protocols are implemented.
C. Within the first 24 hours of admission each patient is screened by a Case Manager for disruptions in functional health patterns. The data are recorded on the Functional Health Pattern Screening form.
D. Based on functional health pattern screening, the case manager identifies the patient's nursing diagnoses.
E. Realistic, measurable goals are established with the patient and family/significant other and nursing orders are written by the Case Manager.
F. The patient's comprehensive care plan contains provisions for meeting learning needs and discharge planning needs. The family/significant other is involved as appropriate.
G. Patient response to every nursing order in the comprehensive care plan is documented at least once each shift by the Case Associate/Case Manager.
H. A summary of the patient's progress is documented in the nursing progress notes each shift that the Case Manager works.
I. Periodic quality assurance activities indicate that the nursing care provided has met the objectives identified in the comprehensive care plan.

OBJECTIVE II: PLANNING PERFORMANCE

To maintain an ongoing system of planning in order to ensure effective utilization of human and material resources in delivering quality patient care.
Standards
A. Departmental goals are established annually by the Coordinating Council in collaboration with the Senior Vice President for Patient Care.
B. The Coordinating Council formulates the departmental goals based on the recommendations of each of the four councils.
C. Since the various councils are responsible for implementation of the goals, the role of the Patient Care Manager in implementation is that of facilitator.
D. Capital and operating budgets are developed by the Patient Care Manager of each unit and submitted to the Senior Vice President for Patient Care. The annual budget for the Department of Nursing is submitted by the Senior Vice President for Patient Care to the Chief Executive Officer for approval, prior to its submission to the Board.

E. As a member of the senior management staff, the Senior Vice President for Patient Care represents the Department of Nursing at the organizational level in planning policy and decisions that affect patient care in the hospital.

OBJECTIVE III: LEADERSHIP PERFORMANCE

To maintain a working environment that encourages professional growth through practice, education and research, resulting in quality nursing care and satisfaction for nursing practitioners.

Standards

A. Decisions are made at each level of accountability in the organization, using a decision-making model.
B. The Patient Care Manager of each individual unit is primarily responsible for the nursing activities and personnel in his/her department and is accountable to the appropriate Director of Nursing consistent with the mandates of the Council on Nursing Management.
C. Individual registered nurses are directly accountable to the patient for the nursing care they render in accordance with the objectives of the Professional Nursing Staff, the Council on Nursing Practice, and the individual department.
D. The Department of Nursing and each nursing unit maintain an ongoing in-service program designed to meet the educational needs of its nursing practitioners and approved by the Council on Professional Development. Advice and service for educational programs are obtained from the Department of Training, Education, and Development.
E. All positions in the Department of Nursing are filled by the candidates who best meet the criteria and objectives for the position.
F. Performance appraisal is an ongoing process, with individuals being evaluated in relation to approved departmental standards and individual objectives derived from his/her performance standards.

OBJECTIVE IV: ORGANIZING PERFORMANCE

To ensure that all work is organized and related so that effectiveness and personal satisfaction are maintained.

Standards

A. The organizational chart reflects professional relationships as well as communication mechanisms.
B. Decisions are made at the lowest possible level within the Department of Nursing.
C. Position descriptions and performance standards are maintained for all positions that relate to Professional Nursing in order to facilitate role description and performance evaluation.
D. The organization of Nursing represents a commitment to shared governance at all levels in the department.

OBJECTIVE V: CONTROLLING PERFORMANCE

To measure results against objective criteria with consideration given to acceptable exceptions. To ensure that corrective action is taken immediately where variances are not within acceptable limits.

Standards

A. Written structure, process, and outcome standards define and describe the scope of nursing practice at Suburban Hospital. All standards are reviewed a minimum of once every three years, revised as necessary, dated to indicate the time of the last review, and signed by the Senior Vice President for Patient Care and the chairperson of the appropriate council. A copy of the Nursing Practice Standards Manual is available on each nursing unit. The manual is kept in a place that is accessible to each staff member.
B. Implementation of standards is the responsibility of the members of the Nursing Council from which the standard originated in conjunction with the Patient Care Managers of individual nursing units.
C. Quality Assurance activities are directed by the Council on Nursing Quality Assurance with participation at all levels of the nursing service organization.
D. A time frame is established for corrective action of all unacceptable variances.
E. All exceptions outside of acceptable limits of variance that are not corrected within the predetermined time frame are reported to the Senior Vice President for Patient Care with recommendations for corrective action.

ARTICLE II: THE ROLE OF THE PROFESSIONAL NURSE

Consistent with the rules and regulations of the Maryland State Board of Nursing and national standards of nursing practice, the professional registered nurse (hereafter referred to as nurse) will assume accountability for the delivery of nursing care within the institution known as Suburban Hospital. The professional nurse (R.N.) delivers, coordinates, and integrates all nursing care services related to the identified needs of the patients admitted to Suburban Hospital. Professional nurses (R.N.s) may delegate specific nursing tasks to licensed practical nurses and unlicensed nursing personnel. Legally, however, the registered nurse is responsible and accountable for all nursing tasks that are delegated as outlined by the Maryland State Board of Nursing.

The professional nurse collaborates with other health professionals in fulfilling the health needs of the hospitalized patient. Professional nurses participate in the organized delivery of patient care services through contributions to the following hospital or medical staff committees:

Cancer Committee
Cardiology Center Committee
Collaborative Practice Committee
Critical Care Committee
Disaster Committee
Infection Control Committee
Institutional Review Board
Medical Records Committee

Nutrition Committee
Operating Room Committee
Patient Advisory Committee
Pharmacy and Therapeutics Committee
Pulmonary Function and Inhalation Committee
Quality Assurance Committee
Safety Committee
Trauma Committee
Utilization Review Committee

Professional nurses also have the opportunity to participate in the decision-making function within the Department of Nursing through membership on nursing governance councils, nursing committees, and task forces.

Each practicing professional registered nurse is accountable for the care he/she renders to the patient. The Board of Trustees, through the institution's organizational structure, expects the accountable execution of the nursing professional's role in the delivery of nursing care at Suburban Hospital.

ARTICLE III: MAJOR CLINICAL NURSING SERVICES

There are four (4) major clinical services within which nursing care is rendered at Suburban Hospital. In addition to the major services, nurses also practice in the Addiction Treatment Center and the Skilled Nursing Facility.

Section 1—Critical Care Services

Critical Care Services include Critical Care, Cardiology, and Emergency/Shock Trauma nursing. Critical care services are rendered by nurses who have highly specialized knowledge and skill in crisis intervention during an episode of critical illness. The critical care nurse is responsible for nursing assessment, planning, intervention, and evaluation of patients in the critical care setting.

Section 2—Medical/Surgical Nursing Services

The medical/surgical nurses are accountable for the assessment, planning, intervention, and evaluation of nursing care of medical/surgical patients. The nurse accepts responsibility for interpreting prescriptive measures of other health professionals and incorporating the activities of the health care team into the ongoing care needs of the individual patient. Discharge planning needs are incorporated into the role of the professional nurse in the medical/surgical clinical service. Medical/Surgical Nursing Services include specialities such as Oncology, Urology, Orthopedics, and Pulmonary Nursing in addition to general medical/surgical nursing.

Section 3—Psychiatric Nursing Services

Psychiatric nursing services are rendered by nurses with specialized knowledge and skill in managing patients with acute psychiatric illness. The nurse is accountable for assessment, planning, intervention, and evaluation of the patient's nursing needs. In addition, the nurse is expected to contribute to the multidisciplinary treatment plan. Members of the psychiatric nursing service are expected to maintain the therapeutic milieu on the psychiatric unit.

Section 4—Perioperative Nursing Services

The nurse in the perioperative environment is accountable for the appropriate care and safety of the patient who is undergoing operative intervention. The nurse is responsible for the assessment, planning, intervention, and evaluation of all preoperative, intraoperative, and postoperative nursing care needs. This nurse communicates and integrates the care prescriptions of other health professionals into the patient's operative plan of care, and coordinates nursing care activities directed to meeting the operative care needs of the patient.

ARTICLE IV: NURSING STAFF MEMBERSHIP
Section 1—Definition of Membership

Nursing staff membership is a privilege that is extended to those who meet qualifications, standards, and requirements as set forth in these bylaws and in accordance with Nursing Practice standards and the personnel policies of Suburban Hospital.

Section 2—Professional Nursing Staff

A. Members of the professional staff must be registered nurses, licensed to practice in the state of Maryland, who can give evidence of their background, experience, and education and can demonstrate professional competence with the appropriate supporting credentials. No professional registered nurse shall be entitled to membership on the nursing staff or to the exercise of specific clinical nursing privileges in the hospital solely by virtue of licensure to practice in the state of Maryland without presenting evidence of the previous additional requirements.

B. The professional nurse applying for privileges and appointment to the nursing staff shall be a graduate of an approved school of nursing and be legally licensed to practice nursing in the state of Maryland. This individual must meet all of the criteria and requirements indicated in these bylaws and in the unit to which the nurse is applying for specific privileges.

C. Nursing staff privileges shall be granted within the context of these bylaws and shall not be granted or denied for any other reason.

D. Acceptance of membership on the professional nursing staff shall constitute agreement to abide by the nursing standards that are promulgated by the Professional Nursing Organization.

Section 3—Conditions and Duration of Appointments to the Professional Nursing Staff

Initial appointment and reappointment to the nursing staff shall be made through the nursing personnel appointment process and shall be consistent with the hospital's personnel policy.

A. The initial appointment to the professional nursing staff shall be for a period of 3 months (90 days) for the probationary status. Permanent appointment shall be determined by the credential review process of the Department of Nursing pending a satisfactory performance evaluation by the Patient Care Manager of the unit to which the nurse is assigned. Probationary status can be extended by the Patient Care Manager for up to 90 days.

B. Appointment to the professional nursing staff shall confer on the appointee those clinical privileges and levels of nursing practice appropriate to the competence of the professional nurse.

C. Every application submitted for consideration for privileges on the nursing staff, when signed by the applicant, shall specify in writing the applicant's acknowledgment of the obligation to provide to the patient continuous nursing care that is consistent with nursing standards and the policies of the hospital. The applicant agrees to abide by the nursing staff bylaws and all other rules and regulations promulgated by the nursing staff.

D. The applicant for privileges within a specified clinical service or nursing unit of the Suburban Hospital shall present the following information and credentials supporting the application for clinical privileges.

1. A current copy of the applicant's registered nurse license is submitted to the recruiter for nursing.

2. The applicant's intention to obtain a license to practice in the state of Maryland prior to initial appointment is confirmed.

3. All license renewals and/or changes must be communicated, along with a copy for the file, to the Staffing Specialist in the Nursing Office within 3 working days of receipt in order for practice privileges to remain in force.

4. Application for privileges must include the following supporting data: academic preparation, special certifications, national certification, membership in professional organization(s), previous experience and appointments, leadership positions(s), applicable continuing education, publication(s), honors, experience in teaching inservices, special skills and abilities, professional goals.

5. The applicant will be available for a personal interview with the Patient Care Manager and at least one practicing nurse peer in the clinical service for which the applicant is seeking privileges.

6. The applicant will provide appropriate references and supporting information to validate the clinical practice experience indicated on the current application for privileges.

E. Those nurses seeking consulting nursing staff privileges will be granted consulting privileges if they are registered professional nurses duly licensed in the state of Maryland, who will provide per diem consultation or temporary practice services to the Department of Nursing upon request. Each consulting nursing staff applicant must apply for privileges in the same method and manner as all other applicants for privileges to the nursing staff within the Department of Nursing. Consultants to the nursing staff are classified but not limited to the following categories:

- Nurses employed by physicians as extensions of their practice within the hospital (must also be reviewed through the Medical Staff credentialing process as required; i.e., nurse practitioner).

- Clinical instructors employed by other agencies or institutions.
- Specifically skilled practicing staff nurses.

F. Temporary nursing practice privileges shall be obtained for a period of time that immediate services are to be rendered, not to exceed 24 hours. These privileges are extended to individuals appropriately licensed to practice in the state of Maryland. Temporary privileges may be extended beyond the 24-hour period by mutual agreement of the hospital, the agency that employs the nurse, and the professional nurse. All nurses who are granted privileges must be oriented to the Nursing Practice Standards of Suburban Hospital prior to receiving a patient assignment. Periodic performance evaluations using pre-established performance criteria must be completed by members of the institution's professional nursing staff of all temporary staff members used in the hospital. The performance evaluations are to be forwarded to the Nursing Office, where they are reviewed and filed. Temporary staff privileges may be granted only to those nurses employed by an agency with whom the hospital contracts for specific services. These privileges may be suspended at any time without prior notice to the agency.

G. All professional nurses who are applying for permanent privileges must submit all appropriate credentials to the recruiter for Nursing. This individual will forward the credentials to the Patient Care Manager of the area where the applicant is seeking privileges. The Patient Care Manager will forward the application of all applicants who have been selected to the Chairperson of the Credentials Review Board. Nursing credentials review will be consistent with these bylaws and the nursing credentials process. Privileges to practice nursing at Suburban Hospital will be confirmed by letter from the Chairperson of the Credentials Review Board upon successful completion of the physical examination and the credentials review process.

Section 4—The Probationary Nursing Staff

A. All initial appointments to the nursing staff will be provisional for 3 months (90 days). An additional extension, not to exceed 90 days, may be granted upon recommendation of the Patient Care Manager at the time of the probationary evaluation. After the initial 90-day period and/or at the end of the period of extension, the failure to advance from probationary to permanent staff status shall be deemed as termination from the nursing staff. The probationary appointee to the nursing staff whose membership is terminated is accorded whatever appeals, rights, and privileges are specified by hospital personnel policies.

B. Probationary staff members will be given an orientation to the hospital and the Nursing Practice Standards. They will be assigned to the nursing unit of their choice where they will be assigned a preceptor. The preceptor will be a member of the professional nursing staff. This individual will orient the probationary staff member and advise the Patient Care Manager of the appointee's eligibility for professional staff membership and continued exercise of the privileges that have been granted.

C. Acceptable performance of nursing staff responsibilities, as determined by the probationary evaluation, provides the advancement to the professional nursing staff category. Upon satisfactory completion of 90 days in probationary status, the new staff member shall be accorded all rights and privileges of the full professional nursing staff.

Section 5—Credentials Review Process

A credentials review process shall be initiated and maintained in the Department of Nursing, which reviews specific credentials of applicants to the nursing staff for potential membership thereupon. Credentials review shall be based upon, but not limited to, the following items:

A. Evidence that the applying individual has the appropriate licenses, certificates, diplomas, degrees, or other evidence indicating adequate preparation for the role for which the candidate is applying.
B. Applicant has successfully interviewed with the Patient Care Manager of the clinical service in which the applicant is applying for privileges.
C. Applicant has met the criteria of the level of the Professional Advancement System for which the candidate is applying.
D. Applicant has been recommended for approval by the Patient Care Manager of the unit in which the applicant is seeking privileges.

The credentials review process will be invested in a subcommittee of the Quality Assurance Council. This subcommittee is appointed by the Council on Nursing Quality Assurance and is known as the Credentials Committee. It will take up the business of credential review for initial and permanent appointments.

The Credentials Committee may be called into session by the chairperson any time it is necessary to fulfill the business of the Committee. However, the Committee will meet at a minimum of once a month. After establishing a framework for credentials approval within the nursing organization, and consistent with these bylaws, the Credentials Committee shall invest responsibility in the recruiter for Nursing for the following:

- Review and accept credentials supplied by the applicant to the nursing staff
- Obtain appropriate approval of the Patient Care Manager of the unit the candidate is applying for
- Accept the candidate as a probationary member of the nursing staff, subject to the 90-day probationary period

As the credential review officer, the recruiter for Nursing shall meet with the Credentials Committee at all its scheduled meetings. Final approval of all applicants to the institution's nursing staff, once the credentials have been reviewed and the physical examination has been cleared by Occupational Health, rests solely with the appointed credentials committee.

ARTICLE V: GOVERNANCE STRUCTURE OF THE NURSING STAFF

The governance structure shall be clearly identified through and within which the nursing staff will organize, integrate, and manage the delivery of nursing care services. The governance structure will recognize participation from all nursing staff members and will give evidence of shared decision making within the formal structure of the nursing staff.

Section 1—Governance Councils

There shall be four (4) governance councils that will assume responsibility for the management, operation, and integration of the Department of Nursing. They shall be identified as follows:

- Council on Nursing Management
- Council on Nursing Practice
- Council on Nursing Quality Assurance
- Council on Nursing Professional Development

Each council will be clearly identified in the bylaws and will operate consistent with the mandates of its roles and responsibilities as articulated in the bylaws.

Section 2—Council on Nursing Management

A. Membership. The Council on Nursing Management shall consist of all those nurse managers holding line management positions at the department head level. Membership shall consist of at least the following:

- Nursing Administration/Senior Vice President for Patient Care
- Directors of Nursing
- Assistant Director(s) of Nursing
- Patient Care Managers
- Recruiter for Nursing
- One staff nurse representative from the professional nursing staff

Each member of the Council on Nursing Management has one position on the council and may hold one vote. Unexcused absences will be reflected in the annual performance review. Excused absence will be granted for vacation and other reasons determined acceptable by the council. Membership on the Council for Nursing Management will be consistent with tenure in one of the above positions.

B. Role of the Council. The council on Nursing Management is responsible for human, material, and support resources within and affecting the continued operation of the Department of Nursing. All matters relating to the allocation, distribution, and assignment of resources to the individual units and the department as a whole, shall be determined, defined, and undertaken by the Council on Nursing Management.

C. Responsibility. The Council on Nursing Management shall devise, maintain, and control financial budgets, staffing schedules, materials acquisition and allocation mechanisms, and interdepartmental communication for effective utilization and support of nursing services. Further, the Council on Nursing Management shall determine the adequacy of support for clinical activities and shall maintain policies, procedures, rules and regulations of the hospital, and bylaws of the nursing staff, consistent with the management role.

D. Officers. The Chairperson of the Council on Nursing Management shall be a nurse manager. The term of the Chairperson begins in January and lasts for one (1) year. The Chairperson may be elected to serve a second consecutive one (1)-year term. A chairperson may not serve more than two consecutive terms as Chairperson of the Council on Nursing Management. A Chairperson-elect is elected each year in December. The Chairperson-elect may serve two consecutive one (1)-year terms whenever the Chairperson is elected to serve a second consecutive one (1)-year term. The Chairperson-elect is then eligible to serve two consecutive one (1)-year terms as Chairperson.

The Chairperson shall appoint committee members and task forces and shall convene and manage the business of the Council on Nursing Management. For immediate operational decisions and/or emergency situations and/or between regularly scheduled meetings, the Chairperson may act for the council. Such action must be reported to the council membership at its next regularly scheduled meeting for their review and approval. In the absence of the Chairperson, the Chairperson-elect will carry out these duties.

The Council on Nursing Management shall meet at least once a month at a regularly scheduled time.

If during the term of office, the Chairperson resigns, the Chairperson-elect finishes out the Chairperson's term and serves for the term that he/she has been elected. Within 1 month, a Chairperson-elect must be elected.

Section 3—Council on Nursing Practice

A. Membership. Membership on the Council of Nursing Practice shall be drawn from the professional nursing staff with representation from each of the four major clinical services. Members may be nominated or may volunteer from the professional nursing staff. Applications for membership are to be submitted to the Chairperson of the council. The Chairperson of the Council shall be elected by the membership. Staff nurse membership shall be at least ten (10) members. Additional members must include one (1) voting Nurse Manager IV or V, one (1) nonvoting representative from the Department of Training, Education, and Development, one (1) voting Clinical Specialist, and a nonvoting nursing administrative advisor.

B. Role of the Council. The Council on Nursing Practice will define, implement, and maintain the highest standards of clinical nursing practice consistent with national standards of practice promulgated by the appropriate national nursing specialty organization, regional, and community practice standards and those promulgated by Suburban Hospital. Standards of nursing practice and standards of nursing care shall be clearly defined and shall provide a framework of all nursing clinical activity to which frequent and ongoing reference can be made.

C. Responsibility. The Council on Nursing Practice is responsible for the review and approval of all materials and activities related to clinical nursing practice. Such review shall include but not be limited to the following:

- Review and approval of all standards that relate to or specifically affect clinical nursing practice

- Review and approval of all standards of nursing practice from every clinical specialty within which nursing practice occurs
- Assessment and review of, and response to, all problems, concerns, issues, and other related activities with an impact on the clinical operation of the Department of Nursing at Suburban Hospital
- Determination and dissemination of needed changes in practice to other appropriate councils and committees and to the nursing staff for review, education, and implementation

D. Officers. The Chairperson of the Council on Nursing Practice shall be elected in December of each year from the council membership. The term of the Chairperson begins in January and lasts for one (1) year. The Chairperson may be elected to serve a second consecutive one (1)-year term. A Chairperson may not serve more than two consecutive terms as Chairperson of the Council on Nursing Practice. A Chairperson-elect is elected each year in December.

The Chairperson-elect may serve two consecutive one (1)-year terms whenever the Chairperson is elected to serve a second consecutive one (1)-year term.

The Chairperson-elect is then eligible to serve two consecutive one (1)-year terms as Chairperson.

The Chairperson shall appoint committee members and task forces and shall convene and manage the business of the Council on Nursing Practice. For immediate operational decisions and/or emergency situations and/or between regularly scheduled meetings, the Chairperson may act for the council. Such action must be reported to the council membership at its next regularly scheduled meeting for their review and approval. In the absence of the Chairperson, the Chairperson-elect will carry out these duties.

The Council on Nursing Practice shall meet at least once a month at a regularly scheduled time.

If during the term of office the Chairperson resigns, the Chairperson-elect finishes out the Chairperson's term and serves for the term that he/she has been elected. Within 1 month, a Chairperson-elect must be elected.

Section 4—Council on Nursing Quality Assurance

A. Membership. The Council on Nursing Quality Assurance membership shall be representative of the major clinical services in the Department of Nursing. Represented on the Council on Nursing Quality Assurance shall be at least one member from each of the following:

- Medical Nursing
- Surgical Nursing
- Orthopedic Nursing
- Critical Care Nursing
- Cardiology Nursing
- Perioperative Nursing
- Emergency Nursing
- Any other clinical specialty deemed appropriate by a majority vote of the members of the Council

Membership shall be drawn from the professional nursing staff. Total professional nursing staff membership shall be at least ten (10) members. Also represented on the Council of Nursing Quality Assurance is one (1) voting Nurse Manager IV or V, a clinical specialist with voting privileges, and a nonvoting nurse representative from the Department of Training, Education, and Development. A nursing administrative advisor shall also be a nonvoting member of the council.

B. Role. The Council on Nursing Quality Assurance shall review all current clinical practices to determine compliance with standards and the need to initiate new standards of practice determined through the quality assurance mechanism. The Council on Nursing Quality Assurance shall report to the appropriate council, committee, department head, or division head any outcome data that affect compliance with standards of practice, the quality of nursing care, and the potential for implementing new standards, processes, and practices related to nursing care activities.

C. Responsibilities. The Council on Nursing Quality Assurance shall devise measurement tools for monitoring ongoing nursing care activities; shall review and compile data reflecting compliance with activities; shall make and forward recommendations to the appropriate council, committee, department head, or division head for action regarding care as revealed by current state-of-the-art literature and nursing research. The council will be responsible for disseminating information in order to ensure continued compliance with appropriate and defined levels of nursing practice within Suburban Hospital's Department of Nursing. This council shall also mandate standing committees for the review of nursing staff credentials, and approval/rejection/appeal of applications for promotion through the Professional Advancement System.

D. Officers. The Chairperson of the Council on Quality Assurance shall be elected in December of each year from the council membership. The term of the Chairperson begins in January and lasts for one (1) year. The Chairperson may be elected to serve a second consecutive one (1)-year term. A Chairperson may not serve more than two consecutive terms as Chairperson of the Council on Quality Assurance. A Chairperson-elect is elected each year in December. The Chairperson-elect may serve two consecutive one (1)-year terms whenever the Chairperson is elected to serve a second consecutive one (1)-year term. The Chairperson-elect is then eligible to serve two consecutive one (1)-year terms as Chairperson.

The Chairperson shall appoint committee members and task forces and shall convene and manage the business of the Council on Quality Assurance. For immediate operational decisions and/or emergency situations and/or between regularly scheduled meetings, the Chairperson may act for the council. Such action must be reported to the council membership at its next regularly scheduled meeting for their review and approval. In the absence of the Chairperson, the Chairperson-elect will carry out these duties.

The Council on Quality Assurance shall meet at least once a month at a regularly scheduled time.

If during the term of office, the Chairperson resigns, the Chairperson-elect finishes out the Chairperson's term and serves for the term that he/she has been elected. Within 1 month, a Chairperson-elect must be elected.

Section 5—Council on Nursing Professional Development

A. Membership. Every nursing unit shall have representation on the Nursing Professional Development Council. Each nursing unit shall have one (1) voting professional staff representative on the Professional Development Council. Professional nursing staff membership shall be limited to the number of nursing units. The council will not exceed 18 staff nurse members. There shall be representation by one (1) nonvoting nurse representative of the Department of Training, Education, and Development, one (1) clinical specialist voting member (may have two {2}) and one (1) voting Nurse Manager IV or V. A nursing administrative advisor shall also be a nonvoting member on the Council on Nursing Professional Development.

B. Role. The Council on Professional Development shall review all continuing education programs prior to instituting the education process. The council shall further define education needs on a division and department basis and shall review and approve those educational offerings submitted for review by each nursing unit representative. All nursing educational programs are integrated and approved for implementation by the council. The council is accountable for maintaining the highest levels of nursing care through education that is related to the ongoing portion of the responsibility of the professional practice of nursing in the hospital.

C. The Professional Development Council is responsible for the review of all annual, monthly, and special education programs undertaken within the Department of Nursing and/or under the Department of Training, Education, and Development on nursing's behalf. Specific educational needs, as identified by the Council on Nursing Practice, the Council on Nursing Quality Assurance and the Council on Nursing Management, are also reviewed, approved, and undertaken by the Council on Nursing Professional Development. Maintenance of the institution's ongoing education recording and documentation is assured through the activities of the Council on Nursing Professional Development.

D. Officers. The Chairperson of the Council on Nursing Professional Development shall be elected each year from the council membership. The term of the Chairperson begins in January and lasts for one (1) year. The Chairperson may be elected to serve a second consecutive one (1)-year term. A Chairperson may not serve more than two consecutive terms as Chairperson of the Council on Nursing Professional Development. A Chairperson-elect is elected each year in December. The Chairperson-elect may serve two consecutive one (1)-year terms whenever the Chairperson is elected to serve a second consecutive one (1)-year term. The Chairperson-elect is then eligible to serve two consecutive one (1)-year terms as Chairperson.

The Chairperson shall appoint committee members and task forces and shall convene and manage the business of the Council on Nursing Professional Development. For immediate operational decisions and/or emergency situations and/or between regularly scheduled meetings, the Chairperson may act for the council. Such action must be reported to the council membership at its next regularly scheduled meeting for their review and approval. In the absence of the Chairperson, the Chairperson-elect will carry out these duties.

The Council on Nursing Professional Development shall meet at least once a month at a regularly scheduled time.

If during the term of office, the Chairperson resigns, the Chairperson-elect finishes out the Chairperson's term and serves for the term that he/she has been elected. Within 1 month, a Chairperson-elect must be elected.

Section 6—Meeting Times

All nursing councils shall meet at least monthly and each shall be responsible for the respective work consistent with these bylaws. Minutes must be taken and recorded in the format accepted by the Department of Nursing. Minutes are distributed to all nursing units for review. Eight hours are allotted for all council meetings except for the Management Council which meets for 4 hours. One half (½) of the total representation of a council or a constituent committee shall constitute a quorum and shall be deemed appropriate for conducting business of the council or committee.

Section 7—Selection of Governance Council Membership

Members to any one of the governance councils shall be selected from the designated departments, clinical services, or management roles. Membership is limited to registered nurses (R.N.s) only. Potential members may volunteer or may be nominated by peers, recommended by current council members or managers, or suggested by staff for council membership. All suggested and recommended potential members must be approved by majority vote of the council in which the candidate is seeking membership.

Section 8—Service of Council Members

Membership shall be rotated 1 year from the date of appointment. Members may be reappointed for no more than two consecutive one (1)-year terms. One exception to this rule is the Chairperson-Elect, who has already served one or two terms as a council member. This individual is eligible to serve two (2) years as Chairperson-elect or two one (1)-year terms as the Chairperson. Members are required to attend three fourths of all scheduled council meetings. Members not complying with attendance requirements may be removed and replaced through a majority vote of members attending the meeting at which the decision is rendered. Other than the Management Council, members may not serve another consecutive term on any governance council. After 3 months of not serving on a governance council, the registered nurse is again eligible for council membership. Possible exceptions to this rule are the Clinical Nurse Specialist and Education Specialist. The Councils on Nursing Practice, Quality Assurance, and Professional Development each require a Clinical Nurse Specialist as a voting member. The Chairperson will not also serve as the unit representative. An Administrative Advisor shall be appointed by the Senior Vice President for Patient Care to serve as a nonvoting member of each council. The Administrative Advisor shall serve a term of not longer than 2 years.

Section 9—Standing Committees

Standing committees are established in Nursing to meet long-term, broad goals and objectives that support ongoing nursing programs within the hospital. A committee will be established only after it has been determined by the Coordinating Council that the stated goals and objectives cannot be met by the appointment of a task force.

Every standing committee in Nursing functions under the auspices of the council to which the respective program is responsible. At least one member of the committee shall also be a member of the council to which that committee reports.

Minutes are kept at every committee meeting and these minutes shall be sent to the appropriate council chairperson within 2 weeks of the date that the committee meeting has taken place. An annual report of the work of each committee is forwarded by the committee chairperson to the chairperson of the council each year in November. At the December meeting of the Coordinating Council, all committee reports are reviewed and a recommendation may be made whether to continue or to abolish the group as a standing committee.

The composition of a committee, as well as the frequency of meetings, is determined by the council to which the committee reports. The chairperson of the council will appoint the chairperson of each committee. This is done annually in January. The term of a committee chairperson is not to exceed 2 years. The Coordinating Council may request, however, that a committee chairperson extend beyond a 2-year term in order to maintain continuity in the committee's work.

ARTICLE VI: DISCIPLINE, APPEALS, PEER REVIEW PROCESS, REVIEW, AND REMOVAL FROM THE NURSING STAFF
Section 1—Discipline and Appeals

All members of the professional nursing staff, regardless of category, are subject to Suburban Hospital's standards of employment practices and disciplinary and appeals process, as mandated through the policies and procedures of the Personnel Department. All nursing staff members have the same rights and privileges and access to protection policies and procedural support regarding the discipline and appeals processes as all other employees of Suburban Hospital.

Section 2—Peer Review Process

In addition to evaluation of competence by self and one's manager, all members of the professional nursing staff who work at least 40 hours a pay period shall participate in the peer review process a minimum of once a year at the time of the annual evaluation. The methods used to select the peer may vary from unit to unit. An evaluation by only one peer is required, although some units may choose to have two peer evaluations.

Every member of the professional nursing staff who applies to move from one level to another through the Professional Advancement System must be evaluated by a minimum of two peers. In selecting the peers, the manager will submit to the professional nurse a list of not fewer than five names. From this list, the nurse will select the names of two peers. The manager will notify the peers and have them submit the completed evaluation forms which the manager will place in the nurse's promotion packet. These evaluations will be presented as a part of the promotion packet.

Section 3—Removal From the Nursing Staff

When a member of the permanent, probationary, temporary, or consulting staff does not meet the standards provided for the individual's role in Suburban Hospital's Department of Nursing, removal from the Nursing staff may be undertaken through initiation of the hospital's disciplinary process. When performance indicators, peer review, evaluation processes, or developmental counseling by the manager reveals that a member of the nursing staff is not acting within the bylaws or consistent with the standards of practice acceptable at Suburban Hospital, the appropriate nurse manager will initiate the disciplinary process. If, after due process, termination is the result, the member of the nursing staff must be informed in writing that privileges have been withdrawn and that the nurse has been terminated from membership on the nursing staff. As herein indicated, all rights of appeal may be accessed by the disciplined or terminated nurse, consistent with the policies and practices of the Personnel Department.

ARTICLE VII: COORDINATION OF THE DEPARTMENT OF NURSING
Section 1—Administration

The Senior Vice President for Patient Care and her delegates are responsible to the President of Suburban Hospital for the coordination, integration, and administration of nursing. In this role, the Senior Vice President for Patient Care shall be accountable for ensuring that these bylaws are promulgated to all of the nursing staff members of Suburban Hospital and that members adhere to the articles and mandates of these bylaws, consistent with all existing rules, regulations, policies, and practices of Suburban Hospital.

Section 2—Coordination of Governance Activities

A Nursing Coordinating Council shall be composed of the elected Chairpersons and Chairpersons-Elect of the four governance councils: Nursing Practice, Quality Assurance, Professional Development, and Nursing Management. These individuals shall be identified as the officers of the nursing staff and shall serve no longer than five (5) years from the date of appointment. The Senior Vice President for Patient Care and the immediate past Chairperson of the Professional Nursing Staff shall also sit as voting members of the Nursing Coordinating Council. Each year in January, the professional nursing staff shall elect the Chairperson-elect of the nursing staff from among the governance council chairpersons. That person will serve as Chairperson-elect for one (1) year and Chairperson for the following year. The Chairperson of the nursing staff shall conduct the business of the Nursing Coordinating Council and the business of the quarterly nursing staff meetings.

Section 3—Role and Meeting Time

The business of the Nursing Coordinating Council shall be directed to coordinating, communicating, and facilitating integration of the work of the nursing staff. The Nursing Coordinating Council shall meet at least monthly and may be called to meet at other times, at the discretion of the chairperson.

Section 4—Quarterly Professional Staff Meetings

Quarterly meetings of the nursing staff shall be held in January, April, July, and October. They shall undertake the business of the nursing staff and shall review and approve such matters as are brought before it by the Coordinating Council. On matters submitted for staff vote, a majority of those present shall be sufficient for passing the voting issues. At the January meeting, a Chairperson-elect of the Nursing Staff shall be elected from the Chairpersons of the Councils. This election will be done by secret ballot. At this meeting, the annual goals of the Professional Nursing Staff will also be approved.

The business meetings will be chaired by the Chairperson of the Nursing Staff. Reports from the governance councils and their designated task forces shall be made. Issues and motions from the staff can be addressed in this meeting following the accepted protocol.

ARTICLE VIII: BYLAW REVISION
Section 1—Annual Review

These bylaws shall be reviewed annually in October by the Coordinating Council and presented to the nursing staff in January.

Section 2—Amendments

Any professional staff member may recommend changes in the bylaws by submitting any such changes to any nursing council Chairperson. The council Chairperson will present the proposed change to the Nursing Coordinating Council for review and consideration. Revised bylaws shall be presented to the Vice President for Patient Care for review and approval.

ARTICLE IX: RULES AND REGULATIONS

The nursing staff through its constituent councils shall adopt such rules and regulations as may be necessary to implement and maintain these bylaws. All new or changed rules and regulations shall be approved by the Nursing Coordinating Council prior to their implementation. Such changes shall become effective upon approval of the Nursing Coordinating Council.

_____   _____

President   Chairperson,
Nursing Staff

_____

Senior Vice President for Patient Care

9 Shared Governance and Collective Bargaining; Integration, not Confrontation

David G. Crocker
R. Michael Kirkpatrick
Laura Lentenbrink

Collective bargaining evolved as a peaceful method to transfer power from employers to employees. In most cases it involved a for-profit employer and employees who could be replaced with little training. The employer was concerned with maximizing profits and the union with maximizing wages, benefits, and job security.

The laws that allowed collective bargaining in the for-profit industrial setting are now applicable to hospitals and professional nurses. The total self-interest on the part of the employer and employees that drove the collective bargaining process into the industrial environment has been weakened in the hospital-nurse relationship. The majority of hospitals are not-for-profit institutions. Registered nurses are skilled professionals. The product is not a car but a human life.

A professional nurse is concerned with the total patient care environment, not simply wages, hours, and working conditions. A union can require that a hospital negotiate with respect to wages, hours, working conditions, and the terms and conditions of employment. A hospital is not required to bargain with regard to staffing, services provided, quality of care, and other areas of importance to the professional nurse. Even if a hospital was willing to negotiate these issues, a collective bargaining agreement is an unsatisfactory vehicle to use in resolving them. Patient census and mix change daily, government payments and demands for services fluctuate, new procedures are implemented and the old discarded. Patient care cannot be adequately addressed on a triennial basis as can normal collective bargaining concerns. The adversarial process, with unmet demands enforced by lockouts and strikes, requires a period of labor peace to work properly. Therefore collective bargaining cannot be continuous, but must result in a written agreement that will govern the relationship of the parties in certain limited areas for a specific period.

239

Shared governance addresses the concerns of hospitals and professional nurses that cannot be adequately embodied in the static terms of a collective bargaining agreement. The implementation of shared governance impinges on such traditional management rights as staffing and nurse performance. It also must not evolve into a replacement of the union as the exclusive collective bargaining representative of its bargaining unit nor take away the rights of the individual professional nurses. Because of the reasons for the collective bargaining process, the state and federal legislature and courts have been more protective of employees than employers. Unions and employees are prohibited from engaging in certain conduct and contracting away certain rights in order to preserve a balance of power at the bargaining table. This chapter examines the legal implications of implementing a shared governance model in a collective bargaining environment. Because of variations among hospitals, the assistance of a labor attorney will be needed for successful implementation.

HISTORICAL PERSPECTIVE

The National Labor Relations Act (the Act) is the federal law that controls labor-management relations in the private sector of our nation's industries. Inequality of bargaining power between employees and employers; denial by some employers of the right of some employees to organize and collectively bargain; and certain practices by some labor organizations, their officers, and members were all found by Congress to burden or obstruct commerce (Section 1).

Congress therefore declared it to be the policy of the United States to eliminate the causes of certain substantial obstructions to the free flow of commerce by encouraging the practice of collective bargaining (Section 1).

Section 7 of the Act grants employees the right to form labor organizations, to deal collectively through such organizations regarding terms and conditions of employment, and to engage in concerted activities in support of these and other rights.

The Act has evolved in four major cycles: the Wagner Act in 1935, the Taft-Hartley Act in 1947, the Landrum-Griffin Act in 1959, and the Health Care Amendments of 1974.

In the early nineteenth century, concerted labor activities were treated as common law conspiracies and were met with criminal prosecution. Later, the civil injunction became the favored method of combating unionization. The injunction was more effective against labor activities than the criminal proceeding because an injunction could ordinarily be secured from a state court on the basis of affidavits presented to the judge, without notice to the employees (Gorman, 1976).

The federal courts also became active through diversity-of-citizenship jurisdiction and federal antitrust laws. The Sherman Act of 1890 declared illegal "every contract, combination . . . or conspiracy, in restraint of trade or commerce among the several states" (Section 1). It provided for government injunction, criminal prosecution, and private treble-damage action. It was applied more frequently by the lower federal courts to labor unions than to corporate conspirators. Any strike that might shut down a major plant could be treated as a conspiracy interfering with interstate trade (Sherman Antitrust Act. 26 Stat. 209, 1890).

The National War Labor Board, created during World War I, was the first federal body to announce the principle of employee freedom to organize in and bargain collectively through trade unions, free from employer interference.

The Clayton Act of 1914 was designed to withdraw the power of the federal courts to regulate labor activities through the antitrust laws. Section 20 of the Clayton Act listed the conventional concerted activities such as strikes, picketing, and boycotts, and declared these to be nonenjoinable and not violative of the Sherman Act. However, Section 20 of the Clayton Act was very narrowly construed by the Supreme Court in *Duplex Printing Press Co. v. Deering* (1921). Congress took an additional step in 1932 by enacting the Norris-LaGuardia Act. That statute declared it to be the public policy of the United States that employees be permitted to organize and bargain collectively, free of employer coercion, and sought to achieve that goal by regulating, and in most cases barring, the issuance of injunctions in a labor dispute. Peaceful strikes, picketing, and boycotts were sheltered against the injunction. The Norris-LaGuardia Act imposed severe limitations on the use of restraining orders and provided for full and fair hearings before the issuance of preliminary injunctions.

In 1940 the Supreme Court limited the reach of the Sherman Act as applied to labor unions in *Apex Hosiery Co. v. Leader*. Closely following that decision, in *United States v. Hutcheson* (1941), the Court held the broad protection of the Norris-LaGuardia Act not only barred injunctions against labor activities but also immunized such activities from antitrust actions for treble damages and criminal relief.

Congress enacted the Wagner Act, or National Labor Relations Act of 1935. This act enumerated certain rights, privileges, and proscriptions regarding both employers and employees.

The Wagner Act also established the National Labor Relations Board (NLRB). The NLRB was authorized to order the employer and the union to remedy unfair labor practices, with such orders enforceable or reviewable in the United States Courts of Appeals. The Wagner Act was sustained by the Supreme Court against a constitutional attack in *NLRB v. Jones & Laughlin Steel Corp.* (1937). The Wagner Act embodied the spirit of the new age of labor-management relations and served as a basis on which later acts and court cases would build and evolve into our nation's labor relations policy.

As a response to the rapid increase in union membership, greater use of the strike, and some corruption and undemocratic practices in internal union affairs, Congress enacted the Taft-Hartley Act in 1947. As a result, the prosecutorial and quasijudicial functions of the NLRB were separated. Supervisors and independent contractors were removed from the coverage of the Act. Limitations were placed on the NLRB in handling election cases, and the federal courts were given greater authority to review and set aside findings of the NLRB. The Taft-Hartley Act reintroduced the labor injunction, but limited it to use against unfair labor practices and only at the behest of an official of the NLRB. It also provided federal court jurisdiction over suits to enforce labor contracts, while giving unions the right to sue or be sued in federal actions. Congress also enumerated several unfair labor practices by labor organizations: restraining or coercing employees in the exercise of their Section 7 rights; causing an employer to discriminate illegally against employees; refusing to bargain in good faith; striking or inducing a strike in support of a secondary boycott; demanding recognition when another union is certified as the employee representative; demanding the assignment of work that is the subject of a jurisdictional dispute; and causing a employer to pay for services not performed.

The Act was further amended in 1959. The Landrum-Griffin Act, also known as the Labor-Management Reporting and Disclosure Act, was enacted to address the problems of corruption within union leadership, which was addressed by elaborate union reporting requirements, and of undemocratic conduct of internal union affairs, which resulted in a "Bill of Rights" for union members in such matters as union meetings and elections, eligibility for office, and union disciplinary procedures.

Not-for-profit hospitals were excluded from the Act until Congress passed the Health Care Amendments of 1974, which eliminated the statutory exclusion for not-for-profit medical institutions. Supporters of the Amendments noted that the exemption of not-for-profit hospitals from the Act had resulted in numerous instances of recognition strikes and picketing. Coverage under the Act should, it was thought, completely eliminate the need for any such activity, since the procedures of the Act would be available to resolve organizational and recognition disputes.

Congress attempted to meet the needs of the hospitals' patients by adding certain notice requirements and mediation before strike. No other recognition of the unique product of all hospitals or health care facilities has been enacted. Thus the Act, which was designed to encourage the peaceful settlement of disputes in the industrial sector by economic warfare (i.e., strikes and lockouts), has been extended to hospitals and professional nurses essentially unchanged.

ORGANIZED NURSES AND PROFESSIONALISM

A concern raised by the history of collective bargaining is the flexibility allowed by the law within which to exercise the responsibilities of professionalism. The federal statutes that protect union activities are designed for the nonprofessional worker. The areas specified as being of legitimate concern to these employees by the law were limited to wages, hours, and other terms and conditions of employment. These same rights are now the limitations on the professional nurse in the union setting.

Nurse managers and staff registered nurses are members of the same profession. A profession is defined as self-governed and self-determining (Cleland, 1978). A profession controls its own credentialing process, exerts influence on professional behavior, and strives to expand its body of knowledge.

Autonomy and control are major components of professional practice. Professionalism requires control over practice to include entry, recruitment, and self-evaluation or discipline (Jacox, 1980; Sheridan, 1982; Stern, 1982). Autonomy is a prerequisite to self-governance, professional independence, and self-regulation (Jacox, 1980; Kiereini, 1980; McGilloway, 1980; Stern, 1982).

The elements of professionalism are not usually attainable in the normal collective bargaining process. Autonomy and control of the nursing environment are not the same as wages, hours, and working conditions. Because of this limitation, collective bargaining as a process to maintain and enhance the professionalism of organized nurses has been criticized. One view is that the predominant efforts of the unions representing professional nurses in bargaining have been directed toward salaries, fringe benefits, working conditions, and job security at the expense of a service ideal (Colangelo, 1980; Rotkovitch, 1980). Personal gain seems, apparently, to be placed before professional service in the adversarial process of bargaining.

The mandatory subjects of collective bargaining—those subjects that may be bargained to impasse and can be the reasons for lawful strikes—do not include many issues that should be addressed by organized nurses to maintain their professionalism. Hospitals are cautious about bargaining on nonmandatory subjects, such as staffing, patient mix, staff mix, peer review, and self-evaluation or discipline of the profession by its members, for at least two reasons. First, these issues are perceived as traditional management rights that must be protected for the well-being of the hospital. Second, the system of collective bargaining normally ends in a written agreement that is not subject to change for its term, which may be 3 years. The attempt to specify such topics as staffing, patient mix, staff mix, and others of a similar nature in the changing hospital environment is considered futile or counterproductive.

There are several methods that could be used to address the subjects vital to nurses. Bargaining on the professional issues could be continuous during the term of the contract. This approach may not be acceptable to hospital management because of the consumption of resources by the process and the possibility that the normal no-strike clause could be nullified. This would result in unrest and insecurity on the part of both management and nurses. Some hospitals and unions have specified committees that are charged with considering and recommending solutions to professional issues. These committees may normally only make recommendations that management may elect to ignore. No actual power is transferred by the usual committee process.

Another approach is to recognize that nursing managers and staff nurses are part of the same profession, filling different roles within a hospital. A collective bargaining agreement could empower the hospital's professional nurses, both management and staff, to resolve the professional nursing issues with the solutions limited only by the constraints of the hospital budget. Committees composed of nurse managers and staff nurses could be given control of issues such as staffing, patient mix, staff mix, peer review, and self-evaluation or discipline of the professional nurse. Such an arrangement does not result in a total transfer of power from the hospital to the organized staff nurse, but is a sharing of power.

There are legal issues raised by this sharing of power or shared governance approach by the Act and the interpretations of the Act by the NLRB and the courts.

LEGAL ISSUES RAISED BY SHARED GOVERNANCE IN AN ORGANIZED HOSPITAL

An agreement between a hospital and a union of staff nurses to empower the professional nurses employed by the hospital to resolve professional nursing issues crosses the grain of the Act and the historical management-union traditions. Because of the usual imbalance of power between an industrial employer and a non-professional work force, the law protects the rights of unions and the individual employees. This protection has most clearly surfaced in the protection against unions that are tools of management or that violate the trust of their members for other reasons, such as leadership self-interest or ties with organized crime. These concerns are commonly abbreviated as "employer-domination," "exclusive representation," and "the duty of fair representation."

Employer Domination

Section 8(a)(2) of the Act prohibits an employer from assisting or dominating a labor organization. This section was enacted to protect employees from the possibility that their union would "sell out" to their employer. However, labor organizations are not limited to unions as commonly understood. Section 2(5) of the Act has defined labor organization to include any employee representation committee or plan in which employees participate and that has as one of its purposes dealing with the employer concerning grievances, labor disputes, wages, rates of pay, hours, or other terms and conditions of employment.

One of the legal issues facing the creation and implementation of shared governance by agreement between a hospital and union is the question of whether the committees or councils inherent in such sharing of power are separate labor organizations and whether such organizations are employer dominated. The drafters of the Act envisioned a system in which the norm would be labor against management. A pure dedication to the self-interest of management and unions was understandable to these legislators—employers dedicated to maximizing profits and unions dedicated to higher wages, fewer hours, and better working conditions. It was not envisioned at the time that conditions would change to the degree that would require, or at least create a situation that was conducive to, a less adversarial model of labor-management cooperation. Neither was it foreseen that the members of a union would have a higher professional calling than merely better wages, or that an employer would not always be concerned solely with higher profits.

In several cases the NLRB has ruled that a labor organization exists if a group of employees deal with their employer even if there are no officers, no charter, no dues paid, or no regular meetings held. The NLRB also has said a labor organization can exist even if there are management members on the committee that is determined to be a labor organization (*Labor Relations Week,* 1990).

The courts have taken a more liberal view than the NLRB of what constitutes a labor organization and have found that some joint labor-management groups, such as quality circles, are not always illegal. The courts have looked at the free choice of employees to determine if participation is voluntary, and if the employees looked on the operation of the committee with favor, and did not view it as a substitute for a union. The courts also have studied whether the involvement of employees in committees is in representative capacities, whether committee members are elected, or if management designates members (*Labor Relations Week,* 1990).

These contrasting views have created uncertainty regarding the status of shared governance committees and other cooperative labor-management programs.

In a February 1990 conference, NLRB member Mary Miller Cracraft noted that the move toward labor-management cooperation counters the underpinning of the Act and traditional adversarial labor relations. Cracraft said "the New Deal was built on the centrality of collective bargaining, formal grievances, and a tacit agreement that strategic business decisions would be left to management. Employees were to organize in their own independent units and conflict was viewed as natural" (*Daily Labor Report,* 1990, p. A-11). Cracraft also noted that cooperative programs are supported by the Department of Labor as a way to enhance the nation's competitive edge. Although cooperative labor-management programs are increasing, Section 8(a)(2) of the Act may also prohibit some such programs. Cracraft said "the central issue seems to be whether such committees are employer-dominated and initiated. The tension between the Act and the cooperative programs will have to be resolved so that they can be more uniformly adopted" (*Daily Labor Report,* 1990).

Section 2(11) of the Act defines a supervisor as "any individual having authority in the interest of the employer to hire, transfer, suspend, lay off, recall, promote, discharge, assign, reward, or discipline other employees, or responsibly to direct them, or to adjust their grievances, or effectively to recommend such action, if in connection with the foregoing the exercise of such authority is not of a merely routine or clerical nature, but requires the use of independent judgment." This section is to be read as though supervisory elements are separate so that possession of any one of the enumerated attributes of management is sufficient to confirm supervisory status (*NLRB v. Edward G. Budd Mfg. Co.,* 1948). This definition includes most nurse managers. Supervisors are management representatives. Their actions and words are attributable to their employers. If supervisors dominate an employee committee, the committee is employer dominated.

The leading court decision regarding employer-dominated employee committees is *NLRB v. Cabot Carbon Co.* (1959). In *Cabot Carbon,* the employer decided to establish an Employee Committee at each of its plants. The employer prepared, in collaboration with employee representatives from its several plants, a set of bylaws stating the purposes, duties, and functions of the proposed employee committees, for transmittal to and adoption by the employees in establishing such committees. The bylaws were adopted by a majority of employees at each plant and by the employer, and the Employee Committees were established.

In essence the bylaws stated that the purpose of the committees was to provide a procedure for considering employees' ideas and problems of mutual interest to employees and management; that each plant committee should consist of a stated number of employees; that each plant committee should meet with the plant management at regular monthly meetings and at all special meetings called by management; should assist the plant management in solving problems of mutual interest; that time so spent would be considered time worked; and that it was the committees' responsibility to handle grievances at nonunion plants and departments according to procedures established at these plants and departments.

A union that represented workers at several of the employer's plants filed unfair labor practice charges against the employer, alleging in part that the employer was unlawfully dominating, interfering with, and supporting labor organizations, called Employee Committees, at its several plants. In its investigation the NLRB discovered the committees made and discussed proposals and requests respecting many aspects of the employee relationship, including seniority, job classifications, job bidding, makeup time, overtime records, time cards, a merit system, wage corrections, working schedules, holidays, vacations, sick leave, and improvement of working facilities and conditions.

Based on these findings, the NLRB found the Employee Committees to be labor organizations within the meaning of the Act, and that during the period involved the employer dominated and supported the labor organizations in violation of Section 8(a)(2).

The employer then petitioned the Court of Appeals to review and vacate the NLRB's finding and order. The Court of Appeals denied enforcement of the NLRB's order and set it aside. It found the employer dominated and supported the committees but held that they were not labor organizations within the meaning of the Act because (1) dealing with, as used in Section 2(5) of the Act, means bargaining with, and these committees avoided the usual concept of collective bargaining, and (2) the provisions and legislative history of the 1947 amendment of Section 9(a) of the Act show that Congress, in effect, excluded such committees from the definition of labor organization. The Board appealed to the Supreme Court.

The Supreme Court held that an employee committee that does not formally bargain with an employer in the usual manner of collective bargaining can engage in dealing with an employer, and, if the committee does deal with an employer concerning grievances, labor disputes, wages, rates of pay, hours of employment, or conditions of work, it is a labor organization within the meaning of Section 2(5). The Court's study of the matter found nothing in the plain words of Section 2(5), in its legislative history, or in the decisions construing it, that supported the Court of Appeals conclusion to the contrary. Certainly nothing in that section indicates that the broad term "dealing with" is to be read as synonymous with the more limited term "bargaining with," the Court held.

The Court found in 1937 that the House of Representatives passed the Hartley bill; proposed items included a new section of the Act to be designated 8(d)(3), providing "(3) forming or maintaining by an employer of a committee of employees and discussing matters of mutual interest, including grievances, wages, hours of employment, and other working conditions, if the Board has not certified or the employer has not recognized a representative as its employees' representative under Section 9," shall not constitute or be evidence of an unfair labor practice under any of the provisions of this Act.

The Court also found the Senate amended the Hartley bill by substituting its own bill, known as the Taft bill. The Senate's bill contained no provision corresponding to the new Section 8(d)(3) proposed by the House, but it did propose an amendment to Section 9(a) of the original Wagner Act by adding that employees have the right to present grievances to their employer and to have such grievances adjusted without the intervention of the bargaining representative, if the adjustment is not inconsistent with the terms of the collective bargaining agreement and the bargaining representative has been given opportunity to be present at such adjustment.

After Senate and House joint conferences, the bill as finally agreed upon by the conferees did not contain the House's proposed new Section 8(d)(3) or any similar language, but it did contain the Senate's proposed amendment to Section 9(a).

The Supreme Court concluded that there is nothing in the amendment of Section 9(a), or its legislative history, to indicate that Congress thereby eliminated or intended to eliminate such employee committees from the term labor organization as defined in Section 2(5) and used in Section 8(a)(2).

Accordingly, the Supreme Court reversed the Court of Appeals and reinstated the order of the NLRB.

The NLRB continues to rely heavily on the principles set forth in *Cabot Carbon*. However, recent court decisions seem to indicate the willingness on the part of some courts to find some employee committees not to be labor organizations.

In *NLRB v. Streamway Division of Scott and Fetzler Co.* (1982), the Appellate Court discussed the effect of *Cabot Carbon* and concluded that an employee committee intended to define and identify problem areas and to elicit suggestions and ideas for improving operations was not a labor organization. The committee in *Streamway* included elected employee representatives with rotating terms and was formed after one unsuccessful union campaign and several months before another such campaign. The company changed its vacation policy after discussions with the committee. The Court stated in *Streamway* that "not all management efforts to communicate with employees concerning company personnel policy are forbidden on pain of violating the Act. An overly broad construction of the statute would be as destructive of the objects of the Act as ignoring the provisions entirely" (*NLRB v. Streamway Division of Scott and Fetzler Co.*, 1982, 691, F.2d, 292).

In support of that rationale, *Streamway* adopted with approval the language of Judge John Minor Wisdom:

An inflexible attitude of hostility toward employee committees defeats the Act. It erects an iron curtain between employer and employees penetratable only by a bargaining agent by a certified union, if there is one, preventing the development of a decent, honest, constructive relationship between management and labor. The Act encourages collective bargaining, as it should, in accordance with national policy. The Act does not encourage compulsory membership in a labor organization. The effect of the Board's policy here is to force employees to form a labor organization, regardless of the wishes of the employees in a particular plant, if there is so much as an intention by an employer to allow employees to confer with management on any matter that can be said to touch, however slightly, their "general welfare." There is nothing in Cabot Carbon, *or in the Labor Management Act, or in any other law that makes it wrong for an employer "to work together" with employees for the welfare of all. It is only when management's activities actually undermine the integrity of the employees' freedom of choice and independence in dealing with their employer that such activities fall within the proscriptions of the Act.*

Streamway, pp. 292-93

Similarly, the 6th Circuit Court of Appeals reversed the NLRB and found that an advisory committee formed to facilitate communication between management and employees was not an illegal employer-dominated labor organization within the meaning of Section 2(5) of the Act (*Airstream, Inc. v. NLRB*, 1989).

The Appeals Court found the committee did not constitute a labor organization because it did not discuss wages, grievances, labor disputes, hours of employment, or conditions of work.

As noted, in contrast to the apparent less restrictive view of the 6th Circuit, the NLRB's view continues, with some exceptions, to be consistent with that first espoused in *Cabot Carbon*.

In *Alta Bates Hospital Institutional Workers Local 250, Service Employees International Union, AFL-CIO and Employee Advisory Committee of Alta Bates Hospital, Party In Interest* (1976), the NLRB considered whether the Employee Advisory Committee of Alta Bates Hospital (Advisory Committee), was a labor organization within the meaning of Section 2(5) of the Act and, if so, whether the employer, in violation of Section 8(a)(2) and (1) of the Act, dominated or interfered with the formation and administration of the Advisory Committee and contributed financial aid or other support to its existence. Also in dispute was whether the employer violated Section 8(a)(5) and (1) of the Act by negotiating with the Advisory Committee over employees' working conditions at a time when those employees were represented by the union.

The hospital's personnel committee created a subcommittee composed of eight employees and four management representatives, all of whom were selected by members of the personnel committee. The purpose of the subcommittee was to recommend to the personnel committee whether it was feasible to have an advisory committee and, if so, what such a committee would do and what its composition would be.

The subcommittee recommendation, as approved, provided for an advisory committee of twelve representatives, eight of whom must be nonsupervisory personnel and four management personnel, and further required that the personnel director have a standing position on the committee as an ex officio member for the purpose of consultation. In connection with the election of these representatives, it was provided that all full-time personnel, including supervisors, were qualified to vote and that the subcommittee would conduct the election.

Employees nominated candidates for positions on the Advisory Committee and the election took place; the ballots were printed and distributed by the employer with the employees' paychecks.

The Advisory Committee approved a set of bylaws drafted by a department head and the personnel director. The bylaws, which were approved by the employer, in pertinent part read:

Article II.

1. (a) To facilitate the discussion of any issues that might concern employees and their work environment and to direct these items to the proper source for resolution. (b) To establish better relations between all employees at Alta Bates Hospital irrespective of job description, title, or department. (c) To provide a mechanism for employees to submit ideas concerning new proposals about the hospital's operation, methods for improving the work environment, and/or the identification of possible problem areas at the hospital to administration. (d) To improve communication between departments, medical staff, volunteers, patients and community (pp. 5-6).

The Advisory Committee had no income and was entirely dependent on the employer in its day-to-day operations. The employer printed and distributed the ballots for the Advisory Committee election. Meetings were held during working times on the premises, and the employees suffered no loss of pay. The employer allowed the Advisory Committee to use a portion of the hospital bulletin board and the hospital newsletter to publicize its activities and permitted the Advisory Committee to use the hospital's mail system to distribute the minutes of the committee meetings and to use a building to display action request forms for employees to fill out and deposit in a box provided by the employer.

Several action request forms submitted to the Advisory Committee, which the Advisory Committee brought to the attention of management, concerned employees' grievances or conditions of work. For example, one action request complained that the food from the vending machines was often unsatisfactory and of a limited variety. Another was from a nurse who complained that the newly constructed nurses' lounges and locker facilities, where the nurses spent their break periods and changed their clothes, were incompletely furnished.

The NLRB found the Advisory Committee to be an organization in which employees participated and which existed for the purpose, in part, of dealing with the employer concerning grievances, labor disputes, and conditions of work. It was a labor organization within the meaning of Section 2(5) of the Act. The Board also found the Advisory Committee to be employer dominated.

The Board considered the fact that the employer created the Advisory Committee with the best of intentions. It was not motivated by any desire to undermine the union or any of the several other unions with which it had bargaining relations. The employer's motivation was based on its belief that if employees had easy access to an Advisory Committee with their unanswered problems or requests, they would be happier with their work environment, and, since satisfied employees tend to do better work, they would provide better care for the hospital's patients. The Board found this not to be a defense, however, because Section 8(a)(2) prohibits an employer from dominating or interfering with the formation or administration of any labor organization. The statute forbids employer interference or domination of a labor organization regardless of its motives—benevolent or malevolent.

However, regarding the alleged violation of Section 8(a)(5), the NLRB found that although the Advisory Committee was dealing with the employer within the meaning of Section 2(5) of the Act, such dealing did not reach the level of collective bargaining contemplated by Section 8(d) and 8(a)(5) of the Act.

The NLRB ordered the Employee Advisory Committee of Alta Bates Hospital to be disbanded.

Similarly, a hospital's Nursing Advisory Committee, inaugurated at a time when union organizational activities were in progress, and having as its purpose discussion with the hospital executive director of problems of staffing, salary increases, scheduling, weekends off, and lack of supplies, was determined, in *NLRB v. South Nassau Communities Hospital* (1980), to be an employer-dominated labor organization within the meaning of the Act. At various meetings within this committee, the employees had raised questions concerning such matters as the wage increase that they might be receiving, overtime pay, call-in pay for time spent performing professional functions, access to the cafeteria, work shifts, weekend work, and parking. It was clear to the administrative law judge that the Nursing

Advisory Committee was an organization in which employees participated. It was similarly clear, given the range of subjects discussed by the Committee with the hospital's executive director, that the parties were dealing with each other concerning the subjects delineated in Section 2(5) of the Act. That the committee may also have been concerned with discussing professional matters not related to wages, hours, and working conditions did not, in the mind of the administrative law judge, negate the role of the committee in dealing with the employer on those statutory subjects.

Finally, in *NLRB v. E.I. DuPont de Nemours & Co.* (1990), the Board found DuPont violated Sections 8(a)(2) and (1) of the Act by dominating and supporting the Design Team, a labor-management committee that included supervisors and rank-and-file workers represented by a union.

The *Daily Labor Report* (1989) noted that the Design Team was composed of 25 to 30 volunteers chosen by DuPont from a larger pool of applicants and that half were managers and the others were bargaining unit employees.

The Design Team was intended to implement organizational techniques to improve workplace safety, innovation, teamwork, open communication, involvement in problem solving, and sensitivity to customers' needs, ultimately making the company more competitive.

The Board found DuPont bypassed the union and fostered a competing organization by soliciting solutions to workplace problems from the Design Team and adopting the Design Team's proposals before introducing them at the bargaining table. In some cases, the company implemented Design Team proposals that had been rejected when the union proposed them. The administrative law judge found the company gave workers the subtle message that change could more effectively be implemented by the rival entity than by the designated bargaining agent.

If a hospital and its staff nurses, through their collective bargaining representative, wish to implement shared governance, with the necessary management-employee committees, the committees must not be labor organizations and the structure must not be employer dominated.

A clear statement creating the shared governance structure and delineating its authority should be set forth in the collective bargaining agreement. The provision empowering nurse managers and staff nurses to deal with professional issues must recognize the primacy of the terms of the collective bargaining agreement and preserve the status of the union as the nurses' bargaining representative. Individual rights of the nurses should be protected through preservation of access to the grievance procedure. Care must be taken to avoid domination of the committees by nurse managers. Power must be shared in the professional areas, but the rights of the union and the individual nurse must not be infringed upon.

Exclusive Representation

A union is empowered to act as the exclusive representative of all employees within the bargaining unit under Sections 8(b) and 9(a) of the Act (*Richardson v. United Steelworkers of America,* 1989). Section 9(a) states that "a representative . . . designated or selected for the purposes of collective bargaining by the majority of the employees in a unit . . . shall be the exclusive representative of all the employees in such a unit for the purposes of collective bargaining. . . ." Section 8(a)(5) of the Act requires the employer to bargain with the chosen representative. Under the Act, a union representative is chosen through election and certification by the NLRB.

The rationale underlying exclusive representation is one of majority rule. Thus, although an employee is not required to vote for union representation, that employee is bound by the majority. It is believed that majority rule results in collective strength and bargaining power, thereby subordinating the interest of the minority to those of the majority (Leffler, 1979).

The exclusive representation concept requires that the employer deal directly with the union concerning wages, hours, and other conditions of employment rather than with individual employees. When this requirement is not met, the union may risk loss of control to dissident groups, resulting in increasing competition, dissatisfaction, and conflict due to diverse results in conflict resolution (*Landers v. National Railroad Passenger Corporation et al.,* 1988). The union as exclusive representative controls processing of grievances and contract administration.

In a shared governance structure in an organized hospital, the union, as the exclusive bargaining representative of its membership, cannot be ignored. The active cooperation of the union in the creation of the committees forming the shared governance structure is essential, not only to comply with legal requirements, but to enhance opportunities for successful implementation. The sharing of power in certain areas by management is disallowed when the union is replaced as the exclusive collective bargaining representative for staff nurses.

Wages, hours, seniority, grievances, and other labor disputes should not be topics considered by the shared governance committee. The traditional adversarial negotiating process between management and the union can effectively deal with those issues. The shared governance system in an organized hospital must work within the limits allowed by law and the terms of the collective bargaining agreement.

Fair Representation

A union has a duty to its membership of fair representation. "A union's duty to represent its members fairly is a judicially created doctrine derived to balance the union's exclusive representation of its members, set forth in Section 9(a) of the National Labor Relations Act, 29 USC section 159(1). With this exclusive authority comes a responsibility to the individual members, whose individual bargaining rights are correspondingly limited" (*Walker v. Teamsters Local 71,* 1989, p. 190).

The union's duty of fair representation extends beyond the negotiation of a contract. It includes day-to-day contract adjustments, working with rules, problem resolution in those areas not covered by the existing contractual agreement, and protection of secured rights (*Conley v. Gibson,* 1957). These duties complement the union's duty to fairly represent its membership in contract negotiation, amendment, and modification.

The union's duty of fair representation in the administration of existing contract rights extends to contract modifications. In *Walker v. Teamsters Local 71* (1989), a union was found to have breached its duty of fair representation when a joint labor-management committee delayed implementation of a contract provision. The court found this action to be a contract modification rather than a contract interpretation; thus the membership should have been offered an opportunity to vote before this modification. By failing to provide this opportunity, the union was found to have failed in its duty to protect the interests of its members. The union breached its duty of fair representation by its failure to diligently seek timely implementation of the contract provision. In effect, the union negotiated away a contract benefit through negligent delegation of its duties to the committee. Furthermore, the delay in implementing the contract provision at issue did not benefit the bargaining unit. The union was criticized by the court for its lack of a review mechanism to ensure contract compliance. The court also noted that the committee had no power under the collective bargaining agreement to modify the contract or negotiate changes.

Employers may be liable when a union breaches its duty of fair representation. "It is well recognized that where an employer has had notice of the lack of authority of the union to enter into an agreement, no agreement is reached. Where the employer has knowledge of the ratification requirement, and this is the basis for the fair representation claim, the employer may also be found liable for breach of the contract or for having joined in the fair representation breach" (*Walker v. Teamsters Local 71*, 1989, p. 193).

The duty of fair representation suggests the inclusion of certain safeguards within a shared governance structure that should be created by contract language. The function and authority of any committees should also be delineated. Committees should not attempt to change contract language beyond the scope of contract authorization. Unions are well advised to maintain a mechanism for review of committee activities. Membership vote for contract modifications should be implemented when questions exist. In areas of peer review and granting of credentials, distinctions that are drawn should be reasonable, relevant, and done in good faith with honesty through use of objective criteria. Access to the grievance procedure by staff nurses must not be impeded.

EMERGING MODELS OF COLLECTIVE BARGAINING

Assuming no changes in the current law, reasonable inferences can be drawn regarding the evolution of collective bargaining encompassing a viable shared governance structure. These are:

1. A union that has been certified as the bargaining agent for registered nurses will be required to continue to perform the functions of exclusive bargaining representative.
2. A union will be required to continue to fairly represent the unit as a whole as well as protecting the individual rights of each of the represented nurses.
3. A union and a hospital will be required to conduct their relations within the law in the implementation and operation of shared governance.
4. A hospital will be required to limit its expenditures for variable and fixed costs to its available funds.

The union will continue to meet its obligations as the exclusive bargaining representative and of fair representation by conducting good faith collective bargaining negotiations with the hospital that result in a written collective bargaining agreement ratified by the bargaining unit, and by taking such actions as may be necessary to ensure that the terms and conditions of the agreement are fully implemented.

The collective bargaining agreement will contain the normal provisions concerning wages, hours, and conditions of employment that affect the bargaining unit uniformly. In addition, the agreement will contain express language authorizing shared governance and empowering the shared governance structure to resolve professional nursing issues. The agreement will require that the resolution of any such issues may not deviate from the terms of the agreement, but will allow referral of necessary changes in the agreement back to the negotiating teams for resolution. If changes in the agreement are then negotiated, they will be presented to the bargaining unit for ratification.

The professional nursing issues expected to be addressed on a continuing basis during the term of the collective bargaining agreement could include staffing, patient mix, peer review, and granting of credentials.

If staffing is used as an example, the collective bargaining agreement will contain the overall methods to be used in increasing and decreasing staff. If staffing is also specified as an issue for shared governance, the specific formulas to determine the number of registered nurses necessary to provide the appropriate level of care within a specific unit and in compliance with budgetary constraints will be provided by the professional nurses using the shared governance structure. The shared governance structure will allow consideration of the individual peculiarities of a nursing unit such as physical configuration, availability of support services, location, type of services provided, and other facts that could not realistically appear in a collective bargaining agreement. In addition, the focus on the individual unit will allow the professional nurses involved to react to unexpected changes in the relevant facts much faster and with more appropriate responses than can be expected from the hospital and the total bargaining unit.

The collective bargaining agreement will contain a mechanism for dispute resolution such as a grievance procedure. The individual nurse, aided by the union, who considers that the change or elimination of the nurse's job as a result of the staffing formula developed by the professional nurses through shared governance and implemented by the hospital is a violation of the collective bargaining agreement, will have access to the grievance procedure to protect the nurse's individual rights.

The models for collective bargaining that should emerge in conjunction with shared governance should allow flexibility to the professional issues. The traditional collective bargaining negotiations will occur on a periodic basis. The issues that will be negotiated should be those that are universal to the bargaining unit. The agreement will specify the universal issues to be at least wages, seniority, union security, methods for use in increasing or decreasing the number of staff nurses employed, work interruption, recognition of the union, shared governance, dispute resolution, and contract term. The shared governance language in the contract will specify those professional issues to be determined by the professional nurses. This empowerment will allow and encourage continuous self-directed attention to and resolution of the professional issues in a timely, appropriate manner.

The hospital will use and implement the shared governance decisions while complying with the collective bargaining agreement. The union will closely monitor the shared governance procedure and decisions and the hospital implementation thereof. The union will stand ready to protect individual rights through the use of the grievance procedure and by appropriate input to its members who are working in the shared governance structure. The shared governance structure will not be allowed to change the collective bargaining agreement, but can recommend necessary changes to both negotiating teams. The hospital and union teams will meet and conduct good faith negotiations concerning the recommendations even though the contract term has not expired. If agreement is reached, it will be subject to ratification by the bargaining unit.

The anticipated models for collective bargaining will thus recognize the unit-wide issues and incorporate them into the collective bargaining agreement. This agreement, with respect to those issues, can be anticipated to be somewhat static for its term. The professional issues specified for shared governance will be subject to a more dynamic process and will be addressed as necessary by the professional nurses in a less structured, more flexible setting. Action can be expected to replace reaction. A more efficient organization that provides quality patient care should result because of the professional nurse expertise and empowerment to determine professional nursing issues.

SUMMARY

Hospitals may share power with their professional nurses in an organized setting. The use of a shared governance structure to empower nurses to handle the issues of professionalism is feasible. The hospital and the union must recognize that there are binding legal rights and obligations placed on both parties. Compliance with the law is most likely if the shared governance structure is created as follows:

1. The shared governance structure should be sanctioned by the collective bargaining agreement between the hospital and union.
2. The committees created to accomplish shared governance should consider professional issues only and should not deal with issues concerning grievances, labor disputes, wages, rates of pay, hours, or other terms and conditions of employment.
3. The power of the committees must be limited by the budget of the hospital.
4. The membership of the committees should be equally divided between nursing managers and staff nurses, or have a majority of staff nurses.
5. The staff nurses who are members of the committees should be elected by the staff nurses or appointed by the union. The hospital should appoint the nurse managers. All committee members should have specified terms.

6. The decisions of the shared governance committees should not be subject to veto by the hospital.

7. The committees cannot alter, modify, or deviate from the terms of the collective bargaining agreement. If the committees determine that a change is necessary in the agreement to further shared governance, the change should be recommended to the hospital and the union. If, after negotiation, the hospital and the union agree to change the agreement, the change should be submitted to the bargaining unit for ratification.

8. Any shared governance structure must not impede the rights of individual nurses to use the contractual grievance procedure.

9. Peer review, granting of credentials, staffing, and other professional issues are proper areas of concern for the committees if authorized by the collective bargaining agreement. However, the decisions of the committees should be reasonable, relevant, and done in good faith with honesty through use of objective criteria. Adverse impacts on individual staff nurses must be subject to challenge through the use of the contractual grievance procedure.

10. Even though there is language in some decisions concerning the unimportance of the motivating factors of the hospital in creating such joint committees, a hospital should not enter into such an arrangement to circumvent the union as the exclusive bargaining representative or to cause the union to be decertified.

11. The union should implement a method to monitor the committees to ensure that the activities of the committees do not violate the terms of the collective bargaining agreement.

If used properly, the shared governance structure can address those issues of professionalism in nursing that are not easily resolved in the adversarial process of collective bargaining or reasonably subject to inclusion in a collective bargaining agreement. The resolution of these issues can be accomplished within the nursing profession with allowance for economic realities and deference to the terms of the collective bargaining agreement.

REFERENCES

Airstream, Inc. v. NLRB. 131 LLRM 2899; 877 F2d 1291 (1989).

Alta Bates Hospital Institutional Workers Local 250, Service Employees International Union, AFL-CIO and Employee Advisory Committee of Alta Bates Hospital, Party in Interest. 226 NLRB 485; 93 LLRM 1288 (1976).

Apex Hosiery Co. v. Leader. 310 US 469 (1940).

Clayton Antitrust Act. 38 stat. 730 (1914), as amended, 15 USC Sections 15, 17, 26 (1970), 29 USC Section 52 (1970).

Cleland, V.S. (1978). Shared Governance in a Professional Model of Collective Bargaining. *Journal of Nursing Administration,* May, 39-43.

Colangelo, M. (1980). The Professional Association and Collective Bargaining. *Supervisor Nurse,* 11(9), 24-32.

Conley v. Gibson. 355 US 41 (1957).

Daily Labor Report. 1989, (15), A-6.

Daily Labor Report. 1990, (30), A-11.

Duplex Printing Press v. Deering. 254 US 443 (1921).

Gorman, R.A. (1976). *Basic Text on Labor Law.* St. Paul, Minn.: West Publishing Co.

Health Care Amendments. 88 stat. 295 (1974); 1974 PL 93-360.

Jacox, A. (1980). Collective Action: The Basis for Professionalism. *Supervisor Nurse*, 11(9), 22-24.

Kiereini, E.M. (1980). Professional Autonomy and Corporate Responsibility. *Journal of Advanced Nursing*, 5(1), 107-108.

Labor Management Relations Act. 61 stat. 136 (1947), as amended by 73 stat. 519 (1959), 83 stat. 133 (1969), 87 stat. 314 (1973), 88 stat. 396 (1974); 29 USC Sections 141-97 (1970).

Labor Relations Week, (1990). Feb. 28, 4; 207.

Landers v. National Railroad Passenger Corporation et al. 485 US 652 (1988).

Leffler, F.C. (1979). Piercing the Duty of Fair Representation: The Dichotomy Between Negotiations and Grievance Handling. *University of Illinois Law Forum*, (1), 35-65.

McGilloway, F.A. (1980). The Struggle at the Clinical Level. *Journal of Advanced Nursing*, 5(2), 105-107.

National Labor Relations Act. 49 stat. 449 (1935), as amended by 61 stat. 136 (1947), 65 stat. 601 (1951), 72 stat. 945 (1958), 73 stat. 541 (1959), 88 stat. 395 (1974); 29 USC Sections 151-69.

NLRB v. Cabot Carbon Co. 306 US 203 (1959).

NLRB v. Edward G. Budd Mfg. Co. 169 F2d 571; 355 US 908 (1948).

NLRB v. E.I. DuPont de Nemours & Co., Respondent and Chemical Workers Association, Inc., International Brotherhood of DuPont Workers, Charging Party and the Design Team, Party-in-Interest. 1989 NLRB LEXIS 736 (1989).

NLRB v. Jones & Laughlin Steel Corp. 301 US 1 (1937).

NLRB v. South Nassau Communities Hospital. 247 NLRB 527; 103 LRRM 1175 (1980).

NLRB v. Streamway Division of Scott and Fetzler Co. 691 F2d 288 (1982).

Norris-LaGuardia Act. 47 stat. 70 (1932), 29 USC Sections 101-15 (1970).

Richardson v. United Steelworkers of America. 864 F2d 1162 (5th Cir. 1989).

Rotkovitch, R. (1980). Do Labor Union Activities Decrease Professionalism? *Supervisor Nurse*, 11(9), 16-18.

Sheridan, D.R. (1982). The Season for Collective Bargaining. *Nursing Administration Quarterly*, 6(2), 1-7.

Sherman Antitrust Act. 26 Stat. 209 (1890) as amended, 15 USC Sections 1-7 (1970).

Stern, E.M. (1982). Collective Bargaining: A Means of Conflict Resolution. *Nursing Administration Quarterly*, 6(2), 9-20.

United States v. Hutcheson. 312 US 219 (1941).

Walker v. Teamsters Local 71. 714 FSupp 178 (WDNC 1989).

10   *Shared Governance: Looking Toward the Future*

Tim Porter-O'Grady

This book has outlined the characteristics and elements influencing the development of shared governance. The focus has been on the current strategies that have emerged over the past 10 years that facilitate the successful unfolding of a nursing shared governance model. If the considerations and discussions ventured by the authors are faithfully applied in the implementation process, success should be ensured regardless of where this approach might be implemented.

In addition to the growing data base regarding successful implementation processes, there is mounting evidence of the successful outcomes of the shared governance process. From objective data supporting the reduction in turnover and increase in retention to the qualitative data that show higher levels of nursing satisfaction and investment in the work and the workplace, shared governance as a professional model is benefiting those who struggle to make it work (Ludemann and Brown, 1989).

The status and role of nursing change in this model from the inside out. First, the nursing organization begins to feel better about itself and to relate differently both within and outside the service. Soon others note that there is something different in their relationship with the nursing organization and begin to assess their response and react to the changes in operation and relationship. This reaction is sometimes positive and at other times this change in nursing generates some concern. The behaviors and self-perception of a profession as pivotal to the provision of health services as nursing cannot avoid having an impact on those who relate directly to it. Some will be thrilled with the enthusiasm and growing sense of self that nurses project; others will be uncertain about what such a change means to their relationship with nurses and the adjustments the system will have to undergo to accommodate these changes. Some may be obstreperous about the changes in the behavior and role of nurses and may not wish to accommodate such changes into their relationship, thereby creating a period of transitional stress between themselves and their nurse colleagues. Such situational occurrences must be expected in a challenging and politically intensive environment such as health care. These are the conditions and risks of change, maturation, and reaching a point where others must accept the new and those who see and act as though they deserve consideration and equity. This is what shared governance demands and produces.

SHARED GOVERNANCE AS A TRANSITIONAL MODEL

The world is in constant change. What was appropriate yesterday is passé today. The values of yesterday yield to the challenges of tomorrow. What was appropriate for one time is inadequate for another.

Although shared governance is a highly successful vehicle for building a truly professional nursing organization and strengthening the profession and the role of nursing in the health care system, it too must undergo change as time and conditions warrant. The times and conditions of the health care environment will demand newer considerations and approaches that will more adequately advance nursing to the forefront of health care, calling for newer arrangements and structures to do so (Haddon, 1989).

If shared governance becomes an end in itself or a point of arrival, it will have failed to serve its intended purpose. Shared governance has always been a transitional model—a means to reaching a new point as a profession and as a vital health service. It is better characterized as a journey than a point of arrival. Its value diminishes as defined goals are achieved. Retaining the structure as though it were the place to stay is to fail to continue the work of maturation and transformation that is always the work of a profession in the fulfillment of the public trust for which it is empowered and licensed.

The concept of describing the structures and work of nursing more as a vehicle than an event is sometimes difficult for the profession. Gains in political, social, role, relational, and equitable outcomes have been long awaited, challenging in process, and uncertain in benefit. In these circumstances the temptation to retain what is gained in the form in which nurses receive it is strong and tantalizing. Unfortunately, to do so is to hold tight to an illusion that soon dissipates into another set of circumstances and conditions that change the experience, defy the perception, and call us all to a new reality (Peters, 1987).

CHANGING TIMES

Life conditions and world circumstances are changing at a quantum rate. Reality seems to be continually adjusted, even before there is time to get accustomed to that new state of being. Although more sensitive to the changes around us, they are so life changing we are not certain we know how to respond to them. From fundamental moral values to political relationships, the world seems to daily reflect an entirely new set of variables demanding response. Those things we have come to count on and trust as constants in our lives change before our eyes and, unfortunately, leave us few tools to cope with what replaces them (Morris, 1990).

The emerging changes in our world are not simply transitional events. They are transformation processes that are changing the very fabric of human existence and calling us to a future radically different from anything we know. As Figure 10-1 illustrates, we are indeed moving from one age to another age—out of the industrial age into a social technocracy whose character and circumstances are still unclear and our picture of it is opaque at best. It is approaching with such speed that we truly do not know how to understand it, or to cope with it (Toffler, 1990).

In the midst of these changes nurses are working to unfold a shared governance

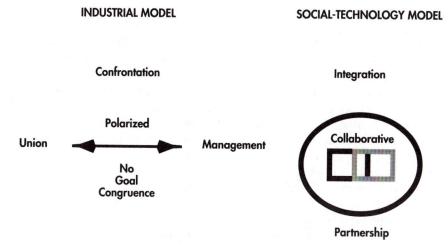

FIGURE 10-1. The industrial model versus the social-technocracy model.

model. Ostensibly, the model prepares the profession and individual nurse for essential new roles and behaviors. Nurses will need to be proactive in efforts to write the emerging script in ways that are beneficial for those whom nurses serve and for the continuing effectiveness and viability of the nursing profession in meeting health care needs in a system in transition. Shared governance serves as a baseline or foundation on which further adaptive structures will be designed and constructed for the future. It is the appropriate redesign and restructuring of the health care system and nurses' responses to it that will be increasingly important as a key task of nursing and nurses. Although shared governance acts as a formal bridge to a new sense of self and a stronger set of relationships and power within the profession, this context provides a foundation for even further change and providing some form and focus in order to have a meaningful impact on the delivery of health care in the future. It is for this purpose that the next steps beyond shared governance must be directed. As those steps are taken, they must allow nurses to design new forms and forums to govern those newer circumstances and contexts within which nurses will work and make their contribution to those they serve.

The health care system of tomorrow will be as different as the world that reflects it. There will be entirely new approaches to provision of health care services. Nursing resources will be used in many new ways and provide nursing services in ways not yet conceived. These roles are not yet altogether clear, nor can they be. The delivery system will undergo much transition before its form and nurses' roles are clear. However, this concern is the crux of the current issue of change with regard to the nursing profession. Just what will the role of nursing be in writing a new script for the future of health care and nursing's role in it? If nurses are not involved in writing this new script, what roles will they be destined (or assigned) to carry out, if any?

Clearly, during transitional times, whoever writes the scenario for tomorrow will no doubt dictate the roles. If nurses are not at the policy table where the deliberations and determinations of how health care will be provided, there may be a good chance that the value nursing can bring to the discussions and the pivotal role that nurses play in the process can be underrated, skewed, or forgotten. The outcomes could thereby be severely compromised because a key player in the health care process is either missing or underrepresented.

Expectations born of a strong shared governance system should lead the nursing profession to expect a role in shared decision making, especially regarding issues that affect what nurses do. Assertive skill building and a clear agenda facilitate the contribution nurses make to deliberations affecting the future of health care delivery. A structure that supports and expects a nursing role to be included in policy and strategic processes that decide the direction and fate of the health care entity or enterprise is vital. The level of maturity contributes to the effectiveness of the health care system and allows a broad range of considerations to emerge and be supported as an important part of the nurse's responsibility for defining and living the future. The overriding sense of contributing to that future provides nurses a stronger sense of ownership related to the solutions and to the work necessary to implement them.

AN ORGANIZATIONAL PARADIGM SHIFT

It is surprising that employee involvement and ownership processes have been so late in the United States. Here, where democracy is the standard bearer for the free world, the rigidity and authoritarianism of the workplace challenge the Americal ideal. However, the realities of a changing global economic stage and competitive marketplace are driving American companies to redesign. Included in the redesign is the effort to create a more involved and invested workplace that incorporates the worker into the decision-making process.

The effort to accomplish this redesign is new and initially appears clumsy and overwrought. There is an awkward overindulgence and even paternalism in the effort that is a part of moving toward creating truly involved relationships. It is the relationship that ultimately will make all the difference in making the "new" workplace successful.

The "noise" and stress of the transition will serve a valuable purpose. First, the superficial and trendy programs that teach total quality management and environments of excellence (and other such "packages") must be experimented with and then, in typical American fashion, discarded because they cannot produce what they promise. The idea that personal and professional values can, by mere act of will or organizational process, be melded mindlessly into an amorphous multidisciplinary team committed to an abstract ideation such as quality is not only silly, it is untenable. Such processes violate the essentials and hard work associated with professional investment and ownership, relational integrity, collaborative agreements, and role and functional parameters driven by the emergence of a "knowledge worker" class in American society (Toffler, 1990).

Rather than give up professional obligation and identity, such character needs to be maximized for a meaningful investment in the outcomes of work to be achieved. The professional worker has a maturing sense of self and commitment to what she or he is doing, bred into the role through years of preparation and application. In today's fragmented work, it is one of the values that can be identified with as contiguous and consistent and maintained. In essence, this knowledge and professional identity is the one thing the professional worker takes home and carries wherever she or he may go. With an increasingly fragmented, decentralized workplace, the individual's professional identity and knowledge base is one of the few life constituents to link with others and create any sense of human and professional connection.

In many of the emerging service-based programs that focus on the service receiver—the product or quality—the perspective of the individual worker is sometimes either lost or relegated to some other level of consciousness. For any quality connection to be made, there must be equated investment in both the worker as provider and the patient as receiver. They enter into a relational exchange in the health care frame of reference, and the exchange will require the efforts of both parties if a desirable outcome is to be achieved. The connection is therefore a living experience that incorporates the life processes, skills, and openness of each to the other in order to work or to move to a "higher" or more esteemed level of either interaction or healing. No value can be meaningfully expressed if the relationship of both is not balanced and attended to, regardless of the power of the drive for a quality outcome or product or cost effectiveness.

None of this suggests that a renewed focus on the product, customer, or patient is not desirable. It is. Nothing can serve the health care field better than a concerted, informed, and legitimate emphasis on the patient, consumer, and/or outcome by all those who provide service. It is suggested that this objective is not achievable over the long term if both the needs of the worker and the needs of the consumer are not equally addressed and attended to. The assumption that the professions, and thus professional workers, are not interested in the best shortchanges the commitment of the worker and fails to create the requisite partnership between the organization and its professions to a process whose outcome is mutually beneficial.

Equally important is the need to teach the process of achieving measurable outcomes that can provide a level of confidence with regard to the quality of one's work and the quality of the work of the enterprise as a whole. When professional skills and values are incorporated into this process and individual investment is nurtured, the organization will surely benefit as evidenced by its own measurement related to the achievement of its goals or quality standards. The partnership, in this case between nurses and the organization, cannot exclude the equitable infusion into the effort of the values, commitment, and concerted action of the professional group in the exercise of its role.

The professions, including nursing, must recognize the need to validate the effect of their work on both the consumer and system. Professional groups have too long escaped reasonable scrutiny to determine the real value and benefit of the services they provide. It has almost appeared that they were afraid to focus on their value because such an emphasis may reveal the group's shortcomings and that the supposed contribution did not match the real outcomes. In other words, there is an unspoken fear that the profession and its work are truly not worth the price paid for its services and thereby subject to inevitable judgment and possible decline in both value and numbers.

The chances are good that this scenario is simply not true and that nursing will find that its value has historically been underrated and that the full value of the profession in the healing process has not been thoroughly explored (Passau-Buck, 1988). Adopting models that focus on the consumers of health care and on service outcomes should provide a stronger base for validating nursing contribution. Therefore nursing should not be reticent to explore opportunities to assess its role and value and to attach the determinations from that assessment to the management of the nursing resource. The issue is the willingness of the profession to do the work necessary to determine its place and legitimate role and function in the delivery of health care services. Because it is likely that the role is broad-based and is the foundation of the contribution nursing makes to health care delivery, the profession should move with confidence in concert with activities to facilitate the determination of its value and contribution. Nursing leadership should be willing to:

1. Evaluate objectively the process of value determination as fully as possible. This process includes the development and familiarity with statistical processes such as those associated with standard data analysis: flow charts, histograms, data diagrams, variance analysis, cause-and-effect data tools. Algorithmic processes that help objectify specific processes must also be incorporated into measurement of services provided. All levels of the nursing service must be comfortable with these processes.
2. Better define quality. Nurses must refrain from use of generalized descriptors of their work and focus more fully on units of service, patient care elements that relate to the payment methodology, and establish a stronger relationship between outcome and the process that achieved it.
3. Better describe and directly identify the relationship with the client or patient. Nurses must move beyond the "second step" service role (agent of the doctor or hospital) to a primary identification with the patient directly and establish roles and relationships within the context of nursing's own paradigm, not the reflection of someone else's role.

MOVEMENT FROM HIERARCHICAL STRUCTURES

Recognition of the transition to more collateral approaches to structuring the decisional process is emerging in health care (Naisbitt and Aburdene, 1985). This move is not without trauma. The hospital health care system has historically developed with a rigid hierarchy and a solidly structured decisional pyramid. The doctor has generally been assumed to be at the top of the medical pyramid because of the socially promulgated myth of informational and clinical ascendancy (Kalisch and Kalisch, 1988). It is difficult to change the structure that supports the physician. The medical model has been the generalized approach to the offering and payment of health care in America for this century.

Now it is more strongly recognized that there are a number of ways to offer health care services outside of a medical model fixation. Increasing evidence supports the efficacy of such practices, raising questions about the viability of maintaining a high-cost, high-intervention system for the delivery of health care in America (Fagin, 1990). Policymakers and legislators in the public sector are beginning to alter the service and payment infrastructure to allow the provision and payment of a different array of services provided by a different kind of provider.

The traditional hospital structure is being threatened continually by increasing cost-control measures. The intent has been to move the patient through the hospital system quickly or to have the patient not enter the system at all, if it can be avoided. Such a strategy has worked admirably, reducing the annual rate of hospital cost significantly through the 1980s and early '90s (Evans, 1989).

Services normally provided by hospitals are now being provided in other settings. Those procedures performed in doctors' offices have increased at the same rate as hospital costs have declined. To counteract this effect, Congress has introduced cost caps to physician payments; the private sector is following with its own efforts to control doctors' payments (Grimaldi, 1990). In effect, the health care system is being forced by economics to change its service characteristics. Paying solely for sickness is quickly becoming outmoded and begs for a different service and payment arrangement in the future. Incentive payment structures will focus on emerging proposals that keep costs as low as possible or, ideally, do not ever generate those costs.

Efforts to produce health giving or maintaining services or to provide services at the lowest point of service cost will continue to develop. As the population ages and as chronic issues become the dominant health concerns of the population, nonacute and noninterventive strategies will ensue at an accelerated rate. The data that support the early intervention or prevention of the conditions or circumstances of illness have long-term benefits, not only on patients' health but also on the costs of providing health care over the long term. Recent data show that emphasis on early nutrition, adequate housing, education, and prevention all contribute to the reduction in health problems in later life. Failure to do this results in high-cost illness (Program, 1990).

The effects of this refocusing will soon emerge in the service delivery system and be reflected in the payment structures as the data increasingly support the transition. How services are provided also will change radically. The hospital as the traditional location of all intervention services of an acute nature will become less central to the delivery of many services provided in the system. Emerging models of service delivery will take precedence and newer, more cost-effective ways to treat patients will develop outside of the hospital. Connection to the hospital will be maintained as the community's link to a more intense diagnostic or therapeutic environment.

Many community or noninstitutional services will be provided by nurses in nontraditional settings. Their practice will reflect the requirements of the client and be offered where the client can more easily access them and remain as independent as possible for as long as possible. The nurse in such situations will often become a primary provider of health care, referring to the physician only when a medical plan of care needs to be incorporated in the patient's care. This change in the structuring of health care will change the role and relationship of the nurse to others in the health care system (Hudson, 1990). Because the structure in the example above indicates a high degree of decentralization, the nurse will be less loosely tied to the institution than today. Nurses will also interact more often with other health professionals as an independent part of their work than they have in the past. The therapeutic relationship will include consultation and advice from a number of health professionals, based on the needs of the patient and what the health professional has to offer the patient.

Patient problems will become less acute and more chronic than in the past. Because of this reality and fueled by an increasingly aging population, the nurse may often be the case manager or key primary care provider. This will begin in the low-income, high–service need arena where the nurse's service and economic value will be well evidenced. As the data related to the efficacy of nursing expand into the policy and payment area, adjustments in the payment structure will accelerate and direct payment for services rendered will result. The nurse's viability in the "mainstream" also will be encouraged by successes in managing the underserved.

In the hospital, newer care structures and relationships will continue to emerge. Experimentation with a broad range of models and designs for care delivery will be undertaken. From case management to multidisciplinary teams and from unit-based designs to redesigning the patient care service, a transformation of service delivery approaches will occur. At the center of the new models will be the nurse, well prepared to manage the continuum of care. Regardless of the approaches created, nurses will most often emerge as the integrators and linkages in the care delivery process.

This shift will create a different relationship both within and outside of the profession. The organizational ties that bound the nursing organization in the past will be altered. Newer ways of connecting with the profession and maintaining a nursing frame of reference and support will be the major work of the profession over the next two decades.

Anticipating this change, nursing leaders in service and management will have to dialogue with each other to create organizational structures to support these newer relationships and service arrangements. The current organizational models, including shared governance, will have to adapt to these newer realities. Indeed, much of the structure of the nursing organization may assume a different look in the new health care system (see Figure 10-2).

Nurses will continue the need to be flexible and available to offer health care services in a variety of ways. Some exchange of value must result for the newer, direct health care provided by nurses. As the relative value of a nurse and the nurse's time are calculated within the system, newer ways to manage the nurse and connect with other nurses and the system will be developed.

Important in this consideration is the reality that the health care system is becoming increasingly decentralized and noninstitutional in its service framework. As the institutional services in health care become increasingly constrained, offering services in other ways and in other settings must increase. Home and community-based service structures will continue to emerge to address the need for services no

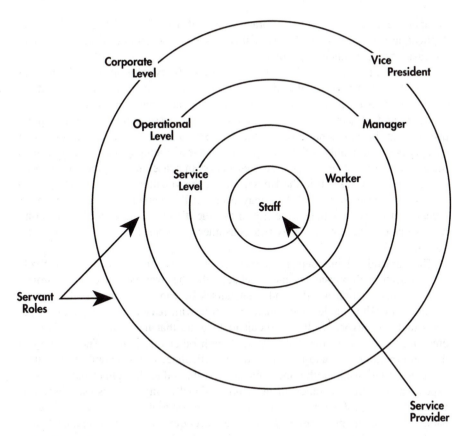

FIGURE 10-2. The organic model for the twenty-first century health care organization.

longer provided by hospitals. The opportunities for nurses to provide a growing array of services will be magnified almost yearly. Most new employment of nurses is not within the hospital structure but rather in other settings. How will nurses and nursing as a profession stay connected when its members are working in a variety of service arrangements in the communities and neighborhoods of America? How will nurses of tomorrow maintain their identity with the profession when they may spend more time working with other disciplines than with other nurses? Indeed, nurses may not see other nurses in their practice and may identify more strongly with their own work settings than with nursing colleagues.

Current organizational models do not accommodate this newer (older?) kind of nursing practice. The values of the profession and the unique contribution of nursing to the health of the community may become lost if there is not a mechanism to conform to the new framework for nursing practice.

The shift in nursing practice will require a new look at an old issue. What is the appropriate base of education for nurses who must manage their own practice and who will be devoid of the extensive supervision and policy control in the decentralized setting? Indeed, the system will not be able to provide enough managers to supervise all the new arenas of practice even if it so desired. The overhead and duplication necessary for such supervision would overwhelm the system and could not easily be economically justified.

To provide both the practice expertise and credibility with other disciplines, an advanced level of nursing education will be needed to ensure viability in a different competition for services. As other professions are increasing their educational expectations for their practitioners, nursing is still reacting to the entry into practice issue at the functional level of practice. Still a more than adequate supply of cheaply prepared highly technical registered nurses is being prepared in the United States. As the numbers of less educated nurses increase and become the majority of the nursing profession in the United States, the vocationalization of the profession will proceed over time. This may occur as the demand increases for nurses prepared at higher levels of expertise to assume direction and control of the complex array of health-based activities consumers will need if costs are to be reduced.

The demands of interdependent practice are based on the need to effectively communicate with physicians and to relate with other well-educated health professionals. This relationship demands that nurses be capable of meaningful professional relationships, able to articulate their role with reason, and prepared for patient- and self-advocacy. It is difficult to imagine that nurses with associate degrees may progress to the dialogue stage with other disciplines. The inequity of their information base and their inability to articulate, in comparable terms, their value and relationship within the same context that other disciplines have come to expect can cripple the achievement of professional equity. This is especially true when the other profession's minimum provision for professional practice is comparable to graduate preparation. If nurses expect equity in role and treatment, they must manifest the accoutrements of equity and exhibit comparable evidence of equivalence before the relationship can develop. In preparing for the future, nursing leaders must be cognizant of the need to change the educational focus from basic preparation to advanced education in those service areas that will be in greatest demand: community health, psychosocial, gerontology, women's health, midwifery, nurse practitioner, family practice, etc.

The new paradigm for health care is emerging in ways not previously imagined. The "old script" is not adequate to the needs and the current valuation of a non–illness-based health care system (Lamm, 1990). The traditional players are subject to the vagaries of a radically changing time. Physicians have long escaped the controlling characteristics of a limiting dollar and are now facing that reality with ever-increasing trepidation. Nurses have been directly insulated but no less affected by the changes and will have to soon directly account for their value in the delivery system. This entails translating their work value and economic value into concrete data to support the health system's continued investment in their services. Nurses must not expect responses to their demands for compensation, benefits, and other perks that are not somehow related to the result of nursing activity. A changed understanding and relationship between health care leadership and nurses is a certainty, but there will also be a changed character in the relationship between nurses and others. Expectation on demand is not sufficient.

The collective bargaining process so valued by organized nursing will also be subject to a change in role and character in the near future. As the challenges of the workplace change, the very nature of work relationships and the processes associated with collective bargaining cannot remain unaffected. At a time when polarization in the workplace serves no purpose, logistics that depend on polarized positions can only be failure strategies (Porter-O'Grady, 1990). When the opportunity to seek increasing shares of the economic pie is no longer viable because there is no increasing size to that "pie," efforts to maximize one's advantage at the expense of the other cannot succeed. All who share work in the enterprise are stakeholders in the work and the workplace. Seeking unilateral advantage without consideration of the outcome is simply an example of organized suicide. Neither management nor labor can "win" in a time of constraint if both parties cannot compromise, use the same language, mutually invest in the well-being of the workplace, and consider the impact of each party's decision on the viability of the other. Neither will survive with this flexibility. When the enterprise fails, there is no one to pick up the pieces and all the players are losers. The issues of rights, prerogative, due process, etc. pale when there is nothing to negotiate and no one is left to do the work because the place is no longer in business (Maraldo, 1990).

Some may argue that this scenario is simply an overdramatic representation of the current situation in health care. It must be noted that in the United States hospitals and health care facilities are closing at an average annual rate of more than 100 a year. It might be wise to ask nurse leaders in rural communities what it felt like when their hospital could no longer remain open and their roles were no longer available to them. Whether nurses are regarded as "labor" or "management," it behooves all nurses to consider how they can move from the periphery of the relationship with each other to the center, where the best interests of the profession and the enterprise are a mutual concern to nurses regardless of role and where the nurse can undertake consensus building processes. Nursing's collective future will depend on it.

Just as the relationship among nurses will be affected in the future, regardless of role, the role of management will change as well. Perhaps the most-changed role in nursing will be that of the nurse manager.

Management has undergone significant role redefinition in this century, but the fundamental expectations of the manager in the organization have not substantively changed for generations. Much of the manager's traditional role is based on a set of beliefs about the worker and the workplace that has remained unchanged. Many characteristics of the hierarchical structure in most workplaces reflect an almost primordial mistrust of the worker and a fundamental belief that the worker has little place in policy formation and direction setting for the organization. The worker has been viewed primarily as the person assigned to *do,* not to think, strategize, plan, or make decisions about work and how it is done. In fact, much of the research reflecting the modern view of the worker (the so-called scientific view) is based on work done in manufacturing settings and assembly line work environments (Hersey and Blanchard, 1989).

As indicated earlier in this chapter, the emergence of the knowledge worker has greatly changed the workplace and the attitude about the role of the worker in policy formation and direction setting. As Toffler and others have indicated, the success of the organization may chiefly depend on its ability to incorporate all of its participants to varying degrees in formulating and implementing the organization's strategic plan (Toffler, 1990).

The emergence in nursing of a professional consciousness will change the way nurses view their role and participation in the organization. In an age of equity, it is not surprising that the woman of today who is also a nurse is less accepting of arbitrary or third-party determinants of what she does and how much control she will be allowed to exercise in her role. Having reached a certain level of maturity (the average nurse's age is 41 years), she is more balanced and aware of both her own contribution and expectations. At the same time, the nurse entering practice today is much less accepting of predetermined parameters and is more willing to set her own. What is frustrating and also liberating about these "new nurses" is that the parameters are constantly shifting and they are willing to shift their circumstances to suit the changing condition of their lives. For nurses in the baby-boom generation who now seek some stability in the environment, these new nurses can be discomforting and destabilizing and appear noncommitted and selfish. Having been raised with plenty and few restrictions on their possibilities, the new nurses represent an entirely different view of their world. Although this may appear, in the short term, as a cultural clash, it is really a complementary process. After all, it is the mature nurse whose children are now entering the profession. She inculcated the higher levels of expectation and demand now exemplified by the new nurse. Although the new nurse may yet be naive about her place in the world, her levels of expectation regarding her life and its direction represent a new mode of thinking and behaving that will invariably have to be accommodated (Muff, 1988).

For the foreseeable future, nurses will seek a greater role in influencing what they do and exercising control over their lives. It is widely known that the shortage of nurses is not a temporary condition. Nurses know their value and will increasingly wish to see that value expressed in substantive ways. Nurses recognize how difficult it would be to operate a health care venture without their presence in the system.

There is also an increasing demand for nurses in other health care settings. The hospital is no longer the most viable option for planning a future in nursing. Indeed, the greatest new demand for nurses is outside the hospital: community-based programs, HMOs, insurance companies, private sector companies, private practice, per diem services, etc. These demands will increase as hospitals compete with these attractive options.

As a result of these changes, the best-educated and brightest nurses will abandon the hospital, leaving behind a majority of highly skilled but technically focused staff whose frame of reference for practice will be primarily intervention. These functionally focused nurses will have a narrow range of practice and will operate specific to the hospital environment. In the nonhospital setting as well, these same nurses will provide primarily functional, task-based, and supportive roles to the more broadly prepared nurse. The move to creating a technical/professional framework for the continuing transition of nursing education in America will, therefore, have to be accelerated. Indeed, this differentiation is already a concerted need. Anticipatory changes in the education and use of nurses will be required to adequately address the real need for them in the near future.

Many nurses currently prepared and in practice at a wide variety of levels see their future role as a threat to the current paralleling of all nurses regardless of basic preparation or real ability. Differentiation by skill base will create a significant reality-based alignment of nurses that appears on the surface to disadvantage those prepared primarily for technical roles while it advantages those with baccalaureate and advanced degrees. Although this differentiation is a common mechanism for distinguishing roles in the professions, the cultural and behavioral shift in nursing is rife with political conflict and organizational transformation beyond the willingness of the profession to assume it in a significant or meaningful way.

There is one certainty in the next decade. The need for advanced practice in the health care marketplace will continue at an accelerating rate. If the nursing profession cannot respond proactively to the need, the system will respond in other ways and the nursing role will continually become more functional, vocational, and managed outside of the constructs of a professional frame of reference. Nurses with advanced preparation may simply move into another social descriptor for themselves and nursing will lose whatever equitable professional delineation it currently has or will have obtained in the future.

THE NEED FOR A STRUCTURAL MODEL

No major change or social transformation can occur without a structure to provide form and direction. At a time when historical structures are continually being questioned with regard to their efficacy and effectiveness, newer models are being proposed almost monthly. The question raised during this time of transition is: What is the most appropriate kind of structure needed by nursing organizations or organized nursing to assist it in bringing form to the changes nurses must undergo to prepare themselves for an ever-changing health care system?

Regardless of the structures designed or selected by nurses, they must be internally integrating, capable of presenting an image of solidarity, involve all those who practice nursing in decision making, and respond to the increasing demands on nurses to lead change in reformatting the American health care system. The model for change should reflect the need for change and be service based, reflecting the cultural circumstances of each of the organizations from which they will emerge. Increasingly, these models will have to reflect involvement of smaller units of nursing activity to include nurses at all levels of activity in the organization. This process will have to invest all nurses directly by affecting nurses where they live their lives and make changes in the way in which they relate, problem solve, and work. Failure to adjust circumstances and relationships at the work level of the organization means failure to make any substantive change in important areas in the practice places where most nurses spend the majority of their nursing experience (Porter-O'Grady, 1988).

Perhaps the most significant issue affecting shared governance today is the fact that many organizations that *claim* to have shared governance do not. One of the

issues that often develops in nursing service circles is reflected in the wide disparity between what nurses say they are or do and what actually exists. Unfortunately, in such situations, people believe only what they see. Health care leaders
outside of nursing often chide nurses for talking grander than they live. To them,
such talk often appears more dream than truth. Credibility is directly affected by
such situations. This same circumstance affects the perceptions of others with regard to the development of nursing shared governance (Porter-O'Grady, 1989).

Shared governance creates a significant shift in both the structuring and empowerment of the nursing organization. It makes some fundamental changes in the
way the professional workplace is conceived and operated. It is not an old message in new clothes. It is not a new way to be nice to workers. As the preceding
chapters clearly illustrate, shared governance is a major undertaking that does not
occur overnight and cannot be undertaken by either management control or fiat. It
creates an organizational and operational system that reflects the values of professional accountability and builds structures to ensure that such accountability is obtained and maintained. Shared governance creates the form and process that leads
to a level of equity behavior in the nursing organization such that it relates to itself
and to other disciplines in a manner reflecting its value, commitment, role, relationship, and leadership in the provision of health care services.

Shared governance is not an end in itself. It is a means to an end. It demands
that those who undertake it have a notion of where they are going and are willing
to undertake a concerted and collective effort to attain their goals. It is, therefore,
ever-shifting and changing in both form and structure. One does not arrive at
shared governance. One travels along the road of shared governance to move to
newer places and roles as the health care system and the American public demand.

Nursing must be able to confront the changes that affect it in ways that are at
once both challenging and responsive: challenging, insofar as an appropriate proactive response must be constructed; responsive, insofar as the needs of those who
seek response are addressed. The structures within which nursing's work unfolds
must permit the broadest possible investment and dialogue but also an accountability that ensures adequate response that leads directly to effective action. This cannot be accomplished successfully without much transformation and work in the
nursing service.

The structural models addressed in Chapter 4 serve as a framework for discussion of current approaches to formatting shared governance in those organizations
initiating such approaches to create a professional organization (McDonagh,
1991). Most of this book is devoted to issues of implementing shared governance
in a variety of settings. The issue for future consideration is: What about tomorrow? Will this model as described herein serve the profession well as it moves into
the twenty-first century? The answer is a resounding *no!* No model of organization
is fixed in time. The social and relational realities are always changing. Organizations of professional workers, especially, must always be free and ready to meet
the needs of a changing society and service framework. Included are the responses
undertaken by a profession to the changing demands on the profession itself.

Newer delivery models will emerge that reflect a different sense of community
in the delivery of health services. Integrated, multidisciplinary, joint-ventured

models of care delivery and professional relationships will continually unfold, creating entirely new ways of serving patients. Openness to inviting others who are not nurses into a stronger relationship with nursing will be a clear characteristic of the health care enterprise. In many ways, nurses are leading the way into these newer models by creating them as a response to a demand for more effective and cost-efficient service models.

Health care will continue to move toward a community-based approach to the delivery of health care services. Driven by cost considerations and the continuing changes in the demographics of health care, much of what is offered will not be centrally institutionally based. The question raised by this reality is: How will nurses stay integrated and professionally connected in increasingly diverse service settings and nursing roles?

Newer kinds of service and organizational structures must be formatted to address the changing frame of reference for nursing practice. The wide diversity of practice and disparity of practice settings and roles will drive nursing to organize and structure itself in ways not previously considered appropriate or legitimate. Economics will continue to influence the types of service structures and the business relationships that exist in health care. Regardless of whether a universal payment structure emerges in the American health care system, one thing can be assured: there will be fewer dollars available for intervention at the high-tech and terminal end of care services, and more dollars will be moved to address both prevention and chronic health needs as the population ages.

To ensure the necessary service integration and continuity and to build on those structures already present in the system, hospitals and health centers will continue to play a key role. The relationships, control, and services in these centers will adjust considerably over the years, but their role will still be central to effective delivery of health services.

In these "health service centers" a high level of control and coordination will be exercised, even though much of the services provided will be offered outside the institutions. Through complex computer networks, hospitals will control everything from patient data, service characteristics, pricing, and charging. Human resource use will be monitored just as patient care reporting, providing both care and cost information to every provider regardless of service location. Payment for services will be more directly related to the service provided; therefore salary or fee rates can be more accurately documented and matched to the services provided by the professional and the cost/benefit relationship can be clearly described for both institution and provider. Thus both the cost and income obtained in nursing services can be more clearly calculated and tied with other important data to determine the value and contribution of both the service and the nurse to the viability of the enterprise. This information can help nurses maintain data with regard to the cost of providing services, their value in the situation, their contribution to the organization, and its contribution to them.

These information networks will become more user friendly and more valuable over time. As they become better-operating and can provide some direct support to the nurse, they will be more successful not only as tools for reporting but also as mechanisms for better managing care and integrating the workplace.

These mechanisms will not be sufficient to provide the kind of integration and identity that members of a profession indicate they need. The connectedness of each to the other is one of the requisites of professional relationship. The ability of the profession to ensure it is meeting the demands placed on it by society is just as important as anything else nursing might do. To do this, however, nurses must be able to connect with each other and study the work of the profession beyond simply the level of individual work. As a profession, nurses have some collective obligation for the broader issues affecting not only what nurses do but also the effect of what they do on the whole health care system.

The work of shared governance is to increase the act of partnership between the profession and the organization in the provision of health care services. In the initial stages, however, this partnership has more to do with creating the structure and behaviors in the nursing organization essential to partnership than actually creating real partnership within the work context. The initial effort of the nursing organization in shared governance is attempting to create organizational models that emphasize mature adult-adult relationships in the workplace. Because of the tradition of ascendant behaviors on the part of the medical staff and administration with regard to the roles of any other practitioners in health care, the real contribution of others was never fully evidenced or acknowledged in the health system. Often, as in the case of nursing, its own internal and external behaviors did not reflect well or equitably on itself or with either of the "power groups" in health care. This was a reinforcement of the perception in the system that nursing and other groups were and should be subordinated to the physician and administrator, whether legitimate or not. Because it has been so much a *circumstance* of the relationship between the groups in health care, time and history have made it now a *condition* of the relationship.

As health care evolves toward new models that reflect a different paradigm, relationships and the prevailing assumptions about them are subject to question. As emphasis in the care and treatment in a health care model, when contrasted to an illness care model, changes dramatically, so too do all the relationships previously entered into or perceived in the "old" model. It is within this circumstance that many of the future roles, structures, and relationships of nursing will unfold (Kinzer, 1990).

The reasons for and conditions supportive of inequity in health care are quickly changing. Improvements in education and opportunity for women and thus nurses have accelerated at an unparalleled rate during the past three decades. As more information becomes more broadly generated and as specific kinds of information become more valuable, the nature and character of relationships change. As health becomes more important than illness and health care is refocused and restructured to value this reality, nurses will assume roles and relationships that will require a different self-perception and relationship with others in the health care system.

Nurses in community settings—from home to community center, from clinic to hospital—will play primary roles in delivering health care services. Often it will be the nurse who is the identifier of needs and the gatekeeper of clinical services. It may be the nurse who refers the client/patient into and through the system and on whom the physician may depend for referral and access. It will be the nurse who may connect the patient to the service network and will work with the social service professionals to determine how various service processes can be best used to the patient's benefit.

The nursing role will become more central to the delivery of services in noninstitutional settings and will become increasingly involved in decentralized settings. As a result, the nurse's ability to identify with colleagues and to maintain the integrity of the nursing service and profession will be progressively more difficult. The current move to product line and service line structures and interdisciplinary care models is just a small sample of the kinds of new structures and relationships that will be necessary to provide services in a more efficient and cost-effective manner. In addition, the modification of total quality management principles from the industrial and manufacturing sectors of the economy will influence how people are used and related in providing services in the future (Minerva-Melum, 1990). The ability of the professions to do what they do best and to maintain their identity and their value in society will be directly related to their adroitness in establishing newer relationships within their ranks that can prevail in the existing atmosphere. The structures they create, however, must be powerful enough to participate in the design of new systems, yet flexible within the ever-adjusting models of providing services.

The real work of creating professions' internal structures will be important and at the same time delicate. The professions are not islands. The nature of their representative processes and political context heightens their public visibility. It will be imperative that they not be shortsighted or self-serving in their efforts to restructure their organizations. In this effort there is a fragile balance between the needs of the profession and its members and the needs of those it serves. It may initially appear that efforts to gain increasing control over the activities of the profession can operate at the expense of increased service availability and collaborative relations with other disciplines who see a major role for themselves in the delivery of health care services. Boundary development often appears to constrain others' work or even be self-serving. Over time it will also be more difficult for one profession to work independently without the participation of other involved or affected groups.

To reach the point where the relationships of other disciplines are affected by nursing boundary developments in any but a significant way, nursing as a profession must gain stronger control over the activities of its members. Nursing must control its relationship to both the work and the workplace. Nursing practice must have as much influence on the design and choice of service provision to which it has a significant role as any other group with a major role. Because this requires considerable retooling of the workplace and the nurse as worker, much internal rearrangement must occur. All activities that reflect nursing obligations and roles under a service structure that is led and operated by nurses are included.

To accomplish such a change is not easy. Not only must nursing leaders be concerned with how nonnursing leadership responds to this effort, they also must be concerned with nursing colleagues' fear of this undertaking. Many nurses have long sought to be individually or sectionally empowered at the expense of the empowerment of the profession as a whole. Nurses have cooperated with other administrative leaders in fragmenting the nursing organization or profession in the work setting into a number of functional organizational components responsible to administrative leadership that is either not committed to the work of nursing or unprepared to understand the commitment of a profession in the accomplishment of its mission. These circumstances have resulted in the increasing vocationalization of nursing, the definition of nursing work in strictly functional terms, and the institutionalization of the perception and operation of the role of nurses and nursing in health care delivery. Often, individuals in nursing leadership in such situations have advanced their own personal power but at great expense to the profession and its power to make aggregate and integrative change for the organization and the patients nurses serve.

In its current form shared governance responds positively to this situation. It creates a desirable organizational model that operates at the benefit of both the organization and the profession. It builds on the beliefs associated with creating work partnerships between the profession and the institution. Shared governance strengthens the relationship between nurses and reactivates the desire for "connectedness" between all nurses in the enterprise regardless of where they may work and to whom they may "report." Benefit is seen by nurses in their collective relationship, not in a polarized sense as often occurs in union settings, but instead as a part of the policy-making structure, as a partner or investor in the enterprise. In this way influence is seen as a part of the collective effort with the organization rather than one that operates as fully independent of any obligation to the success of the enterprise. Success, in this frame of reference, causes the desire to be a part of it and extends success to other members of the success group wherever they may be located. This desire to be "a part of it" operates in opposition to the prevailing behavior in nursing not to be a part of the whole, evidenced in the breakup of the nursing service into a number of nonrelated, nonintegrated nursing groups.

Although shared governance creates this opportunity to again "rejoin" nurses, it does not and has not created a forum that can be better self-described and self-controlled. Nursing is still conceived primarily as an employee group and remains within the delineation of employee status both legally and operationally. This delineation limits the ability of the profession to behave as a true partner in health care delivery with the credibility and obligation that accompany that designation.

This reality does not improve the broader sense of obligation to health care on the part of the practitioner of nursing. As long as nurses focus simply on their component of the work and not on the whole exercise of health care providing roles, their consciousness remains functionally or task focused. This pertains to the institution and its perception of the nurse as well. Thus, today in shared governance there is a more committed, satisfied nurse with a stronger sense of self and role in relationship to others and a stronger sense of power over those things that affect nursing. There remains only to develop the role of the nurse so that the nurse sees, both individually and collectively, the obligation to set direction for health care, produce a financially viable product, tie productivity to reward, and negotiate equitably accountability for specified health care services. To do this demands a move to the next step of shared governance: nursing corporate reorganization.

TRANSITION TO THE CORPORATE VENTURE

The movement to a new organizational model for nursing that is not institution specific is clearly a radical change. It creates a new paradigm of thought with regard to the organization and operation of the nursing service. In fact, the conception of a strategy that leads the profession in the direction of self-determination and self-sustaining behaviors is, in some circles, not in the best interests of nursing nor of benefit to the health care system.

It can be conceived that another interdependent player in the health care system would only add to the confusion and sectionalism of the professions and create communication and relationship problems. The assumption in these remarks is that there are no problems present in the current set of relationships and interactions among the various players in the system. Perhaps had nursing been at the table when policy and direction were set for the American health care system, it would not have its current problems. Historical denial of nursing access to the process of setting policy has clearly impeded success in providing adequate health care to the American public. Therefore it should be relatively easy for nurses to suggest a new approach to formalizing their activities and their relationship to the other players in the health care system.

Most of the work, however, will have to be done by and with nurses. They will have the greatest number of arguments and fears with regard to forming a new kind of structure and relationship with the health system. To separate as an entity from the current models will require much courage and engender a high level of risk. Some might conclude that to form large-scale corporate entities in nursing may take revolutionary activity with very little support in the system. This may be true, but it is more probable that it will be less revolutionary and more evolutionary than first perceived.

Nursing is doing well in the public forum and at the national level. As nurses become better educated and more astute in the political process, they are competing better for the attention of those who make policy and generate dollars to the service sector. The data on nursing efficacy are overwhelming and thoroughly validate the contribution nurses make to health care in America at a fraction of the cost of other providers, notably physicians. That process will continue.

Whereas growing national prominence and success are vital to the future of the profession, real change must occur in the service setting—where nurses practice and where the consumers of their services touch their lives every day. If behaviors and expectations do not change there, all the public effort at the national level will do nothing to substantively change the experience and role of nurses. It is in this setting that most of the changes must occur. It is also here where such changes will be more difficult and transforming.

CREATING STRUCTURE

Shared governance as currently configured does much to change the internal operating structure of the nursing organization. It does not do much to change the overall relationship of the profession with the institution and the health system as a whole. There is an experience of change in the organization with others' relationship to nursing, but mostly within the context of affiliation and problem solving. These internal changes are more mechanical than substantive. Often in these settings other professionals want to have some of the same operating characteristics and liberties as nursing appears to have. Generalized interest in empowerment emerges in a number of professional services and a generic desire to exemplify the characteristics of shared governance ensues.

These efforts to expand the influence and organization of shared governance should not be discouraged. The process is not *owned* by any one discipline, and the behavioral characteristics are beneficial to all. Indeed, nurses should work diligently to promulgate the values of shared governance within the organization to improve relationships, facilitate problem solving, and generate organizational consistency among the various work groups. Exclusivity and unilateral ownership create discord and ascendant behaviors, and alienate various groups in the workplace. It is the nature of nursing's work to be facilitating and empowering. Anything in the organization that benefits that process should be supported and encouraged. Many hospitals are developing institutional models of shared governance to create organizational integrity and consistency. Nursing should be encouraging, indeed, leading the way to develop this effort in all shared governance organizations.

Although it is important to fulfill the organizational obligation to create general stability, growth, and functional integrity, nursing must also recognize that its role in the health system demands that it continue to change into newer models. Because of the significance of the current economic and service shifts in the health care system, nurses must respond differently than they have in the past in order to participate in correcting both the excesses and inadequacies of the health system. This will require a different kind of relationship in the service setting and a different set of operating characteristics for nursing as identified above.

To achieve parity and partnership in the health system with policymakers, physicians, and administrators, nursing must have a different kind of relationship with them. This relationship must be one with both service and economic characteristics that directly affect the appropriate functioning of the health system. It must represent the economic and social characteristics of equity. The exchange between nursing and the health system must reflect a character of equivalence that includes the risk of both opportunity and failure. In addition, nursing must be able to articulate its service value in real economic terms so that the economic value can be both described and operated in a manner understandable to the payer. Simply, nursing must be able to define its service and have it compensated.

To accomplish this goal, however, a different process will be needed. Nursing is generally a service that has an aggregate of providers who furnish a multiple range of services in a collective venture. In hospitals, for example, units are staffed by several nurses who provide services to a group of patients. This model of service extends a different set of variables from the one patient–one provider fee for service model. All costs associated with nurses must reflect a more corporate undertaking than current unilateral provider-based fee for service arrangements could adequately address.

There are concurrent changes in the system that will create a growing number of venues within which highly decentralized services will be provided. These nursing services must also be addressed by some entity that would be accountable for the delineation and management of the nursing resources that provide them. The organizations using nursing services must also be assured that the funds they are spending on these services are achieving the outcomes agreed upon at the outset of the relationship. Contracting this relationship will become increasingly more important in highly decentralized environments. If only to maintain continuity and standards of care, individual entities will require some way of ensuring that staff members who provide nursing services are capable and are meeting agreed upon standards for the delivery of nursing originated services.

How can the nursing profession prepare for the future by using models that not only assure nursing autonomy but insure nursing contribution to the service characteristics of the health system and also the outcomes promised in the original contracted relationship? Tying the service to agreed-upon outcomes and matching nursing performance to the achievement of those outcomes builds a different approach to the access and use of the nursing resource (Porter-O'Grady, 1990).

Shared governance models provide a solid underpinning for movement into newer organizational configurations. The accountability base of shared governance as identified in Chapter 2 provides the underpinnings of an organization that more clearly defines what it offers and evaluates what it accomplishes. The standards-based, quality-moderated approaches of most shared governance organizations built on the five professional accountabilities of practice, quality assurance, education, research, and resource management provide a strong framework for corporate formation. In those settings the process of nursing activities, when correlated with the outcomes achieved, builds bridges among work done, outcomes achieved, and the cost of the service. Charging and contracting nursing services thereby becomes a relatively straightforward proposition. The agency contracting for the service simply asks what it will receive for the funds expended and the nursing organization simply explains what it will do to fulfill the obligation, and a negotiated agreement with regard to service and payment is reached. Although not quite as simple as an agreed negotiation between independent parties, it does bear many of the characteristics of such a setup. Moderating the relationship are the payers, other providers, the agencies providing services, and other options in the delivery system. Also affecting the move to corporate formation are the following issues:

1. Review of political and legislative initiatives regarding the payment for nursing services in different ways than currently defined
2. Adjustment of payment formulas that fail to treat nursing as an individuated service (not a part of the "hotel" services) to reflect a more adequate application of dollars for nursing services
3. The option that non-nurse providers may emerge to offer services in a more cost-effective manner in areas once thought the exclusive province of nurses
4. The need to consider replacing high-cost providers like physicians for some services once offered exclusively by them but which could be offered by nurses with the same or improved outcomes at considerably less cost
5. A change in the employment and practice of nurses in a corporate model.

Nurses would seek privileges with the corporate entity instead of the service setting. The corporation would then sell individual or collective services to service entities as contracted.

6. Determination of the cost saving advantage of this approach to nursing organization and service. It can be reasonably assumed that since negotiated roles would reflect dollars available in the system, such nursing cost would not increase any higher than the current rate; indeed, it could be conceivably less.

7. The effect of newer configurations of corporate nursing services on the "master-servent" relationship as currently described in the American legal system. Also affected would be the traditional employee base, influencing the collective bargaining process as applied to the traditional workplace arrangement. Newer models of relationship in a professional corporation would ultimately emerge.

Shared governance has provided a solid base for moving to more independent corporate structures. This can be accomplished over time by degrees: from internal operating structure to collateral corporate entity (a part of a health care holding company arrangement), to independent, freestanding corporate venture comprised of professional nurses.

Bylaws formats provide the first step in the transition. The professional nursing staff that emerges in a shared governance system requires, at some stage of the transition, the formulation and approval of bylaws for the nursing organization (Porter-O'Grady, 1985). Eventually, these bylaws must be approved as the operating characteristics of the professional nursing staff within the context of specific hospitals or health care agencies. The boards of trustees of those organizations must approve them before they have support necessary for them to be credible and a recognition of the professional independence of the nursing staff.

In the bylaws, format (see Chapter 8) and content are the basis for beginning identification of nursing as a corporate and independent entity within an organizational context. The seeds of its own corporate identity are born within the bylaws structure. This may raise concerns for some of the hospital leadership. To some, the idea of an emerging nursing corporate entity not strictly within the exclusive authority base of the institution is a threat to operational control and organizational integrity. This opinion reflects a strong attachment to the unilateral control structures of the industrial age. It is not consistent with the multilateral designs for organizations that reflect the partnership between the organizational system and its knowledge workers.

Most of the effort that will effectively move nurses to corporate arrangements will unfold in newer delivery arenas. As health care moves into the community and nurses assume a greater role in creating, managing, and providing services in these settings, opportunity will abound for new corporate arrangements. Joint ventures, collaborative practice models, community nursing centers, birthing clinics and centers, and gerontologic service centers are just a small sample of the opportunities for nursing-driven service arrangements. As preventive measures assume greater significance in the health system as an effort to reduce cost, there will be even greater opportunity to expand the role of the nurse and extend organizational relationship.

Contracting relationships will create an arrangement that reflects a payment for services provided based on outcomes achieved. The satisfaction with outcomes will have to provide the relational base for nurses in the future. Nurses will need to recognize that there is a direct relationship between what gets accomplished and what people are willing to pay for. Individual nursing income will reflect the nurse's relationship to that reality.

In these settings productivity will also have its own reward. Increased opportunity for investment, income enhancement, and ownership for nurses will be afforded by their agreement to enter more fully into the activities that produce more revenue or income or reduce costs, thus enhancing nursing corporate margins.

Differing models of corporate arrangement will also be reflected in the newer health service arrangements in the future. Professional stock ownership models may materialize that make every member of the corporation a stockholder, investing the worker in the enterprise and its success. Program bonuses relate the nurse to the provision of additional income based on delivery of services that either enhance revenue or reduce costs in the organization. Whatever approach is taken, it will demand a different relationship between the individual nurse and the corporate entity.

There will also be demands on the organization that offers health services to enter into a different kind of relationship to the nursing service. On both sides of the issue, there are some significant concerns and issues affecting the future of the nursing relationship. Of benefit to the health care entity is the ability to contract within the parameters of the relationship clear to them. Outcomes can be identified and some measurement of the relationship between process and outcome can be included in the evaluative processes. Dollars spent can be accounted for and budgets can be reasonably definitive. Nursing benefits by a relative independence regarding how best to use dollars, some freedom regarding use of funding, and movement of funds when necessary to facilitate appropriate outcomes. Service delivery frameworks can be better controlled and adjusted based on their achievements for both the patient and the organization. This mutuality creates a more equitable and thus satisfying relationship for both parties. In such a setting much better outcomes for each patient should result.

Nursing is changed in this relationship in a significant way. The many arguments for status quo and for dependency values fade in an accountability-based relationship. The argument that the profession has a diversity of participants and therefore a justifiable diversity of commitments and outcomes will not be valid after shared governance systems are implemented. If a profession is to have any measure of influence or impact on its constituencies, it must have some measure of certainty with regard to what it can expect from its practitioners. Certain levels of performance, commitment, and expectation must be in place. If the profession cannot rely on the commitment of its members to achieve its agreed-upon outcomes, it should expect that it is seen as nonviable and therefore should be eclipsed by those who are viable.

As the profession enters the mainstream as a corporate partner in health care, it will find that the competition is tough and the expectations on performance are high. Stakeholders in the health system fight hard for their territory, their stake. If they think that it is threatened or compromised, they respond with passion. That is how the game is played in a free and open economy, and indeed, how it should be played. No one will acquiesce to the nursing venture based solely on demand. Evidence of nursing viability, maturity, and performance ability will be the primary factors influencing choice of nursing as a preferred service.

Political savvy will be essential in negotiating a place for nursing and competing with those whose perspective is different but who are just as interested in their viability (Rogers, 1990). Some in the health system have difficulty with this perspective. This is especially true in the age of total quality management in which the difference in work groups is somehow supposed to blend into homogeneous work groups whose sole interest is in the benefit of those they serve. Although collaborative strategies are essential in the emerging workplace, they will not be successful unless they represent the needs of the professional. Service is not a unilateral or unidirectional activity; exchange is involved in the relationship. This exchange demands some level of mutuality and all parties must obtain some value that is both rewarding and meaningful. Professional values will not disappear but must be moderated by the need for relationship and the mutuality that is invariably associated with success.

INFORMATION STRUCTURES

Regardless of the form that nursing service corporations take in the future, they will invariably be linked by computerized data systems. It is inconceivable that nursing leadership will be able to operate multilocational activities in the same way that single institutional services were managed. These entities will have neither the resources nor the time to manage in models that worked in the traditional hospital. The need for informational support also will increase dramatically in the future.

The ability to document clinical activity has already been eclipsed by the activity itself. Nurses can no longer expect that they can even approach the level of documentation necessary today and in the future by using manual methods. Changes in the system and in the patient now occur at a rate demanding immediate response. The tools of information necessary to respond to these circumstances are already needed today and are essential in a distributive delivery system like that envisioned in the corporate framework.

Clinical nurses must be self-managing in ways not previously expected. Because they may never enter the corporate center, they will have to be connected in ways that provide access to both information and direction with regard to clinical and corporate activities. Nurses must be computer literate and be able not only to access appropriate information but to analyze and evaluate it as well.

The system will need the nurses' expertise with computerized systems because both the quantity and quality of their work will affect the nursing corporate venture. Nursing performance and productivity will also be measured by the kind of data that appear in the system relating what has been done with the expectations for the service. Previously redefined quality indices will be built into the system and performance measures will be evaluated against the expectations. Clinical, service, performance, and financial demonstration will be readily accessible to the corporate leadership as well as the involved nursing staff.

Sophistication with the generation, collection, and interpretation of data will be an ongoing expectation of the practicing professional. This will be especially true of nurse leaders in the various service settings. They must be able to make quick judgments and respond appropriately. Because it is the primary tool of communication in highly decentralized settings, nurses must have facility in computer use.

The data produced in a corporate setting by clinical nurses will include operating and finance data related to the service provided. No longer will clinical providers be insulated from the information that affects performance. The computer provides information about the efficacy and viability of nurses' service. The availability of greater amounts of data will enable nurses to respond to changes in situations and how they respond. Nurses can be held accountable for the data and it becomes a management tool without substantial on-site supervision.

The preparation of practitioners clearly reflects the need for more highly prepared nurses. There will be an increasing need for master degree preparation in these decentralized service settings. Educational institutions must be cognizant of the need to accelerate preparation of highly trained specialists for these roles. This will entail continuing emphasis on retooling education to prepare fewer nurses with associate degrees for an environment with a decreasing need for these practitioners and encourage the preparation of nurses with advanced degrees in an era of increasing demand. This will not occur without "noise" both within and outside of the nursing profession. There are as many vested interests within the profession that do not operate in its best interests as there are on the outside. Because of personal value or need, there are many who perceive changes in the status quo as a significant threat. It is noteworthy that nurses who decry patients' or the health system's lack of insight with regard to health-giving behaviors often exhibit those same attitudes and behaviors when changes must be undertaken by the profession to better respond to a new set of demands and retool nursing for a new role in the future. This is further enhanced by these same nurses who are appalled when someone outside the profession suggests changes that respond to a current or future need in a way that threatens the nursing profession but could have been anticipated if nursing had previously addressed the issues.

CONCLUSION

These are exciting times for nursing. The challenges and opportunities are almost overwhelming in their number and intensity. The paradigms for the health care system are shifting even as they are being conceived. There is no real model remaining that can be considered adequate for the future—the rules are changing before the health care system has time to adequately respond. The system costs more every day and provides less meaningful service. There are cracks in the health care system, just as in American society at large, that are indicative of far more serious concerns.

The world is shifting to a new reality (Morris, 1990). There is no conception of what that reality will look like. There is no single script that will clearly define the preferred route to the future. Many scripts continue to be suggested and just as quickly are questioned or replaced by new options and suggestions. The players in the health care system are experiencing the pain of a disseminated system and are afraid of what it portends.

As with all major social change, there are opportunity and danger. Both appear to be couched in the same context. Perhaps both are the same thing viewed from a different perspective. Those who envision a response and are willing to assume the burden of not only creating a meaningful future but also living it will be well positioned to make it reality.

For nursing this time is either constraint or opportunity for arriving at a level of full maturity and partnership in the health care system. Shared governance provides every latitude necessary to develop and live the maturity and creativity necessary to make the health care system effective and meaningful. It provides a framework for nursing and nurses to become equal members of the health care team and to define more clearly their role and contribution.

Shared governance is really a model of professional maturity because it demands a professional, proud of the profession, desirous of being in control of professional life and of making a difference in job performance and quality. Such nurses want to play their role as full partners in decisions that affect their practice and are willing to make the necessary commitment to do so. Nurses in a shared governance model no longer worry about whether their services are valuable to the system. Instead they recognize that they are even more valuable than previously conceived and are anxious to provide form to that value by translating it into an economic and policy reality. Shared governance creates the milieu that ensures a nursing partnership in the health system. The nurse expects to both act and be treated as a partner in decisions that affect the future of nursing and the future of the health care system.

Shared governance creates a framework for even greater transition of both nursing and the health care system. Nurses recognize their unique contributions in relationship to the contributions made by others. They recognize the need to change how nursing relates to others and offers its services. The changing times call nurses to form new kinds of arrangements for doing their work. Corporate arrangements that create parity and newer opportunities to offer nursing services in different ways are the next major step in creating an equitable and viable nursing profession and service in the future.

This book has focused on the characteristics of implementing a shared governance system in nursing or any other discipline. It has emphasized the developmental characteristics necessary to create a successful model. It has not prescribed any specific approach. The authors have recognized that many approaches can work provided the principles guiding belief in shared governance are maintained.

There is no risk-free way to implement shared governance. If readers have implemented shared governance without significant "noise" in the system, then they may need to review whether shared governance is truly in place. To introduce this model into existing systems is inherently threatening to the operation. It changes relationships and the role of nursing and the nurse in the operation of the system.

It matures the nurse and creates an adult-to-adult frame of reference. It raises the expectations for communication and interaction, and sometimes raises questions that are uncomfortable, direct, or difficult to answer. Administration and management must change the way in which they relate and interact with the staff. Secrets are much harder to keep and adult-to-child communication strategies between management and staff are highly unsuccessful over the long term.

Benefits to the organization are extraordinary. Higher levels of satisfaction among the nursing staff and with the nursing organization are normal outcomes of shared governance. Higher levels of involvement by nurses in the organization are reasonable expectations. The maturing of the physician-nurse relationship is also strengthened by the shared governance model.

As with all systems, however, shared governance is not the end of a transition, rather it is simply a beginning. If the model is complete in itself, it has not served its true purpose. As previously indicated, shared governance is a vehicle—no more, no less. It provides an organizational framework for behavioral and systems changes. If it does not transform itself to the next stage of change, it can become an agent of stagnation and decline. Shared governance should provide a forum for safe risking of efforts to change and itself changes as the demand for movement indicates.

It is a time of great hope, great pain, anticipation, and uncertainty. It is a time to seek vision and leadership. The visionaries and leaders must come from different backgrounds and be able to join their visions and energies to create a new reality for the world. Today's nurses are transformational people, neither here nor there but rather perennially on the journey. The future will arrive soon enough. Its appearance depends primarily on what is done with today. Shared governance creates a way to make the future real and provides a vehicle which the nursing profession can use to join with others in taking the health care system where it needs to go. Health care needs what nurses have to offer; nursing needs a way to offer it. Shared governance provides the format for involvement, investment, leadership, and change for nurses and others. What is needed is the simple encouragement of leadership to emerge and join in writing a new script for health care wherever it is offered. That is what nursing was and is and upon which its future will be built.

REFERENCES

Evans, H. (1989). Old Birth Idea Reborn in the Bronx. *New York Daily News,* (February 19), 7 and 44.

Fagin, C. (1990). Nursing's Value Proves Itself. *American Journal of Nursing,* (October), 17-30.

Grimaldi, P. (1990). Will New Fee System Slash Physician Payments. *Nursing Management,* 21(8), 22-23.

Haddon, R. (1989). The Final Frontier: Nursing in the Emerging Healthcare Environment. *Nursing Economics,* 7(3), 155-161.

Hersey, P. and Blanchard, K. (1989). *Management of Organizational Behavior* (6th ed.). Englewood Cliffs, N.J.: Prentice-Hall.

Hudson, T. (1990). Use of Health Professionals Poses Payment, Authority Conflicts. *Hospitals,* 64(19), 46-51.

Kalisch, B. and Kalisch, P. (1988). An Analysis of the Sources of Physician-Nurse Conflict. In J. Muff (Ed.), *Women's Issues in Nursing* (pp. 221-233). Prospect Heights, Ill.: Waveland Press, Inc.

Kinzer, D. (1990). Twelve Laws of Hospital Interaction. *Health Care Management Review,* 5(2), 15-19.

Lamm, R. (1990). *The Brave New World of Health Care.* University of Denver.

Ludemann, R. and Brown, C. (1989). Staff Perceptions of Shared Governance. *Nursing Administration Quarterly,* 13(4), 47-56.

Maraldo, P. (1990). The Aftermath of DRGs: The Politics of Transformation. In J. McCloskey and H. Grace (Ed.), *Current Issues in Nursing* (pp. 387-392). New York: C.V. Mosby.

McDonagh, K. (1991). *Nursing Shared Governance.* Atlanta, Ga.: KJ McDonagh Associates, Inc.

Minerva-Melum, M. (1990). Total Quality Management: Steps to Success. *Hospitals,* (Dec. 5), 42-44.

Morris, C. (1990). *The Coming Global Boom.* New York: Bantam Books.

Muff, J. (1988). *Women's Issues in Nursing: Socialization Sexism and Stereotyping.* Prospect Heights, Ill.: Waveland Press, Inc.

Naisbitt, J. and Aburdene, P. (1985). *Re-Inventing the Corporation.* New York: Warner Publisher.

Passau-Buck, S. (1988). Caring vs. Curing: The Politics of Health Care. In J. Huff (Ed.), *Women's Issues in Nursing* (pp. 203-209). Prospect Heights, Ill.: Waveland Press, Inc.

Peters, T. (1987). *Thriving on Chaos: Handbook for a Management Revolution.* New York: Harper & Row.

Porter-O'Grady, T. (1985). Credentialing, Privileging, and Nursing Bylaws: Assuring Accountability. *Journal of Nursing Administration,* 15(10), 30-36.

Porter-O'Grady, T. (1988). Restructuring the Nursing Organization for a Consumer Driven Marketplace. *Nursing Administration Quarterly,* 12(3), 60-65.

Porter-O'Grady, T. (1989). Shared Governance: Reality or Sham. *American Journal of Nursing,* (March), 350.

Porter-O'Grady, T. (1990). *The Reorganization of Nursing Practice: Creating the Corporate Venture.* Rockville, Md.: Aspen Publishers.

Program, F. and Program, N. (1990). *A Study of the Outcomes of Nutritional Programs on the Cost of Later Medicaid Outlays.* Department of Agriculture.

Rogers, T. (1990). No Excuses Management. *Harvard Business Review,* (July-August), 84-98.

Toffler, A. (1990). *Powershift.* New York: Bantam Books.

Index